An Atlas of
ULTRASONOGRAPHY IN OBSTETRICS AND GYNECOLOGY

THE ENCYCLOPEDIA OF VISUAL MEDICINE SERIES

Reprinted from

An Atlas of
ULTRASONOGRAPHY
IN OBSTETRICS AND
GYNECOLOGY

Edited by
Asim Kurjak

The Ultrasonic Institute
University of Zagreb
Croatia

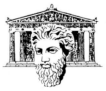

The Parthenon Publishing Group
International Publishers in Medicine, Science & Technology

Casterton Hall, Carnforth,
Lancs, LA6 2LA, UK

120 Mill Road, Park Ridge,
New Jersey 07656, USA

British Library Cataloguing in Publication Data
Atlas of Ultrasonography in Obstetrics and Gynecology. –
(Encyclopedia of Visual Medicine)
I Kurjak, Asim II. Series
61,8
ISBN 1-85070-362-0

Library of Congress Cataloging-in-Publication Data
An Atlas of ultrasonography in obstetrics and gynecology /
    edited by Asim Kurjak
      p.   cm — (The Encyclopedia of visual medicine series)
    Includes bibliographical reference and index.
    ISBN 1-85070-362-0 : $145.00
    1. Ultrasonics in obstetrics – Atlases. 2. Generative organs.
Female – Ultrasonic imaging – Atlases. I Kurjak, Asim. II.
    Series.
    [DNLM: 1 Fetal Diseases – ultrasonography – atlases. 2.
Genital Diseases – ultrasonography – atlases. 3. Pregnancy
Complications – ultrasonography – atlases. 4. Prenatal Diagnosis
– methods – atlases.   WQ   17 A8815]
RG527.5.U48A86   1992
618'.047543 – dc20
DLC
For Library of Congress   91-45571
                                                        CIP

Published in the UK and Europe by
The Parthenon Publishing Group Limited
Casterton Hall, Carnforth
Lancs. LA6 2LA

Published in North America by
The Parthenon Publishing Group Inc.
120 Mill Road
Park Ridge
New Jersey 07656, USA

Typeset by Ryburn Typesetting Ltd, Luddendenfoot,
West Yorkshire

Contents

The Encyclopedia of Visual Medicine Series

Consultant Series Editor: R D Mann

Titles currently planned in this series include:

An Atlas of Oncology

An Atlas of Hypertension

An Atlas of Common Diseases

An Atlas of Osteoporosis

An Atlas of the Menopause

An Atlas of Contraception

An Atlas of Endometriosis

An Atlas of Ultrasonography in Obstetrics and Gynecology

An Atlas of Practical Radiology

An Atlas of Sexually Transmitted Diseases

An Atlas of Psoriasis

An Atlas of Trauma Management

Series Foreword

The art of effective diagnosis is one that relies to a considerable degree – although certainly not exclusively – on the recognition of visual signs and manifestations of disease. The objective of this Series is to provide a practical aid to diagnosis by illustrating and explaining the wide range of visual signs that a physician needs to be aware of in current medical practice.

Whilst the visual manifestations of disease themselves remain constant, the development of new techniques of invasive and non-invasive diagnosis means that new images are frequently being added to the range of visual material that the diagnostician must be familiar with: ultrasound, radiology, magnetic resonance imaging, endoscopy and photomicrography all provide examples of this kind of material. It is the intention of this Series to document, where appropriate, the results of such techniques and to explain and elucidate their relevance – in addition to documenting all the more standard visual images.

The Series is also distinctive in that individual volumes will focus on carefully selected, specific topics, which can be covered in some detail – rather than on generalized and broadly-based subject areas that could not easily be covered so thoroughly.

The authors contributing to the Series have all been selected for their special expertise in their own chosen fields, their access to outstanding visual material and their ability to explain the significance of it in an effective and lucid way. Finally, particular emphasis is being placed on achieving a very high quality colour reproduction in the printing process itself in order to do full justice to the wide variety of visual images presented.

It is hoped that this carefully structured and systematic approach to the visually significant aspects of medicine will make a valuable and ongoing contribution to good diagnostic practice.

List of contributors

Z. Alfirevic
Ultrasonic Institute
University of Zagreb
WHO Collaborating Centre for Diagnostic
    Ultrasound
P. Miškine 64
41000 Zagreb
Croatia

K. Aydinli
Department of Obstetrics and Gynecology
Cerrapaca Tipfakültesi
Istanbul
Turkey

S. Campbell
King's College Hospital Medical School
University of London
Department of Obstetrics and Gynaecology
Denmark Hill
London SE5 8RX
United Kingdom

F. Catizone
Universitá di Bari
Clinical Ostetrica e Gynecologia II Policlinico
70124 Bari
Italy

F.A. Chervenak
Director of Obstetric Ultrasound and Ethics
The New York Hospital
Cornell Medical Center
525 East 68th Street
New York, N.Y. 10021
USA

V. D'Addario
Universitá di Bari
Clinical Ostetrica e Gynecologia II Policlinico
70124 Bari
Italy

V. Dukic
Ultrasonic Institute
University of Zagreb
WHO Collaborating Centre for Diagnostic
    Ultrasound
P. Miškine 64
41000 Zagreb
Croatia

M. Evans
Division of Reproductive Genetics
Department of Obstetrics and Gynecology
Wayne State University School of Medicine
Detroit, MI
USA

A.S. Garden
The University of Liverpool
Royal Liverpool Hospital
Department of Obstetrics and Gynaecology
Prescot Street
Liverpool L7 8XP
United Kingdom

W. Holzgreve
Westfälischen Wilhelms-Universität Münster
Albert-Schweitzer-Strasse 33
4400 Münster
Germany

A. Ianniruberto
Universitá di Bari
Clinical Ostetrica e Gynecologia II Policlinico
70124 Bari
Italy

G. Isaacson
The New York Hospital
Cornell Medical Center
Department of Obstetrics and Gynecology
525 East 68th Street   M713
New York, N.Y. 10021
USA

E. Jauniaux
Department of Obstetrics and Gynecology
University Hospital Erasmus
Free University of Brussels
Brussels
Belgium

D. Jurkovic
Ultrasonic Institute
University of Zagreb
WHO Collaborating Centre for Diagnostic
   Ultrasound
P. Miškine 64
41000 Zagreb
Croatia

S. Kupešić-Urek
Ultrasonic Institute
University of Zagreb
WHO Collaborating Centre for Diagnostic
   Ultrasound
P. Miškine 64
41000 Zagreb
Croatia

A. Kurjak
Ultrasonic Institute
University of Zagreb
WHO Collaborating Centre for Diagnostic
   Ultrasound
P. Miškine 64
41000 Zagreb
Croatia

R. Matijevic
Ultrasonic Institute
University of Zagreb
WHO Collaborating Centre for Diagnostic
   Ultrasound
P. Miškine 64
41000 Zagreb
Croatia

P. Miny
Institut für Humangenetik
Westfälischen Wilhelms-Universität Münster
Albert-Schweitzer-Strasse 33
4400 Münster
Germany

S. Rottem
Department of Obstetrics and Gynecology
Rambam Medical Center
Haifa
Israel

P.A. Stewart
Department of Obstetrics and Gynecology
Academic Hospital Dijkzigt Rotterdam
Dr. Molewaterplein 40
3015 GD Rotterdam
The Netherlands

J. Streltzoff
The New York Hospital
Cornell Medical Center
Department of Obstetrics and Gynecology
525 East 68th Street – M713
New York, N.Y. 10021
USA

H. Takeuchi
Department of Obstetrics and Gynecology
Juntendo Urayasu Hospital
Juntendo University School of Medicine
2-1-1, Tokioka
Urayasu-Shi 272-01
Japan

I. Zalud
Ultrasonic Institute
University of Zagreb
WHO Collaborating Centre for
   Diagnostic Ultrasound
P. Miškine 64
41000 Zagreb
Croatia

J. Zmijanac
Ultrasonic Institute
University of Zagreb
WHO Collaborating Centre for
   Diagnostic Ultrasound
P. Miškine 64
41000 Zagreb
Croatia

Foreword

It is now 40 years since Ian Donald first started to use ultrasound in obstetrics and gynecology. In a relatively short period of time ultrasound has improved in what seems to be a logarithmic progression, and it can with good reason be said to have changed the way of thinking of our age. The magnitude of this step alone is incalculable. Moreover, more than any other modern technique, ultrasound has made it obvious that the fetus is an individual virtually from conception.

Furthermore, technical improvements in ultrasonic instrumentation have opened up new avenues to the visualization and evaluation of normal and abnormal fetal anatomy and normal anatomy and pathological conditions in the female pelvis. They have introduced completely new methods into the diagnosis and treatment of certain fetal diseases (e.g. fetal surgery, uteroplacental blood flow) as well as new applications of ultrasound in the treatment of gynecological diseases, and provided for a better understanding of ovarian physiology (monitoring of follicular growth, ultrasonically guided follicular punctures for *in vitro* fertilization, the assessment of ovarian and uterine perfusion).

The most exciting recent developments are color Doppler and transvaginal sonography. The combination of these two modalities in the same vaginal probe provides for superb simultaneous visualization of structural and flow information and offers new insight into dynamic studies of blood flow within the female pelvis. Most of these exciting developments are illustrated in this book.

The Atlas contains 539 original black and white and 166 color ultrasound pictures, as well as diagrams and photographs of babies after delivery. The book is divided into 22 chapters covering the evaluation of sonoembryology, normal and abnormal fetal anatomy, the use of ultrasound in gynecological diagnosis, color Doppler in obstetrics and gynecology, etc. This major new work in ultrasound diagnosis also comprises an outstanding collection of images produced by the most sophisticated techniques and equipment currently available. We do believe that this book will be of great value to gynecologists, obstetricians and specialists in infertility as well as to diagnostic radiologists. It should serve as a basis for comparison when fetal abnormality is identified or suspected.

A. Kurjak

Section I

Ultrasound in Obstetrics

1 Sonoembryology

H. Takeuchi

THE GESTATION SAC

The gestation sac can be delineated when its diameter has developed to 2 mm in hyperplastic endometrium (Figure 1.1). This time corresponds to around 14 days from fertilization, i.e. to 4 weeks of gestation. This case in Figure 1.1 was considered to be 4 weeks and 1 day of gestation. The diameter of the small vesicle image which seemed to be the gestation sac was precisely 2 mm. After 10 days, a gestation sac of 12 mm diameter and a yolk sac could be observed, but the embryo was not yet recognizable.

While the gestation sac is still small, it is usually delineated as being almost round (Figure 1.2). The position of the sac inside the endometrium indicates the site of implantation. This figure shows the gestation sac with a diameter of 3 mm, which corresponds to 4 weeks and 2 days of gestation. The echogenic ring of the chorion is not yet recognizable. It is difficult to detect the location of implantation from this sectional view. The gestation sac is not always delineated as round, it may sometimes have an ellipsoidal shape (Figure 1.3). The gestation sac in this case is ellipsoidal with a maximum diameter of 3.5 mm. It is considered that the implantation occurred at the anterior fundal site in the endometrium.

Implantation usually occurs in the upper half of the uterine cavity, but implantation into the lower half is occasionally observed. A hypothesis that low implantation is the reason for either low-lying placenta or placenta previa is not fully understood. The case in Figure 1.4 was determined to be implanted into the lower half, but the localization of the placenta was completely normal throughout pregnancy.

By the time the sac diameter reaches 5 mm at 5 weeks of gestation, primary chorionic villi become secondary and later tertiary resulting in an increase of thickness with characteristic echogenicity on the rind of the gestation sac. The thickness is almost uniform on the whole circumference. The case in Figure 1.5 is at 5 weeks and 2 days of gestation. The 6 mm diameter gestation sac can be interpreted as an anterior, right-side implantation. A space with blood flow between chorion frondosum and decidua basalis is observed. Nothing is recognizable yet inside the gestation sac.

During weeks 4 to 6 of gestation, the yolk sac inside the gestation sac is larger than the embryo. Therefore, there may be a time when only the yolk sac is observed before the embryo can be depicted.

THE 3 TO 5 MM EMBRYO

Embryonic configuration can be discernible with cardiac activity as early as 5 weeks and 4 days of gestation. Such an embryonic pole with maximum length of 2–4 mm is observed directly adjacent to the yolk sac in Figure 1.6. From the viewpoint of resolution of ultrasound, measurement of a distance as short as 2–4 mm is not always reliable. In this case the maximum length of the embryo was measured as 4 mm.

The cardiovascular system is the first organ system to reach a functional state. Contractions of the heart begin at 5 weeks and 0 or 1 day of gestation. However, these primitive contractions occur in peristalsis-like waves. Co-ordinated pulsatile contractions can be observed by the end of 5 weeks of gestation. Although no fine anatomical structure can be differentiated in a 3 mm maximum length embryo, cardiac activity can be clearly recognized with exceedingly bradycardic pulsation of around 110 beats/min. At this stage the chorion has almost equal thickness on the whole circumference of the gestational sac.

When the crown–rump length of the embryo exceeds 7 mm, the shape of the embryo can first be delineated as of a triangular appearance in its longitudinal section. Figure 1.7 shows such a configuration of an embryo with crown–rump length of 7 mm in 6 weeks and 0 day of gestation. At this stage of gestation, the yolk sac is still larger than the embryo (Figure 1.8). It is separated from the embryo by its growing stalk and increasing amniotic sac. The size of the yolk sac is measured almost constantly from 3 to 6 mm of diameter.

THE 10 MM EMBRYO

In the early development of the embryo, the formation and differentiation of the central nervous system are the most dominant phenomena. The central nervous system is the first and most important landmark for ultrasonographic observation of structural anatomy in the embryo. Figure 1.9, which was obtained at 7 weeks and 0 day of gestation, shows a small brain vesicle of an embryo with a crown–rump length of 10 mm. The amniotic cavity is small at this stage of gestation and the yolk sac can be clearly depicted.

Three primary vesicles of the brain, namely the prosencephalon, mesencephalon and rhombencephalon develop from the rostral portion of the neural tube in the last half of the 5th week of gestation. Although there are three or five vesicles, only one cavity can be delineated. At the time the brain vesicle starts to be depicted, the neural tube can also be observed (Figure 1.10). When the neural tube is depicted in coronal section, it appears as two parallel lines.

An embryo with 12 mm crown–rump length, which corresponds to 7 weeks and 1 day of gestation, is depicted in sagittal section in Figure 1.11. The appearance of the embryo exhibits clearly its morphologic characteristics at this time, but the structure of organs, like the brain vesicle, is not delineated. An extremely short umbilical cord connects embryo and chorion frondosum.

THE 15 MM EMBRYO

A coronal section was obtained in an embryo with crown–rump length of 15 mm (Figure 1.12). The neural tube of parallel lines and a short umbilical cord between embryo and chorion are depicted distinctly. Also, the chorion frondosum is distinguishable from the chorion laeve. In a transverse sectional view of the head of an embryo with crown–rump length of 15 mm at 7 weeks and 4 days of gestation the appearance of the head has become rounder and the largest sonolucent structure is obtained from the fourth ventricle (Figure 1.13).

In a longitudinal view of an embryo with 16 mm crown–rump length at 7 weeks and 6 days of gestation a large head can be differentiated from the trunk, but the neck region is not yet developed (Figure 1.14). The fourth ventricle still appears as a large sonolucent structure in the occipital region.

At the beginning of 6 weeks of gestation, the prosencephalon will be cleaved, and give rise to the telencephalon and diencephalon. Telencephalon will give rise to the brain hemispheres and the lateral ventricle, resulting in the formation of falx cerebri. At this stage the brain structure can first be seen to be divided into right and left (Figure 1.15).

Limb buds first appear at the end of 5 weeks gestation, and at the beginning of 8 weeks of gestation the limbs extend ventrally with digital rays in the hand and foot plates (Figure 1.16).

THE 20 MM EMBRYO

When the crown–rump length reaches 20 mm at the end of 8 weeks of gestation, the intestines enter the extraembryonic celom in the proximal portion of the umbilical cord, i.e. umbilical herniation, which is a normal event in the embryo. The longitudinal image in Figure 1.17 of an embryo with 21 mm crown–rump length shows a ventral prominence which is though to be the umbilical herniation. The liver also gives rise to the ventral abdominal prominence. By the end of 8 weeks of gestation, the cavity of each hemisphere will form the lateral ventricle, and then the third ventricle. Other brain structures like the thalamus also grow rapidly at this stage of gestation. As a result, detailed brain structures become visible in the cross-sectional view of the head region.

In the longitudinal section of an embryo with 20 mm crown–rump length, the developing brain structures are very clearly delineated (Figure 1.18). Since this fetus was terminated the next day a cross-section of the embryo (Figure 1.19) was made for confirmation of the resolution of the echogram. Extremely good similarity was seen between the real view and the ultrasound image. From the frontal to the occipital region, lateral ventricle, third ventricle, midbrain ventricle and fourth ventricle are thoroughly delineated as a continuous sonolucent structure in the echogram. Physiological herniation of the midgut is visible in both cross-sections.

The caudal portion of the fourth ventricle continues to the neural canal at this stage, but the spinal cord is not yet formed.

THE 25 MM EMBRYO

Figures 1.20–1.22 are three cross-sectional views of the head, taken in different directions, obtained from the same embryo with crown–rump length of 25 mm. In the longitudinal section (Figure 1.20), the lateral ventricle with choroid plexus in the forehead

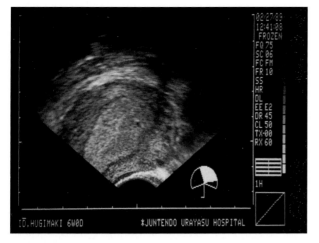

Figure 1.1 A gestation sac of 2 mm diameter at 4 weeks and 1 day of gestation

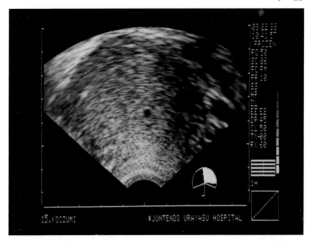

Figure 1.2 The gestation sac at 4 weeks and 2 days delineated in this case as round

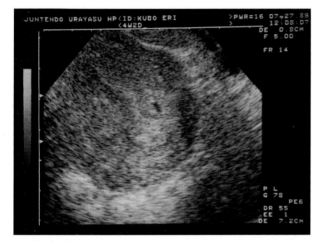

Figure 1.3 A gestation sac showing an ellipsoidal shape with maximum diameter 3.5 mm

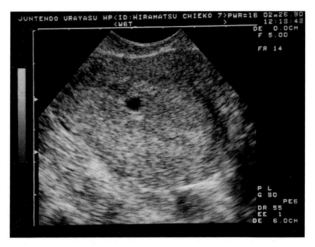

Figure 1.4 Gestation sac implanted in lower half of the uterine cavity

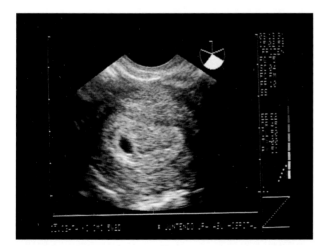

Figure 1.5 Gestation sac at 5 weeks and 2 days showing a space with blood flow between the chorion frondosum and decidua basalis appearing as an arc to the left of the gestation sac

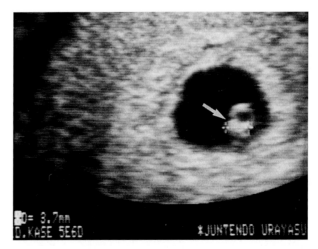

Figure 1.6 Gestation sac at 5 weeks and 4 days, arrow indicates position of the 4 mm long embryo

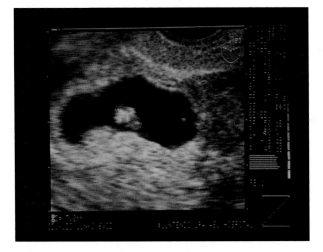

Figure 1.7 Gestation sac and embryo at 6 weeks 0 days. Chorion has almost equal thickness around the whole circumference

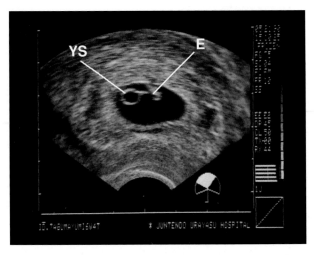

Figure 1.8 Gestation sac and embryo (E) at 6 weeks showing larger yolk sac (YS) attached by growing stalk and amniotic sac

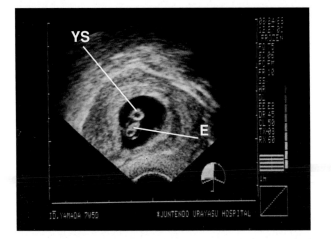

Figure 1.9 Small brain vesicle shown at rostral position in this transverse section of a 10 mm embryo at 7 weeks and 0 day gestation. The yolk sac is clearly depicted above the embryo

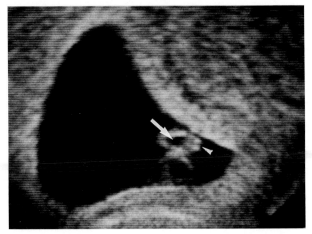

Figure 1.10 Transverse view of an embryo with 12 mm crown–rump length showing the brain vesicle (arrow) and the neural tube on the dorsal side (arrowhead)

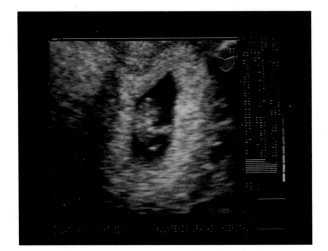

Figure 1.11 Embryo at 7 weeks and 1 day of gestation in sagittal section showing the umbilical cord connecting the embryo and the chorion frondosum

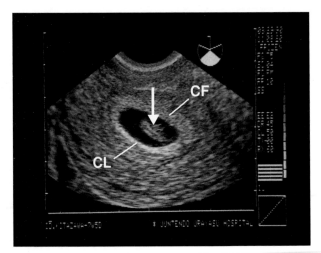

Figure 1.12 Coronal section of embryo with crown–rump length of 15 mm; arrow, umbilical cord; CF, chorion frondosum; CL, chorion laeve

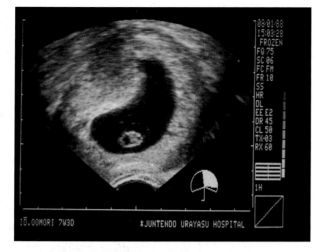

Figure 1.13 Transverse section of the head of a 7 weeks and 4 days embryo showing increased roundness of head. The fourth ventricle appears as the largest sonolucent structure

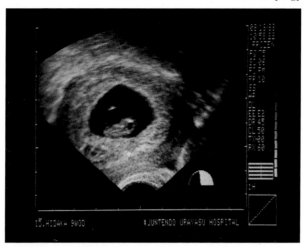

Figure 1.14 Longitudinal section of embryo at 7 weeks and 6 days showing differentiation of head from trunk

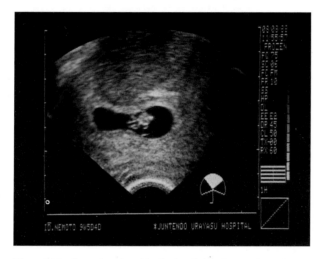

Figure 1.15 Coronal section of the forehead of a 15 mm embryo showing the division of the brain structure into right and left

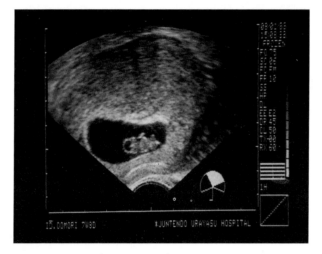

Figure 1.16 Coronal section of a 17 mm embryo showing the four limb buds along the trunk. The fourth ventricle is still clearly visible in the occipital region

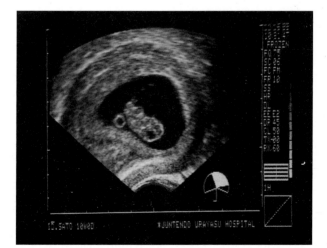

Figure 1.17 Longitudinal image of a 21 mm embryo showing ventral prominence caused by umbilical herniation

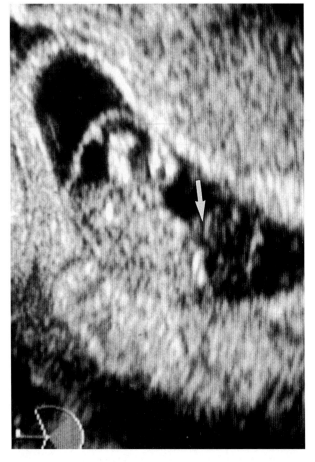

Figure 1.18 Longitudinal section of a 20 mm embryo showing developing brain structures. Arrow indicates umbilical herniation

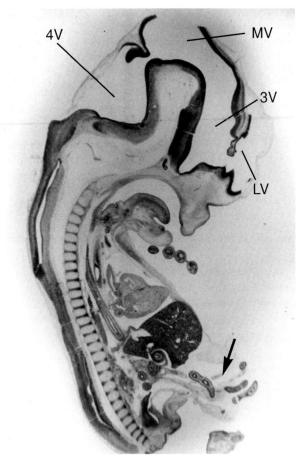

Figure 1.19 Cross-section of embryo in Figure 1.18 confirming the resolution of the echogram. Arrow indicates umbilical herniation; 4V, fourth ventricle; 3V, third ventricle; LV, lateral ventricle; and MV, midbrain ventricle

and a part of the fourth ventricle in the occipital region are delineated. Four choroid plexuses develop in each of the lateral ventricles, in the third ventricle and in the fourth ventricle at the end of 8 weeks of gestation. Among them, those in the lateral ventricles are discernible in echograms from the middle of 9 weeks of gestation. A transverse section of the head (Figure 1.21) reveals the development of the lateral ventricle divided by falx cerebri and echogenic choroid plexus in the lateral ventricle. Thin cranial bone is first discernible in this stage of gestation.

A transverse section (Figure 1.22) obtained slightly downward from the position of Figure 1.21 shows not only the lateral ventricle in the forehead and the fourth ventricle in the occiput, but also the thalamus divided by the third ventricle at the center of the head.

THE 30 MM EMBRYO

At 9 weeks and 6 days of gestation, the head is still disproportionately large, constituting almost half of the embryo. The brain structures described in previous figures are clearly visible. The neck region has now become established. The liver occupies a large portion of abdominal cavity (Figure 1.23) and the intestines are

still within the proximal portion of the cord. Figure 1.24 shows a coronal section of an embryo with 32 mm crown–rump length at 9 weeks and 3 days of gestation. This cross-sectional view through the forehead delineates large lateral ventricles with insufficiently developed choroid plexuses. At the trunk, part of the ventral abdomen is seen. Extremities are delineated and both hands are laid ventrally, one of the characteristics in the embryonic period.

THE 35 MM FETUS

From 10 weeks of gestation, the fetal period begins. By this time the fetus has attained a crown–rump length of 35 mm. All the major organs and systems of the body have already been formed during the embryonic period. Therefore, development during the fetal period is thought to be growth and differentiation of tissues and organs. For instance, progressive development of the lateral ventricle and choroid plexus can be recognized in the head. Figure 1.25 shows remarkably grown choroid plexus in a transverse view of the head of a fetus with crown–rump length of 35 mm at 10 weeks and 5 days of gestation.

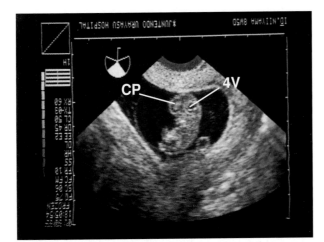

Figure 1.20 Longitudinal section of a 25 mm embryo showing presence of choroid plexus (CP) and the fourth ventricle (4V)

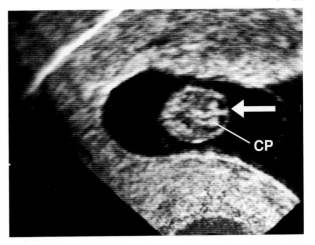

Figure 1.21 Transverse section of same embryo as Figure 1.20 showing the lateral ventricle; arrow, falx cerebri; CP, choroid plexus

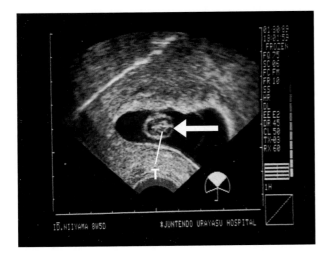

Figure 1.22 Another transverse section of the same embryo as Figure 1.20 showing the thalamus (T); arrow, falx cerebri

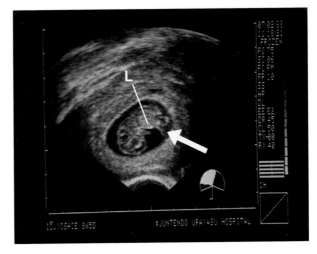

Figure 1.23 Embryo at 9 weeks and 6 days with a crown–rump length of 28 mm. The liver (L) occupies a large part of the abdominal cavity; arrow, herniation of intestine

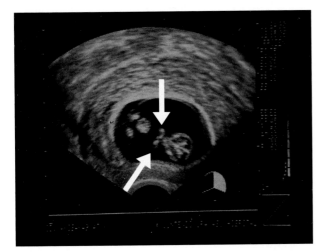

Figure 1.24 Coronal section of a 32 mm embryo with large lateral ventricles but insufficiently developed choroid plexuses; arrows indicate hands

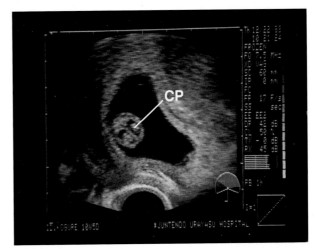

Figure 1.25 Transverse view of 35 mm fetus showing well-developed choroid plexus (CP)

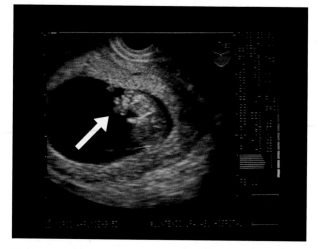

Figure 1.26 Herniation of intestine into umbilical cord (arrow) present at 11 weeks of gestation in this 32 mm fetus

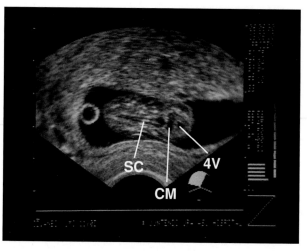

Figure 1.27 Fetus with crown–rump length of 40 mm showing fourth ventricle (4V), cisterna magna (CM) and spinal cord (SC)

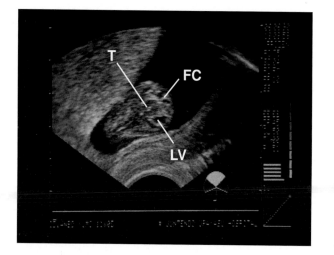

Figure 1.28 Coronal section of same fetus as in Figure 1.27 showing falx cerebri (FC), lateral ventricle (LV) and thalamus (T)

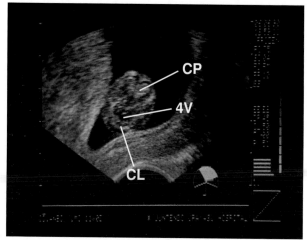

Figure 1.29 Transverse section of head of fetus from Figure 1.27 showing cerebellum (CL), choroid plexus (CP) and fourth ventricle (4V)

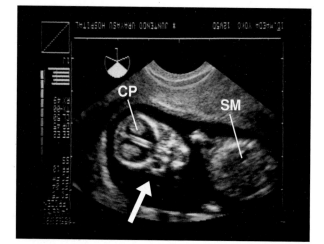

Figure 1.30 Skeletal ossification in a 12 week 5 day fetus; arrow indicates orbit; CP, choroid plexus; SM, stomach

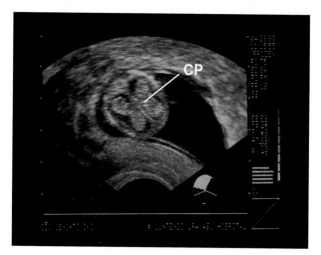

Figure 1.31 Transverse view of 12 week fetus showing large size of choroid plexus (CP) at this stage of gestation

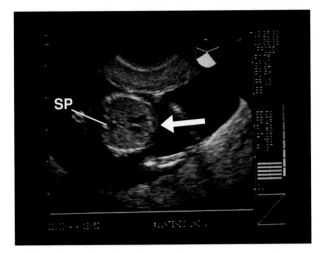

Figure 1.32 Four-chamber view of heart at 12 weeks; arrow indicates heart; SP, spine

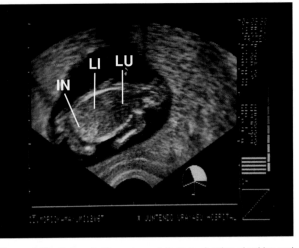

Figure 1.33 Fetus at 12 weeks and 6 days showing shoulder and humerus. The liver, (LI), intestines (IN) and lung (LU) are also visible

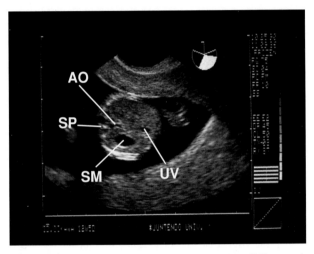

Figure 1.34 Fetus at 12 weeks and 5 days showing aorta (AO), stomach (SM), spine (SP), and umbilical vein (UV)

The stomach is developed as the dilatation of the foregut at the middle of 5 weeks of gestation. In the following 2 weeks, elongation of dorsal wall and 90° clockwise rotation give rise to the characteristic form of the stomach. The fluid-filled cavity of the stomach can be delineated in echograms of fetuses with around 30 mm crown–rump length at 10 weeks of gestation.

Physiological herniation of the midgut can exist until 11 weeks of gestation. Therefore, a distinct view of the herniation of intestine into umbilical cord can be seen in Figure 1.26.

At 10 weeks of gestation, the extremities are still short. The knee is bent from this stage of gestation and, one of the characteristics at this age, the soles of the feet face medially.

THE 40 MM FETUS

When the fetus reaches a crown–rump length of 40 mm, which corresponds to 11 weeks of gestation,

it has a completely human appearance. Figures 1.27–1.29 show different cross-sections of the same fetus. This fetus had a crown–rump length of 42 mm and a biparietal diameter of 17 mm. The coronal view through the dorsal part of the fetus (Figure 1.27) shows, from cranial to caudal, the fourth ventricle, cisterna magna and spinal cord as structures of the central nervous system. The coronal section of the center of the head is shown in Figure 1.28. Thalamus, brain stem, medulla oblongata and spinal cord are well formed and large choroid plexuses in both lateral ventricles are seen concurrently. From 7 weeks of gestation, the cerebellum develops from a very thin roof of rhombencephalon. The rhombic lips bulge into the fourth ventricle and fuse to the ventral portion of the alar plates. Eventually they fuse in the midline to form a dumb-bell-shaped cerebellum. In this 11 weeks fetus (Figure 1.29), the dumb-bell-shaped cerebellum is delineated in a transverse section of the head. Choroid plexuses occupying the lateral ventricles and a relatively large fourth ventricle are also visible.

THE 50 MM FETUS

Ossification of the skeletal system can be discerned as early as the end of 9 weeks of gestation. In this fetus at 12 weeks and 5 days with a crown–rump length of 56 mm and biparietal diameter of 21 mm, cranium, orbits, nasal bone and mandible are clearly depicted (Figure 1.30). Also, the lateral ventricles divided by falx cerebri and choroid plexuses inside the lateral ventricle can be easily observed in this coronal view. The fluid-filled cavity of the stomach is seen in the abdomen.

The extremely large choroid plexus occupying the lateral ventricle is a characteristic view of the head of this age of fetus (Figure 1.31). Relative size of the choroid plexus decreases gradually with increasing

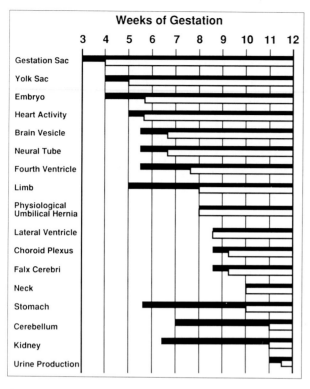

Figure 1.35 Relation between the start of embryological development and ultrasonographical visualization in structures and organs of the conceptus, embryo and fetus. Black bars indicate embryological knowledge of development; White bars show ultrasonographical visualization of each structure or organ by using high frequency transvaginal ultrasound

stomach, umbilical vein, aorta, spine and rib, can be clearly depicted (Figure 1.34). This fetus was measured as having a 21 mm biparietal diameter at 12 weeks and 5 days of gestation.

The ureteric bud and metanephrogenic blastema give rise to permanent kidneys at approximately 6 weeks of gestation. By 9 weeks of gestation, ureter, renal pelvis, callyces and collecting tubules are successively developed. The kidneys attain their adult position by 10 weeks of gestation. After the kidneys begin to produce urine when the fetus is 11–13 weeks of gestation, it becomes easy to interpret the kidneys at both sides of spine.

At the end of 12 weeks of gestation, the lower extremities are still not so well developed as and are slightly shorter than their final relative length. However, they have the general appearance of the adult leg.

READING LIST

1. England, MA. (1983). *A Colour Atlas of Life before Birth*. (London: Wolfe Medical Publications Ltd.)
2. England, MA. (1988). Normal development of the central nervous system. In Levene, M.I., Bennett, M.J. and Punt, J. (eds.) *Fetal and Neonatal Neurology and Neurosurgery*, pp 3–27 (Edinburgh: Churchill Livingstone)
3. Gasser, R.F. (1975). *Atlas of Human Embryos*. (Hagerstown: Harper & Row, Publishers, Inc.)
4. Moor, K.L. (1988). *The Developing Human*, 4th edn. (Philadelphia: WB Saunders Co.)

gestational age. This transverse view of the head was obtained from a fetus with biparietal diameter of 19 mm at 12 weeks and 0 days of gestation.

The heart develops from splanchnic mesenchyme in the cardiogenic area at around 5 weeks of gestation. As the primitive heart tube grows, it bends to the right and has the general appearance of an adult heart by about 7 weeks. Partitioning into four chambers is completed and the heart shows internal structures of the adult heart at about 9 weeks of gestation. Nonetheless, the four-chamber view of the heart is usually difficult to observe at 12 weeks, even using high frequency transvaginal scanning (Figure 1.32).

By the end of 12 weeks, the upper limbs have almost reached their final relative length. In this coronal section of a fetus at 12 weeks and 6 days of gestation (Figure 1.33), the shoulder and humerus are depicted. Although the diaphragm is not clearly shown, the difference in echogenicity can be shown between the lung and liver. There is higher echogenicity in the liver than in lung, and also higher in the intestines than in liver.

In transverse section at the level of liver and stomach, the same anatomical structures that can be seen in second and third trimester, such as liver,

2 Early Malformation Detected by Transvaginal Sonography

S. Rottem

BACKGROUND

Obstetrical ultrasound, more than any other technique, has complemented prenatal diagnosis by permitting the detection of structural anomalies. The contribution of transabdominal sonography to detection of fetal malformations is uncontested. However, due to their relatively low resolution and other physical drawbacks, the currently used transabdominal probes do not permit malformation identification prior to 16 weeks. On the other hand, after 20–22 weeks, when imaging of fetal anomalies becomes easier, the legal and psychological implications of a potential pregnancy termination have to be considered. It is therefore undeniable that an early gestational age is important in the detection of fetal abnormalities. The transvaginal route circumvents almost all physical obstacles of the transabdominal probes and allows for the use of high-frequency transducers to create a clear, high-resolution image.

Consequently, a well-defined fetal anatomy or pathology becomes evident at an earlier gestational age.

Recently, a 6.5 MHz probe was employed for mapping normal embryonic, extraembryonic or fetal structures from 4 to 14 weeks from the last menstrual period. Each structure was considered as first seen when detected in 5% of the scanned fetuses; was considered as significantly seen when detected in more than 75% of the scanned fetuses; and as always seen when detected in all the scanned fetuses. Figures 1A and 1B depict this high-resolution sonographical mapping of 43 organs from 4 to 14 weeks from the last menstrual period and the lag time between the first-seen area (FS) and the always-seen area (ALL). We predict that this organ-age timing chart will serve the reader as a practical guide for early malformation detection by high-frequency transvaginal sonography. Most centers performing extensive malformation investigation feel that 14–15 weeks is an optimal time to take advantage of the high-resolution images of the vaginal probe and that the cost–benefit ratio of this early examination will soon be evident.

Images of normal organs as well as early detected congenital anomalies are presented here.

THE CENTRAL NERVOUS SYSTEM

The contour of the spine on the midsagittal picture becomes clearer as the embryo unfolds from its curled up position at 8 weeks from the last menstrual period (Figure 2.2). Spina bifida spanning across several vertebrae can be imaged as early as 11 weeks (Figure 2.3). Presence of cranial vault can be diagnosed at 11–12 weeks from the last menstrual period and the diagnosis of anencephaly can potentially be made starting from this early age (Figures 2.4 and 2.5).

ABDOMEN AND THORAX

Splanchnic organs, such as the stomach and the liver, are recognizable from 9 weeks together with the fetal lungs (Figures 2.6 and 2.7). During the eighth week the physiological herniation of the midgut makes its appearance as a highly echogenic structure which thickens the umbilical cord at the abdominal insertion (Figure 2.8). This structure may be prominent for the next 2–3 weeks and after 12 weeks 'bowel containing' omphalocele can be diagnosed (Figure 2.9).

The fetal heart resembles a trilocular cavity at the end of the eleventh week (Figure 2.10) and can be seen as a somewhat blurred structure of four chambers at 12 weeks (Figure 2.11). Gross cardiac anomalies may be detected at 14–15 weeks (Figures 2.12).

THE GENITOURINARY TRACT

The kidney can be observed during the eleventh week (Figure 2.13), while the genitalia assume their final phenotypic appearance during the thirteenth

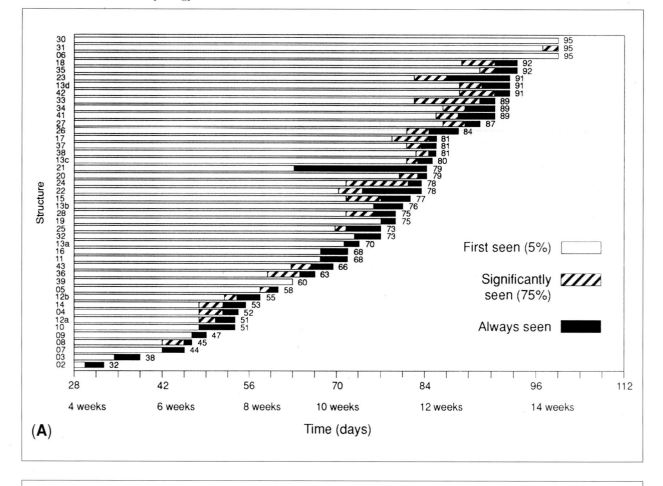

(A)

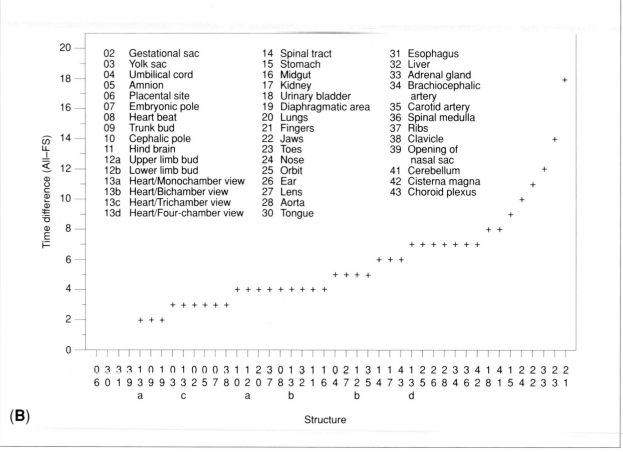

(B)

Figure 2.1 (**A**) The organ-age timing chart and (**B**) sonographic temporal sequence of the organ-age timing chart; All – FS, Always seen – First seen

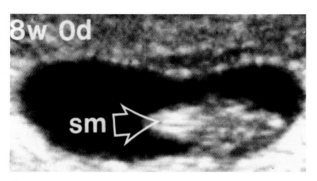

Figure 2.2 Spinal medulla (sm) at 8 weeks 0 days

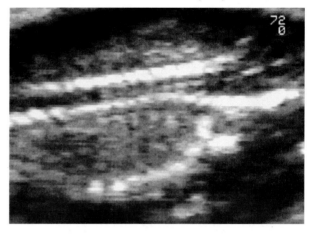

Figure 2.3 Longitudinal scan of the fetal spine at 11 weeks 5 days; an open cervical spina bifida is present

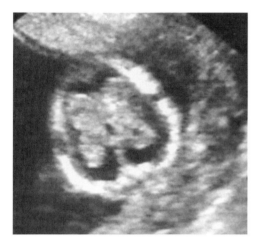

Figure 2.4 Horizontal section of the fetal head (12 weeks) at the level of the choroid plexus

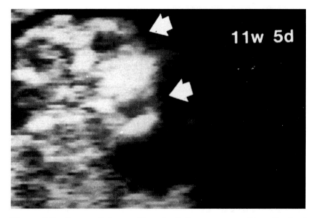

Figure 2.5 Anencephalus at 11 weeks 5 days; arrows point to the fetal orbits

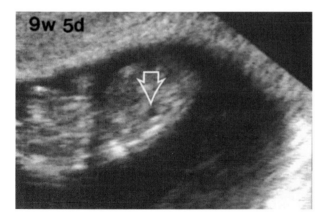

Figure 2.6 The fetal stomach at 9 weeks 5 days is indicated by arrow

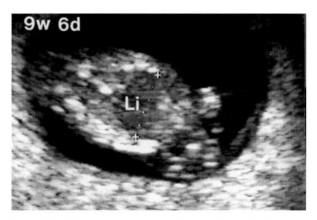

Figure 2.7 Fetal abdomen and thorax at 9 weeks 6 days, Li = Liver

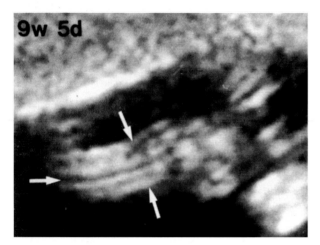

Figure 2.8 Umbilical cord and midgut herniation at 9 weeks 3 days; arrows point to umbilical vessels

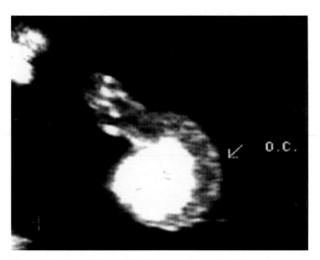

Figure 2.9 Scan of the umbilical cord in a 14-week-old fetus showing an omphalocele (O.C.)

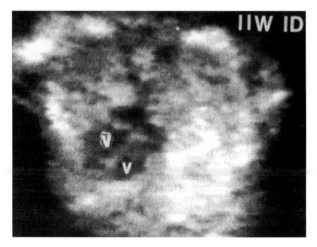

Figure 2.10 Fetal thorax at 11 weeks 1 day; the three-chamber view of the fetal heart is a normal ultrasonographic finding at this gestational age

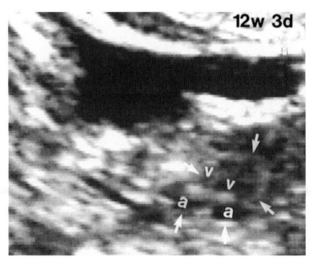

Figure 2.11 Four-chamber view at 12 weeks 3 days; v, ventricle; a, atrium

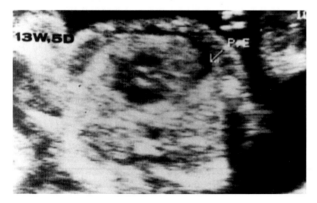

Figure 2.12 Pericardial effusion (P.E.) in a fetus with non-immune hydrops and cardiac hypertrophy at 13 weeks 5 days

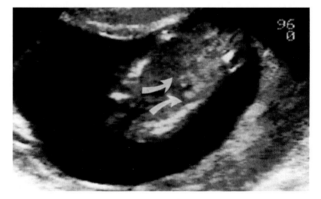

Figure 2.13 Fetal kidney (arrow) at 11 weeks 4 days

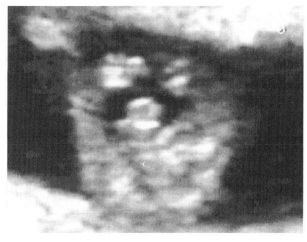

Figure 2.14　Caudal view of the male fetus at 13 weeks 2 days

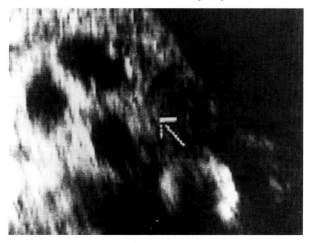

Figure 2.15　An example of multicystic dysplastic kidney (arrow) at 14 weeks

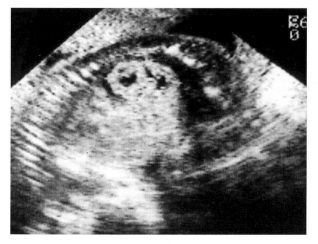

Figure 2.16　Double collecting system at 15 weeks

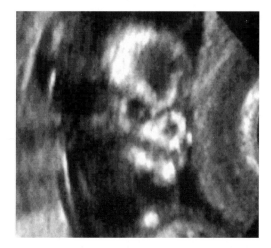

Figure 2.17　Coronal plane of the head at 13 weeks

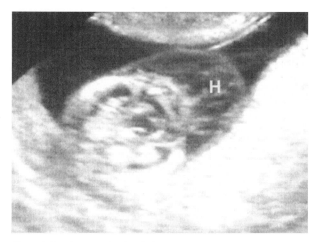

Figure 2.18　An example of nuchal cystic hygroma (H) at 11 weeks 4 days

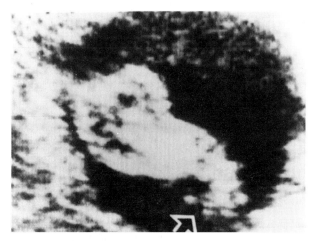

Figure 2.19　Scan of the leg at 16 weeks, showing a pes equinovarus; arrow indicates the toes

week (Figure 2.14). Many renal anomalies can be reliably imaged between 12 and 14 weeks (Figures 2.15 and 2.16).

OTHER ORGANS

The developing fetal face approaches its final shape at 13–14 weeks (Figure 2.17). The palate completes its midline closure only at 13–14 weeks.

The contour of the neck can be depicted at 9 weeks and transvaginal sonography is an advantageous tool for the detection and follow-up of cystic hygromas (Figure 2.18).

High-resolution images of the extremities and possible anomalies can be achieved from 13 weeks or even later depending on the position of the presented part (Figure 2.19).

READING LIST

1. Rottem, S. (1989). *Targeted organ study of developmental anatomy from 4 to 14 weeks using a 6.5 MHz transvaginal probe.* D.Sc. thesis, Technion–Israel Institute of Technology, Haifa, Israel

2. Timor-Tritsch, I.E., Farine, D. and Rosen, M.G. (1988). A close look at early embryonic development with the high-frequency transvaginal transducer. *Am. J. Obstet. Gynecol.*, **159**, 676

3. Rottem, S., Bronshtein, M., Thaler, I. and Brandes, J.M. (1989). First trimester transvaginal sonographic diagnosis of fetal anomalies. *Lancet*, **1**, 444

4. Rottem, S. and Bronshtein, M. (1990). Transvaginal sonographic diagnosis of congenital anomalies between 9 weeks and 16 weeks, menstrual age. *J. Clin. Ultrasound*, **18**, 307

5. Timor-Tritsch, I.E. and Rottem, S. (eds.) (1991). *Transvaginal Sonography*, 2nd edn. (New York: Elsevier Press)

3 Normal Anatomy and Malformations of the Fetal Neural Axis

F.A. Chervenak, G. Isaacson and J. Streltzoff

This chapter focuses on the normal anatomy and the most important malformations of the fetal neural axis. Anomalies in this region are of considerable import, as they often determine survival, physical appearance and function in society. A study of the fetal neural axis as a region necessarily focuses on morphologic abnormalities of the central nervous system, but at the same time considers facial defects and cervical lymphatic dysgenesis. This regional approach is helpful as abnormalities of varied embryological origins may have similar sonographic appearances.

NORMAL ANATOMY

A systematic approach to sonographic examination of the fetal neural axis is necessary to reveal the numerous possible abnormalities in this complex region. This topic is important to each person performing obstetric ultrasound, as a careful evaluation of the fetal neural axis should be considered to be an integral part of all second and third trimester ultrasound examinations.

Head

Historically, serial transverse sonograms have proved very helpful in evaluating fetal intracranial anatomy. These transverse planes are, for several reasons, preferred for antenatal ultrasound over the coronal and sagittal ones used by neonatal ultrasonographers and pathologists. When accessible to ultrasound examinations, the fetal head is most often in an occiput–transverse position (i.e. the side of the head lies parallel to the mother's abdominal wall). Also, the membranous bones of the fetal cranium do not reflect sound waves to the extent that they do when they are more heavily calcified and rigid, in postnatal life. Finally, a transverse plane produces a large cross-section of the brain, in which multiple landmarks may be visualized at one time for orientation. (Figure 3.1).

The lateral ventricles

The lateral ventricles are identified as paired echo-spared areas within the brain substance. The distal ventricle (i.e. the one farthest from the ultrasound transducer) is chosen for study, as reverberation artifacts often obscure the anatomy of the proximal hemisphere. A prominent echogenic area is often seen within the lateral ventricle, which represents the choroid plexus.

In early fetal life, the ventricular system fills a large portion of the developing brain and has the form of two smooth, curved tubes joined above the third ventricle. As gestation progresses, the ventricular system develops a conformation that increasingly resembles that in adult life and occupies a decreasing proportion of the brain's volume. Sonographically, this change is manifested by a decrease in the proportion of the brain's cross-section occupied by the lateral ventricles. This evolution has been documented and nomograms generated that compare the width of the lateral ventricle to the width of the cerebral hemisphere at various gestational ages[1–3].

Although the lateral-to-hemispheric width ratio has been widely used to assess ventricular volume, (Figure 3.2) the 'lateral wall', as seen on ultrasound, may not be the true lateral wall. Assessment of the atrium of the lateral ventricle is well-defined and should measure less than 1 cm[4].

The biparietal diameter

Perhaps the most intensely studied transverse section of the fetus is at the level of the biparietal diameter (BPD) (Figure 3.3). Several intracranial landmarks are located to define a plane 15° above the cantho-meatal line and parallel to the base of the skull. The two landmarks most consistently found are the roughly triangular, paired, non-echogenic thalami and two short anterior lines paralleling the midline, designated the cavum septi pellucidi. Other structures commonly observed in the same plane and near the midline are from posterior to anterior: the great cerebral vein and its ambient cistern sitting above the cerebellum, the midbrain, the third ventricle between the thalami, and the frontal horns of the lateral ventricles. Laterally placed, in the same plane, are the spiral hippocampal gyri posteriorly and the bright paired echoes of the insulae with pulsating middle cerebral arteries.

In this plane, the BPD can be reproducibly measured as the distance from the proximal outer table to the distal inner table of the skull[5,6]. In addition, the head perimeter can be determined by direct measurement or calculated by summing the BPD and occipito-frontal diameter (OFD) measured from the midpoint of frontal and occipital echo complexes and multiplying by 1.62[7]. The ratio of BPD to OFD defines the cephalic index (normal values 75–85). A high value determines brachycephaly and a low value dolichocephaly. With these variants of head shape, BPD may be an inaccurate determinant of gestational age and rarely there may be cranial pathology.

There are several sonographic markers which have anatomic correlates that have been a source of confusion. During the second trimester, the echogenic line, once thought to be the Sylvian fissure, is a reflection from the insular cortex[8]. The area designated as cerebral peduncles in some texts points to the entire midbrain, of which the crus cerebri or cerebral peduncles form only the most rostral parts. Finally, the echospared area caudal to the midbrain, often called the ambient cistern, is in large part composed of the great cerebral vein surrounded by a small amount of cerebrospinal fluid[9].

The cerebellum

The cerebellum may be visualized in a place parallel to the BPD plane. Once located, the cerebellar structures are best studied by rotating the ultrasound transducer 15° farther from the cantho-meatal line. In this plane, the cerebellum (with its brightly echogenic, centrally-placed vermis, and two relatively non-echogenic hemispheres) may be evaluated and measured. Frond-like folia are suggested at the borders of the hemispheres and the midbrain may be seen in front of the vermis. The cisterna magna is seen and can be measured between the vermis and the inner table of the occipital bone[10,11] (Figure 3.4).

The base of the skull

The base of the skull level may be identified by an echogenic 'X' formed by the lesser wings of the sphenoid bone and the petrous pyramid. These bone ridges demark the anterior, middle and posterior fossae (Figure 3.5).

Sagittal and coronal views

Sagittal views of the fetal brain are sometimes helpful to delineate anatomy. The relationship of midline to cranial structures can be seen in Figure 3.6. Coronal views may also be of value (see section on Agenesis of the corpus callosum).

The face

Unlike the cranium and its contents, which may be studied using an orderly progression of well-defined sonographic planes, characterization of the face requires both ingenuity and good luck on the part of the sonographer.

The orbits and eyes

Measurement of the distance between the bony orbits may be useful for determination of gestational age in the search for anomalies characterized by either hypotelorism or hypertelorism. Depending on the position of the fetal head, the inner and outer orbital distances can be measured in coronal or transverse planes and compared to nomograms. The outer orbital distance is the more valuable measurement because of greater normal variation across gestational age as compared with the inner orbital distance. The technique for obtaining these measurements is illustrated in Figure 3.7[12,13].

The lens of the fetal eye may be visualized as a circular area on the front of the globe. On occasion, the aqueous and vitreous humors, the extraocular muscles, and the ophthalmic artery may be recognized[14].

The ears

The pinna of the ear and the development of its cartilages have been observed sonographically. The pinna is initially smooth, but becomes increasingly ridged as gestation progresses (Figures 3.8 and 3.9).

Occasionally, even the basal turn of the cochlea or superior semicircular canal may be visualized within the petrous portion of the temporal bone [16].

The lower face

The nares and the upper lip can be visualized using an oblique transverse scan (Figure 3.10). This plane may be used in the search for cleft lip and cleft palate. The tongue may be observed and its motion in the act of swallowing studied. The fetal profile (i.e. the middle sagittal view) is useful for verifying the position of the nose, the contour of the chin, and the shape of the facial midline.

The neck

The neck should be examined with particular attention to its surface contours as a variety of lesions may protrude from this area. The trachea and carotid bifurcation may be seen within the substance of the neck.

The spine

An appreciation of the variability in the shapes of the vertebral bodies, and the changing sonographic appearance of the spine during gestation is necessary to differentiate small defects in the spine from normal anatomic features [17].

By 16 weeks of gestation, individual vertebrae may be identified by the observation of three echogenic ossification centers in the transverse plane. Two of these are posterior to the spinal canal in the laminae and one is anterior, representing the vertebral body (Figure 3.11). If the spine is scanned sagittally, a line of vertebral bodies and a line of posterior elements may be seen on either side of the non-echogenic spinal canal (Figure 3.12). In the coronal plane, the two echogenic posterior ossification centers are seen to diverge progressively in the cervical region as one moves closer to the base of the skull (Figure 3.13) [18].

During the third trimester, more detail may be seen. The vertebral body, pedicles, transverse processes, posterior laminae and the spinous process may all be identified as echogenic structures in transverse scans. In addition, the spinal canal and intervertebral foramina may be seen as non-echogenic areas (Figure 3.14). In the sagittal plane, a line of vertebral bodies is still seen, but the posterior

echoes are more complex with spinous processes seen jutting from the line of other elements (Figure 3.15) [18].

MALFORMATIONS OF THE FETAL NEURAL AXIS

Anencephaly

Anencephaly is a congenital anomaly in which the cerebral hemispheres and overlying skull and scalp are absent. The incidence of anencephaly, one of the most common congenital disorders in the world, varies depending on geographic location, race and sex. Anencephaly occurs most frequently in areas where spina bifida is also very common. Anencephaly was the first malformation diagnosed with sufficient certainty for which physicians were willing to perform elective abortion based on sonographic findings [19].

The diagnosis of anencephaly is made when the upper portion of the cranial vault cannot be visualized. This bony structure can be seen normally after 14 weeks when the head is not hidden in the pelvis. The area of the cerebro-vasculosa, a vascular malformation seen in this disorder, may appear as an ill-defined mass of heterogeneous density above the level of the orbits (Figure 3.16). Hydramnios may complicate these pregnancies due to poor fetal swallowing.

This diagnosis can be made with accuracy. In the combined experiences of six centers, over 130 cases have been detected with no false-positive diagnoses [20,21].

Anencephaly is a lethal anomaly. The recurrence rate increases with previously affected children as with all neural tube defects.

Hydrocephalus

Hydrocephalus is characterized by a relative enlargement of the cerebro-ventricular system with an accompanying increase of pressure of the cerebrospinal fluid within the fetal head. Hydrocephalus has been successfully diagnosed by a lateral ventricular atrial width greater than 1 cm [4] an abnormally increased lateral ventricle-to-hemispheric width ratio [22,23], a dangling choroid plexus [24], and an asymmetric appearance of the choroid plexus [25,26]. Serial measurements are probably the most useful tool to define hydrocephalus in borderline cases. The location of the obstruction may be determined by observing which portions of the ventricular system are enlarged (Figures 3.17 and 3.18).

Once fetal hydrocephalus is diagnosed, it is essential to search for associated anomalies which

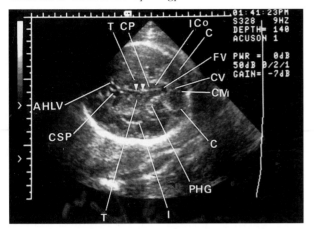

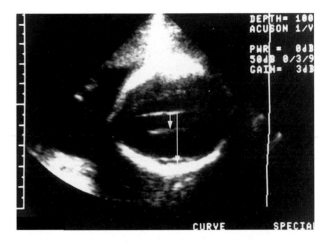

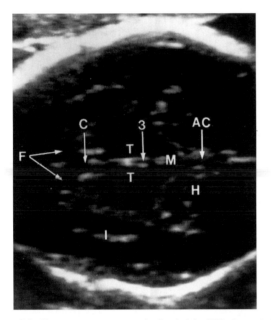

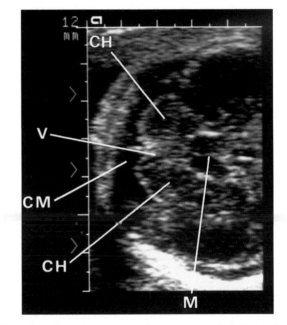

Figure 3.1 Transverse sonogram through fetal skull at the level of BPD but angled posteriorly and inferiorly, demonstrates cerebellum (C), cerebellar vermis (CV), cisterna magna (CM), fourth ventricle (FV), inferior colliculus (ICo), cerebellar peduncle (CP), parahippocampal gyrus (PHG), insular cortex (I), thalamus (T), third ventricle (arrowheads), cavum septi pellucidi (CSP), anterior horns of lateral ventricles (AHLV). (Reprinted with permission from ref. 46)

Figure 3.2 Transverse sonogram through bodies of the lateral ventricles. Arrows demonstrate distance from midline echo to lateral wall of lateral ventricle and distance from midline echo to inner skull table. (Reprinted with permission from ref. 46)

Figure 3.4 Transverse sonogram demonstrates cerebellar hemispheres (CH), vermis (V), midbrain (M), and cisterna magna (CM). (Reprinted with permission from ref. 46)

Figure 3.3 Transverse sonogram at the level of the BPD demonstrates frontal horn of lateral ventricles (F), (3), hippocampus (H), midbrain (M), great cerebral vein and ambient cistern (AC), insula (I). (Reprinted with permission from ref. 45)

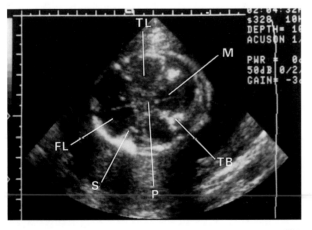

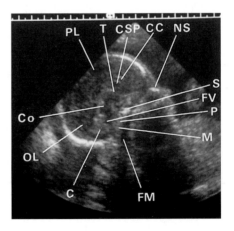

Figure 3.5 Sonogram through base of skull showing frontal lobe (FL), temporal lobe (TL), greater wing of sphenoid (S), temporal bone (TB), pituitary stalk (P), and medulla (M). (Reprinted with permission from ref. 46)

Figure 3.6 Sagittal sonogram which can supply supplemental information for midline cranial anatomy, including nasal septum (NS), body of sphenoid (S), thalamus (T), cavum septi pellucidi (CSP), corpus callosum (CC), parietal lobe (PL), occipital lobe (OL), colliculi (Co), cerebellum (C), fourth ventricle (FV), medulla (M), pons (P), foramen magnum (FM). (Reprinted with permission from ref.46)

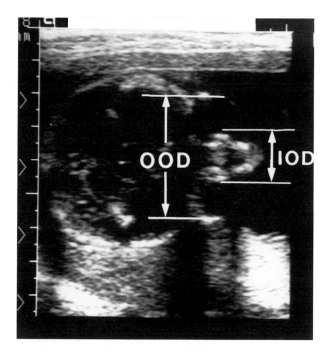

Figure 3.7 Transverse sonogram with outer orbital distance (OOD) and inner orbital distance (IOD) indicated. (Reprinted with permission from ref. 45)

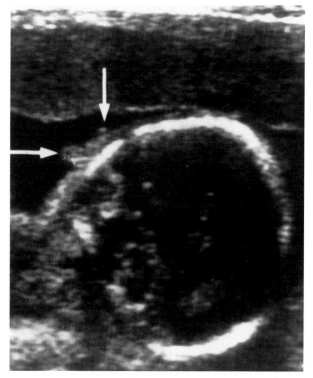

Figure 3.8 Smooth fetal pinna at 18 weeks' gestation (arrows). (Reprinted with permission from ref. 45)

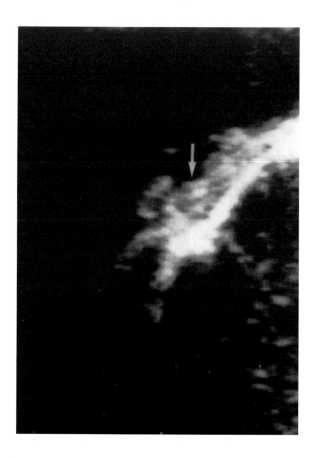

Figure 3.9 Mature, ridged fetal ear at 36 weeks' gestation (arrow). (Reprinted with permission from ref. 45)

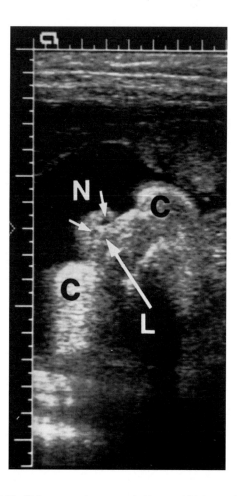

Figure 3.10 Oblique coronal sonogram looking up at fetal upper lip (L), cheeks (C), and nares (N). (Reprinted with permission from ref. 45)

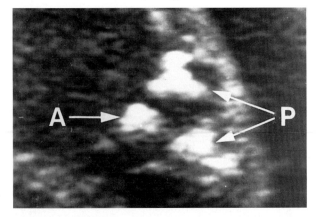

Figure 3.11 Transverse sonogram of fetal spine at 18 weeks demonstrating anterior (A) and posterior (P) ossification centers. (Reprinted with permission from ref. 45)

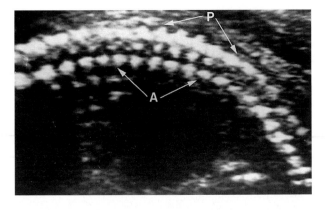

Figure 3.12 Sagittal sonogram of fetus at 18 weeks' gestation showing anterior (A) and posterior (P) perforation elements.

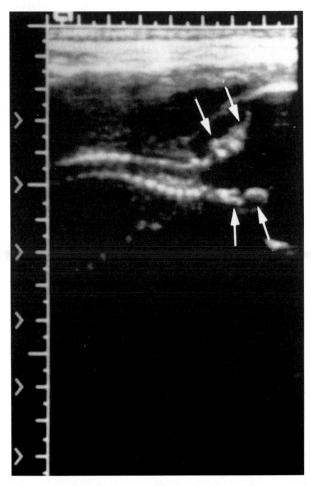

Figure 3.13 Coronal sonogram of fetal spine demonstrates a cervical spine widening (arrows) toward the base of the skull. (Reprinted with permission from ref. 46)

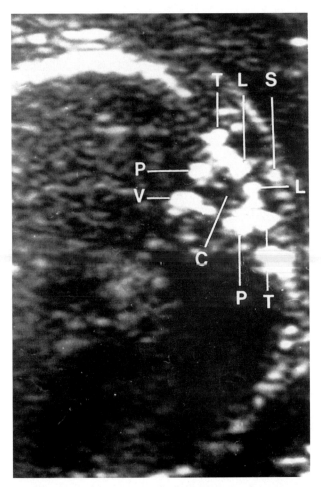

Figure 3.14 Transverse sonogram of mature fetal spine shows vertebral body (V), pedicles (P), transverse processes (T), lamina (L), spinous process (S), and spinal cord (C). (Reprinted with permission from ref. 45)

have been reported to occur in 83% of cases. While spina bifida is the most common associated anomaly, associated structural anomalies may affect any organ system. In addition to meticulous sonographic evaluation, determination of fetal karyotype should be performed[22,23].

The prognosis for hydrocephaly is not dependent upon the severity of the hydrocephalus. Associated anomalies may, themselves, determine a poor

prognosis (e.g. holoprosencephaly, thanatophoric dwarf with cloverleaf skull). For isolated hydrocephalus there is an outcome range from normal to severe retardation.

Microcephaly

Microcephaly means small head. In general, a small

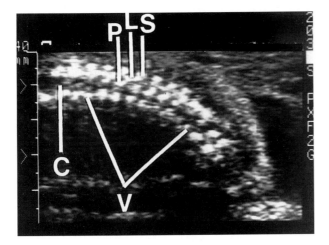

Figure 3.15 Sagittal sonogram of lumbosacral spine shows vertebral bodies (V), spinal cord (C) pedicle (P), lamina (L), and spinous process (S). Note how the spinal cord moves posteriorly in the sacral region. (Reprinted with permission from ref. 45)

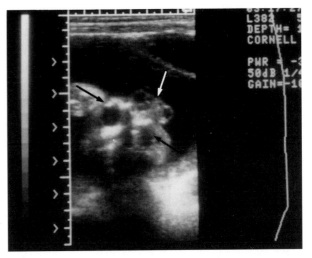

Figure 3.16 Coronal sonogram of fetal head demonstrating anencephaly. Black arrows point to orbits; white arrow points to area cerebrovasculosa

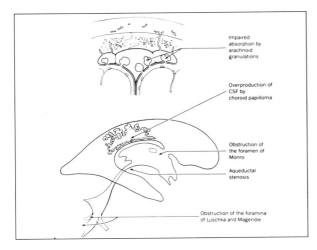

Figure 3.17 Common sites of obstruction of cerebrospinal fluid flow resulting in hydrocephalus. (Reprinted with permission from ref. 45)

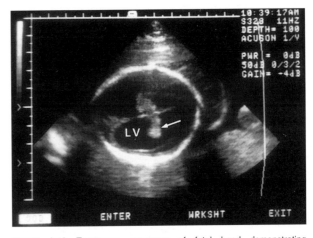

Figure 3.18 Transverse sonogram of fetal head demonstrating hydrocephalus, LV = dilated lateral ventricle, arrow points to dangling choroid plexus

head is the product of an underdeveloped brain, whether as a primary defect or as a part of a more extensive malformation syndrome.

While different biometric standards have been described to define microcephaly in the neonate, a head perimeter 3 or more standard deviations below the mean for age seems workable, and the correlation with mental retardation is very high.

The BPD (the biometric parameter most commonly measured by sonography) is unreliable in the prediction of microcephaly, with a 44% false-positive rate in one study[27]. Compression of the fetal head with resultant dolichocephaly in normal pregnancies accounts for many of these errors. A nomogram of head circumference as a function of gestational age, which corrects for such compressive changes, has proved of greater predictive value. Further aids to diagnosis include nomograms of head circumference to abdominal perimeter and of femur length to head circumference ratios. At the present time, it appears that multiple fetal measurements should be utilized for greater accuracy[28].

The prognosis for microcephaly varies. But, most children will be mentally retarded; in general, the smaller the head the worse the prognosis. As with other malformations, the association with other anomalies increases the likelihood of a poor outcome. Risk of recurrence depends on underlying causes.

Holoprosencephaly

The term holoprosencephaly embraces a variety of abnormalities of the brain and face resulting from incomplete cleavage of the primitive prosencephalon (forebrain) (Figure 3.19). Holoprosencephaly is divided into alobar, semilobar and lobar categories, all determined by the degree of separation of the cerebral hemispheres. The alobar variety shows no evidence of division of cerebral cortex. Thus, the falx cerebri and interhemispheric fissures are absent, and there is a single common ventricle. The semilobar and lobar varieties represent a higher degree of brain development with the semilobar having a partial

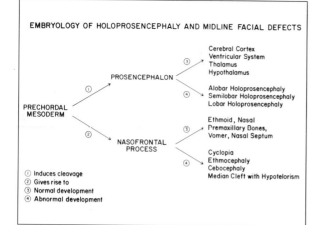

Figure 3.19 Embryology of holoprosencephaly and midline facial defects. (Reprinted with permission from ref. 29)

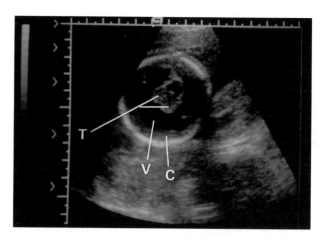

Figure 3.20 Cranial sonogram demonstrating alobar holoprosencephaly, V = common ventricle, T = prominent fused thalamus, C = compressed cerebral cortex

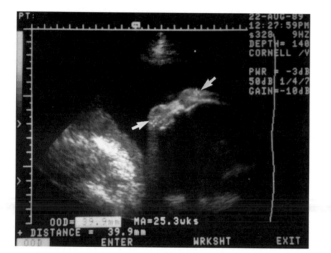

Figure 3.21 Sonogram demonstrating hypotelorism (outlined by white arrows) in a fetus with alobar holoprosencephaly

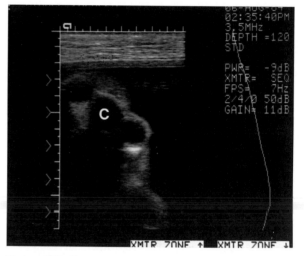

Figure 3.22 Transverse sonogram of fetal head demonstrating cephalocele (C), protruding between bony orbits resulting in hypertelorism. (Reprinted with permission from ref. 32)

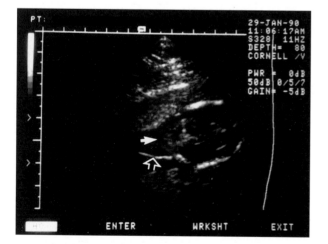

Figure 3.23 Sonogram demonstrating encephalocele (solid arrow) associated with amnion band (bottom arrow)

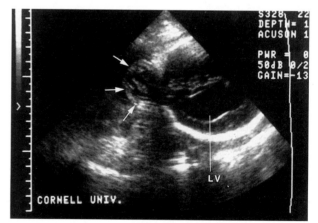

Figure 3.24 Occipital encephalocele (outlined by arrows), LV = dilated lateral ventricle

separation and the lobar having a complete separation of the hemispheres. Microcephaly is usually present because of decreased cortical mass, but macrocephaly may be seen if hydrocephalus develops.

The prechordal mesoderm, an embryonic connective mass between the oral cavity and the undersurface of the neural tube, is thought to be responsible for both the production of the nasofrontal process and the division of the prosencephalon. The nasofrontal process gives rise to the ethmoid, nasal and premaxillary bones, and to the vomer and the nasal septum. Failure of these structures to develop normally can result in the varying degrees of hypotelorism, cleft lip and palate, and nasal malformation that are seen in this disorder. The prosencephalon develops from the most rostral part of the neural tube, and gives rise to the cerebral hemispheres, thalamus and hypothalamus. Failure of its sagittal division can result in a common ventricle, a fused thalamus, and a cortex with neither lobes nor an interhemispheric fissure.

In holoprosencephaly, a spectrum of midline facial anomalies may be seen. Indeed, certain facies predict the presence of the alobar type. Cyclopia, the presence of a single median bony orbit with a fleshy proboscis above it, is the most severe of malformations. In cebocephaly, hypotelorism is associated with a normally placed nose and a single nostril. Hypotelorism with a midline facial cleft also predicts the presence of alobar holoprosencephaly.

Holoprosencephaly may also be associated with milder forms of midline facial dysplasia or normal facies.

Alobar holoprosencephaly may be diagnosed before birth if two criteria are met. The midline echo, generated by the interhemispheric fissure should be absent (Figure 3.20). Hypotelorism can be detected by measuring inner and outer orbital distances (Figure 3.21). The alobar form of holoprosencephaly carries a dismal prognosis. More subtle forms of them may be associated with minimal neurologic deficits[29,30].

Cephalocele

Cephaloceles are protrusions of the meninges and frequently of brain substance through a defect in the cranium. The term includes encephaloceles which contain brain tissue, and cranial meningoceles which do not. In the western world, 75% of these lesions are occipital, but cephaloceles may be parietal, frontal (Figure 3.22), or nasopharyngeal.

Although cephaloceles usually result from a defect in neural tube closure, they may be seen in the amnion rupture sequence (Figure 3.23) or in association with a variety of malformation syndromes, (e.g. Meckel's syndrome).

Sonographically, cephaloceles appear as sac-like protrusions about the head not covered with bone. The diagnosis can be made with certainty only if a defect in the skull is detected (Figure 3.24). Such a defect may be small, however, and difficult to visualize. When present, the position of the defect may be determined using the bony structures of the face and spine and the midline echo for orientation. Ultrasound has not been a reliable technique to differentiate between meningoceles and encephaloceles with a small amount of brain tissue. When brain tissue has herniated, it gives the sac a non-homogeneous appearance. Furthermore, extrusion of a large amount of brain substance may result in microcephaly. Hydrocephalus is commonly associated with cephaloceles[31,32].

Encephaloceles, in general, carry a poor prognosis. Pure meningoceles may have a favorable prognosis and develop normally after surgery.

Facial clefts

Failure of lip fusion, normally complete by 35 days of intrauterine life, may impair subsequent closure of the palatal shelves, leading to cleft lip and cleft palates.

In order to demonstrate a facial cleft before birth, the lower portion of the face must be anterior and clearly visualized (Figure 3.25). Both sagittal and oblique coronal planes of study may be useful. Undulating tongue movements, hypertrophied tissue at the edge of the cleft, and hypertelorism (Figures 3.26 and 3.27) have all been described as useful adjuncts in the diagnosis of a facial cleft[33,34]. Nevertheless, clefts are subtle changes in the face, and their diagnosis is sometimes difficult and inconsistent.

Cystic hygroma

Cystic hygroma are congenital malformations of the lymphatic system appearing as either single or multiloculated cavities filled with fluid. They arise most often about the neck. In fetal life, a more generalized lymphatic disorder exists characterized by cystic hygromas of the posterior triangle of the neck with various degrees of lymphedema. Fetal lymphatic vessels drain into two large sacs lateral to the jugular veins. If these jugular lymph sacs fail to communicate

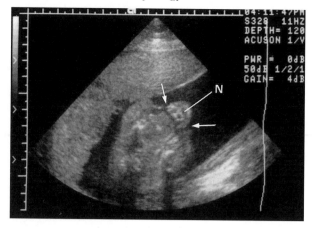

Figure 3.25 Sonogram along an oblique plane through lower part of fetal face demonstrating bilateral cleft lip (arrows), N = nose. (Reprinted with permission from ref. 46)

with the venous system, they may enlarge as they fill with lymph and form cystic hygromas. This failure in lymphatic drainage may also result in the generalized edema of hydrops fetalis[35] (Figure 3.28).

Several sonographic features aid in the diagnosis of fetal cystic hygromas. Hygromas are generally located on the postero-lateral neck, are cystic in appearance, and are frequently divided by random, incomplete septa. As they arise from paired jugular lymph sacs which may enlarge to meet at the posterior midline, a septum representing the nuchal ligament may be visualized (Figure 3.29). Associated hydrops is manifest sonographically as ascites, pleural effusion, pericardial effusion and skin edema (Figure 3.30).

Other cranio-cervical masses that must be differentiated from cystic hygromas include cystic teratomas, cephalocele, branchial cleft cyst and nuchal edema.

The prognosis for cystic hygroma in the second or third trimester is intrauterine death.

Spina bifida/meningomyelocele

Spina bifida refers to a defect in the spine resulting from a failure of the two halves of the vertebral arch to fuse. These lesions usually occur in the lumbo-sacral and cervical regions. If the meninges protrude through this defect, the lesion is designated a meningocele; if neural tissue is included, it is a meningomyelocele.

Sonographically, spina bifida is seen as a splaying of the posterior ossification centers of the spine giving the vertebral segment a U-shaped appearance (Figure

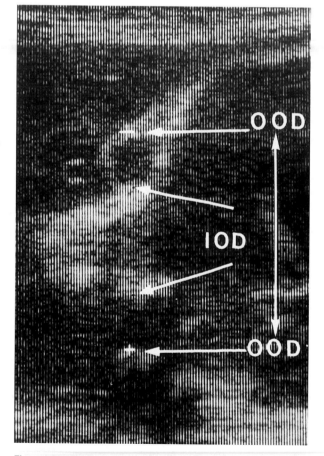

Figure 3.26 Transverse scan through orbits of fetus affected with median cleft face syndrome demonstrating hypertelorism. Inner orbital distance (IOD) and outer orbital distance (OOD) are increased for gestational age of 31 weeks. (Reprinted with permission from ref. 34)

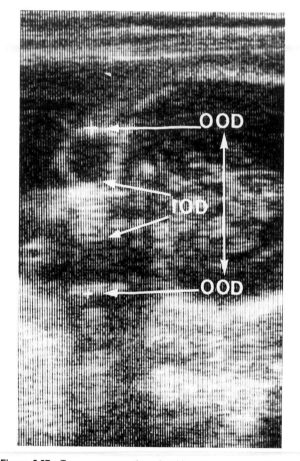

Figure 3.27 Transverse scan through orbits of normal fetus at same gestational age as fetus in Figure 3.26, demonstrating normal IOD and OOD. (Reprinted with permission from ref. 34)

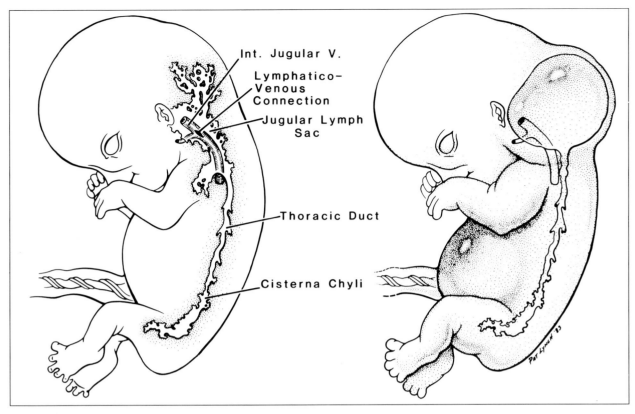

Figure 3.28 Lymphatic system in a normal fetus (left) with a patent connection between the jugular lymph sac and the internal jugular vein and a cystic hygroma and hydrops from a failed lymphaticovenous connection (right). (Reprinted with permission from ref. 35)

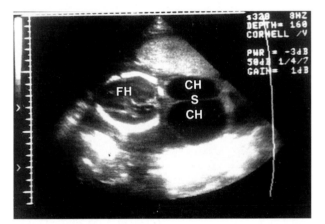

Figure 3.29 Sonogram demonstrating nuchal cystic hygroma (CH), divided by midline septum (S), FH = fetal head

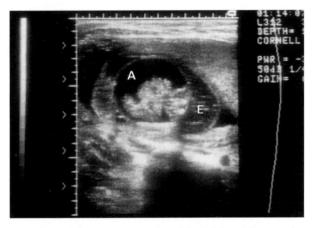

Figure 3.30 Transverse sonogram through fetal abdomen demonstrating fetal hydrops, E = edema of abdominal wall, A = ascites

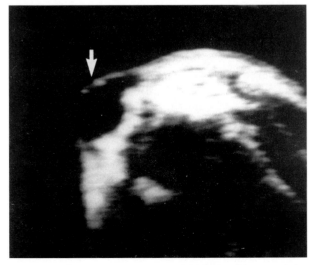

Figure 3.31 Transverse sonogram through fetal spine with arrow pointing to meningomyelocele

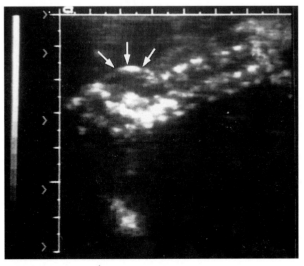

Figure 3.32 Longitudinal sonogram of fetal spine with arrows pointing to meningomyelocele

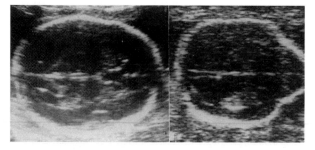

Figure 3.33 Transverse sonogram of a normal fetal head in an 18-week fetus at level of cavum septi pellucidi (left). Transverse section of fetal head at level of cavum septi pellucidi in an 18-week fetus with open spina bifida showing 'lemon' sign (right). (Reprinted with permission from ref. 38)

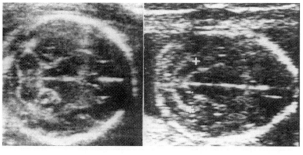

Figure 3.34 Suboccipital bregmatic view of fetal head in an 18-week fetus with a normal cerebellum and cisterna magna (left). Suboccipital bregmatic view of fetal head in an 18-week fetus with open spina bifida, demonstrating 'banana' sign (+) (right). (Reprinted with permission from ref. 38)

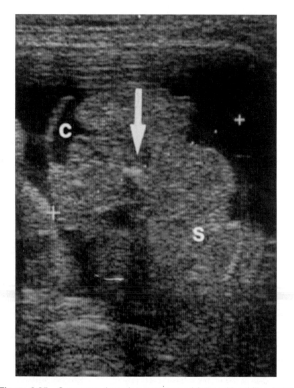

Figure 3.35 Sonogram through a teratoma of fetus with midline facial teratoma demonstrating a complex mass with solid (S) and cystic (C) components. The arrow points to areas of calcification with acoustic shadowing. (Reprinted with permission from ref. 39)

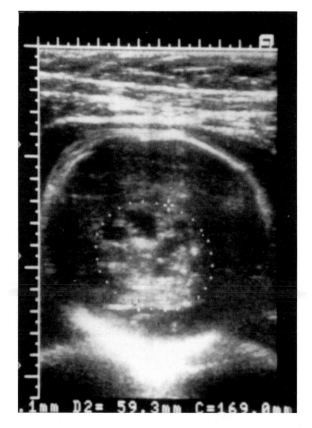

Figure 3.37 Cranial sonogram demonstrating intracranial teratoma outlined by dots with characteristic cystic and solid areas

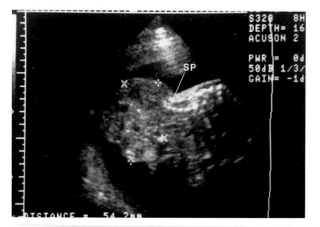

Figure 3.36 Sonogram of sacrococcygeal teratoma, outlined by crosses, protruding beneath fetal spine (SP)

3.31). The posterior ossification centers should be more widely spaced than those in vertebral segments above and below the defect. It should be noted that there is a normal progressive widening of the spinal canal in the cervical region. Although the defect may be visualized on longitudinal scanning, meticulous transverse examinations of the entire vertebral column are necessary to detect smaller defects. When a meningocele or a meningomyelocele is present and intact, a protruding sac may be detected (Figure 3.32). While detection of small spina bifida defects, especially in the sacral area, remains a challenge, sonographic signs of Arnold–Chiari malformation are of adjunctive value[36,37].

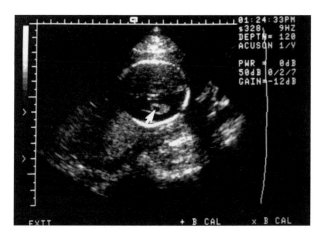

Figure 3.38 Cranial sonogram demonstrating small choroid plexus cyst (arrow)

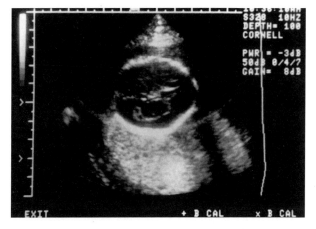

Figure 3.39 Cranial sonogram demonstrating large choroid plexus cyst in a fetus with trisomy 18

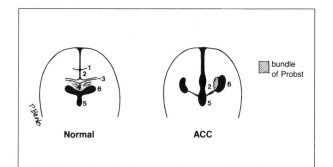

Figure 3.40 Coronal diagrams showing normal anatomy and agenesis of the corpus callosum, 1 = cingulate sulcus, 2 = cingulate gyrus, 3 = pericallosal cistern, 4 = corpus callosum, 5 = third ventricle, 6 = lateral ventricle, hatched area = bundle of Probst. Note that in agenesis of the corpus callosum the third ventricle directly communicates with the interhemispheric fissure and that the lateral ventricle points upwards instead of to the side. (Reprinted with permission from ref. 44)

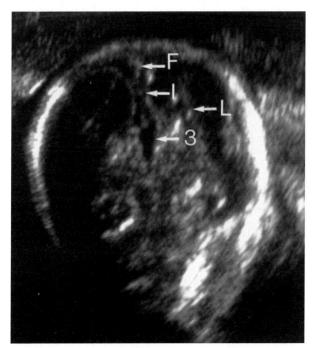

Figure 3.41 Coronal scans of the fetal brain through the level of the third ventricle with agenesis of the corpus callosum, 3 = third ventricle, L = lateral ventricle, F = falx, I = interhemispheric fissure. Note the rhomboid, instead of slit-shaped, third ventricle in agenesis of the corpus callosum. (Reprinted with permission from ref. 44)

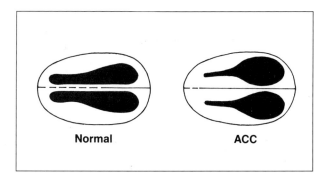

Figure 3.42 Axial views. Normal: the medial walls of the anterior horns lie close to the falx. Agenesis of the corpus callosum: the medial walls are pushed laterally and the posterior horns are dilated (colpocephaly), thus giving the lateral ventricle the shape of a teardrop. (Reprinted with permission from ref. 44)

Although spina bifida may be detected during routine ultrasound examination, many cases are found as a result of careful ultrasound examinations in pregnancies in which elevated maternal serum α-fetoprotein had been detected. Amniotic fluid α-fetoprotein may have an adjunctive role in the diagnosis of smaller lesions.

Prognosis with spina bifida is dependent upon the level of the lesion. Bowel and bladder dysfunction, inability to ambulate and complications due to associated hydrocephalus may occur.

Arnold–Chiari malformation

The Arnold–Chiari malformation is an anomaly of the hindbrain that has two components. The first is a variable displacement of a tongue of tissue derived from the inferior cerebellar vermis into the upper

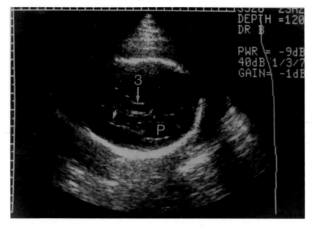

Figure 3.43 Transverse sonogram of fetus with agenesis of the corpus callosum. The medial walls of the anterior horns are pushed away from the falx towards the lateral wall (arrow). The posterior horns are dilated (P) and the third ventricle is dilated and elevated (3). (Reprinted with permission from ref. 44)

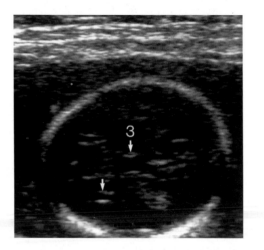

Figure 3.44 Transverse sonogram of the fetus with agenesis of the corpus callosum. Lateral displacement of the medial wall of the anterior horn (arrow) and elevation and dilatation of the third ventricle (3). (Reprinted with permission from ref. 44)

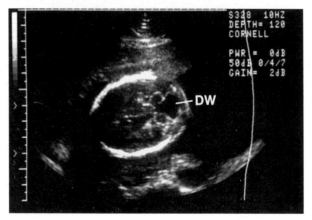

Figure 3.45 Cranial sonogram demonstrating Dandy–Walker cyst (DW) with defect in the cerebellar vermis

cervical spinal canal. The second is a similar caudal dislocation of the medulla and fourth ventricle. It has been stated that most, if not all, cases of spina bifida are complicated by the Arnold–Chiari malformation and that 90–95% of these patients show hydrocephalus.

The Arnold–Chiari malformation can serve,

therefore, as an important marker for spina bifida. Two characteristic sonographic signs (the 'lemon' and the 'banana') of the Arnold–Chiari malformation have been described. A scalloping of the frontal bones can give a lemon-like configuration to the skull of an affected fetus in axial section during the second trimester. The caudal displacement of the cranial contents within a pliable skull is thought to produce this scalloping effect. Similarly, as the cerebellar hemispheres are displaced into the cervical canal, they are flattened antero-posteriorly and the cisterna magna is obliterated, thereby producing a flattened, centrally curved, banana-like sonographic appearance. In extreme cases, the cerebellar hemispheres may be absent from view during fetal head scanning. This characteristic cranial appearance should alert the sonographer to search for spina bifida and has led to its diagnosis in a fetus not previously suspected of having the disorder[38] (Figures 3.33 and 3.34).

Teratomas

Teratomas are neoplasms composed of wide diversity of tissues foreign to the anatomic site in which they arise. They are the most common tumor in neonates, occur in a variety of locations and are usually histologically benign.

Sacrococcygeal teratomas comprise over 50% of these lesions at birth. Those in other locations include intracranial, palatal, cervical, mediastinal, retroperitoneal and gonadal teratomas. The diagnosis of these lesions is of particular importance as they may be resected after birth and the infant cured.

It is not possible to make diagnoses by ultrasound, yet several morphologic features may help to distinguish teratomas from other lesions in similar locations. By ultrasound, teratomas characteristically appear both cystic and solid but the solid components may not be observable (Figure 3.35 – 3.37). The solid components may not be homogeneous in density and may contain calcifications. The cysts frequently have irregular and angulated borders. A variety of anomalies have been reported in association with fetal teratomas including gastrointestinal fistulas. Hydramnios is commonly present. Fetal outcome is generally good with teratomas that are benign and isolated in occurrence. Isolated sacrococcygeal teratomas have a better prognosis than those that arise from vital organs or are found intracranially or along the facial midline[39,40].

Choroid plexus cyst

Small areas of cystic dilatation may be noted in the choroid plexus of the lateral ventricles of the normal, developing fetus (Figure 3.38). Generally they resolve before the end of the second trimester without sequelae. An association with trisomy 18 and bilateral choroid plexus cysts has been described. These lesions are usually transient and without clinical significance but warrant a meticulous ultrasound examination to look for anomalies, especially in larger or bilateral lesions[41,42] (Figure 3.39).

Agenesis of the corpus callosum

The corpus callosum is a bundle of fibers which forms the roof of the third and lateral ventricles. In complete agenesis of the corpus callosum the fibers are still present but they lie in bundles medial to the lateral wall of the ventricles. Their presence pushes those walls laterally and makes them concave in appearance with their tip pointing upward instead of laterally (Figure 3.40). In the coronal sonogram, the widened interhemispheric fissure connected directly with the lateral ventricle (Figure 3.41).

In a transverse sonogram, the medial walls of the anterior horns of the lateral wall lie close to the falx (Figure 3.42). Although the anterior horns are not dilated in agenesis of the corpus callosum, the medial walls are pushed away from their usual midline location. The posterior horns are dilated and, together with the anterior horns, give a tear-drop appearance. The third ventricle is elevated and sometimes dilated (Figures 3.43 and 3.44)[43,44].

It is possible to be entirely normal with agenesis of the corpus callosum but, with undetermined frequency in a fetal population, agenesis of the corpus callosum may reflect a more generalized disorder.

Other malformations of the fetal neural axis

As experience with ultrasound increases and the resolution of the equipment improves, the list of malformations of the fetal neural axis, detected before birth, continues to grow. Several 'cystic' lesions have been detected. Hydranencephaly, appearing as a large, echo-spared area within the head, is distinguished from hydrocephalus by the absence of frontal, temporal and parietal cerebral cortex. Dandy–Walker cyst (Figure 3.45), proencephalic cyst, arachnoid cyst and cerebral atrophy all display echo-spared areas as well. Cranio-facial duplication, vein of Galen malformation, intracranial hemorrhage, fetal goiter and cloverleaf skull add to the list of malformations detected by antenatal ultrasound[45].

REFERENCES

1. Jeanty, P., Dramaix-Wilmet, M., Delbeke, D. *et al.* (1981). Ultrasonic evaluation of fetal ventricular growth. *Neuroradiology*, **21**, 127
2. Johnson, M.K., Dunne, M.G., Mack, L.A. *et al.* (1980). Evaluation of fetal intracranial anatomy by static and realtime ultrasound. *J. Clin. Ultrasound*, **8**, 311
3. Pretorius, D.H., Drose, J.A. and Marco-Johnson, M.L. (1986). Fetal lateral ventricular ratio determination during the second trimester. *J. Clin. Ultrasound*, **5**, 121
4. Cardoza, J.D., Goldstein, R.B. and Filly, R.A. (1988). Exclusion of fetal ventriculomegaly with a single measurement: the width of the lateral ventricular atrium. *Radiology*, **169**, 711–14
5. Shepard, M. and Filly, R.A. (1982). A standardized plane for biparietal diameter measurement. *J. Ultrasound Med.*, **1**, 145
6. Hadock, F.P. Deter, R.L., Harrist, R.B. *et al.* (1982). Fetal biparietal diameter: rational choice of plane of section for sonographic measurement. *Am. J. Roentgenol.*, **138**, 871
7. Jeanty, P. and Romero, R. (1984). *Obstetrical Ultrasound*, pp.87–90. (New York: McGraw-Hill)
8. Jeanty, P., Chervenak, F.A., Romero, R. *et al.* (1984). The Sylvian fissure: a commonly mislabeled cranial landmark. *J. Ultrasound Med.*, **3**, 15
9. Isaacson, G., Mintz, M.C. and Crelin, E.S. (1986). *Fetal Sectional Anatomy: With Ultrasound and Magnetic Resonance Imaging.* (New York: Springer-Verlag)
10. Smith, P.A., Johansson, D., Tzannatos, C. *et al.* (1986). Prenatal measurement of the fetal cerebellum and cisterna cerebellomedullaris by ultrasound. *Prenat. Diag.*, **6**, 133
11. Pilu, G., DePalma, L., Romero, R. *et al.* (1986). The fetal subarachnoid cisterns: an ultrasound study with report of a case of congenital communicating hydrocephalus. *J. Ultrasound Med.*, **5**, 365
12. Mayden, K.L., Tortora, M., Berkowitz, R.L. *et al.* (1982). Orbital diameters: a new parameter for prenatal diagnosis and dating. *Am. J. Obstet. Gynecol.*, **144**, 289
13. Jeanty, P., Dramaix-Wilmet, M., Delbeke, D. *et al.* (1982). Fetal ocular biometry by ultrasound. *Radiology*, **143**, 513
14. Jeanty, P., Romero, R., Staudach, A. *et al.* (1986). Facial anatomy of the fetus. *J. Ultrasound Med.*, **5**, 607
15. Birnholz, J. (1983). The fetal external ear. *Radiology*, **147**, 819

16. Isaacson, G. and Mintz, M.C. (1986). Prenatal sonographic visualization of the inner ear. *J. Ultrasound Med.*, **5**, 409

17. Birnholz, J.C. (1986). Fetal lumbar spine: measuring axial growth with ultrasound. *Radiology*, **158**, 805

18. Chervenak, F.A., Isaacson, G. and Lorber, J. (1988). *Anomalies of the Fetal Head, Neck, and Spine: Ultrasound Diagnosis and Management*, pp.17–36. (Philadelphia: W.B. Saunders)

19. Campbell, S., Johnstone, F.D., Holt, E.M. and May, P. (1972). Anencephaly: early ultrasonic diagnosis and active management. *Lancet*, **2**, 1226–7

20. Murken, J.D., Stengel-Rutkowski, S. and Schwinger, E. (1979). *Prenatal Diagnosis of Genetic Disorders*, pp.94–192 (Stuttgart: Ferdinand Enke)

21. Chervenak, F.A., Farley, M.A., Walter, L. *et al.* (1984). When is termination of pregnancy during the third trimester morally justifiable? *N. Engl. J. Med.*, **310**, 501

22. Chervenak, F.A., Berkowitz, R.L., Romero, R. *et al.* (1983). The diagnosis of fetal hydrocephalus. *Am. J. Obstet. Gynecol.*, **147**, 703–16

23. Chervenak, F.A., Duncan, C., Ment, L.R. *et al.* (1984). The outcome of fetal ventriculomegaly. *Lancet*, **2**, 179–82

24. Cardoza, J.D., Filly, R.A. and Podarsky, A.E. (1988). The dangling choroid plexus: a sonographic observation of value in excluding ventriculomegaly. *Am. J. Radiol.*, **151**, 767–70

25. Benacerraf, B.R. and Birnholz, J.C. (1987). The diagnosis of fetal hydrocephalus prior to 22 weeks. *J. Clin. Ultrasound*, **15**, 531–6

26. Benaceraff, B.R. (1988). Fetal hydrocephalus: diagnosis and significance. *Radiology*, **169**, 858–9

27. Chervenak, F.A., Jeanty, P., Cantraine, F. *et al.* (1984). The diagnosis of fetal microcephaly. *Am. J. Obstet. Gynecol.*, **149**, 512

28. Chervenak, F.A., Rosenburg, J.C., Brightman, R. *et al.* (1984). A prospective study of the accuracy of ultrasound in predicting fetal microcephaly. *Obstet. Gynecol.*, **69**, 908

29. Chervenak, F.A., Isaacson, G., Mahoney, M.J. *et al.* (1984). The obstetric significance of holoprosencephaly. *Obstet. Gynecol.*, **63**, 115

30. Chervenak, F.A., Isaacson, G., Hobbins, J.C. *et al.* (1985). The diagnosis and management of fetal holoprosencephaly. *Obstet. Gynecol.*, **66**, 322

31. Chervenak, F.A., Isaacson, G., Mahoney, M.J. *et al.* (1984). Diagnosis and management of fetal cephalocele. *Obstet. Gynecol.*, **64**, 86

32. Chervenak, F.A., Isaacson, G., Rosenberg, J.C. and Kardon, N.B. (1986). Antenatal diagnosis of frontal cephalocele in a fetus with ateleosteogenesis. *J. Ultrasound Med.*, **5**, 111

33. Christ, J.E. and Meininger, M.G. (1981). Ultrasound diagnosis of cleft lip and cleft palate before birth. *Plast. Reconstr. Surg.*, **6**, 854

34. Chervenak, F.A., Tortora, M., Mayden, K. *et al.* (1984). Antenatal diagnosis of median cleft face syndrome: sonographic demonstration of cleft lip and hypertelorism. *Am. J. Obstet. Gynecol.*, **149**, 94

35. Chervenak, F.A., Isaacson, G., Blakemore, K.J. *et al.* (1983). Fetal cystic hygroma. Cause and natural history. *N. Engl. J. Med.*, **309**, 822

36. Hobbins, J.C., Grannum, P.A.T., Berkowitz, R.L. *et al.* (1979). Ultrasound in the diagnosis of congenital anomalies. *Am. J. Obstet. Gynecol.*, **134**, 331

37. Pearce, J.M., Little, D. and Campbell, S. (1985). The diagnosis of abnormalities of the fetal central nervous system. In Saunders, R.C. and James, A.E. (eds.) *The Principles and Practice of Ultrasonography in Obstetrics and Gynecology*, 3rd edn., pp.246–8. (Norwalk: Appleton-Century-Crofts)

38. Nicolaides, K.M., Campbell, S., Gabbe, S.G. and Guidetti, R. (1986). Ultrasound screening for spina bifida: cranial and cerebellar signs. *Lancet*, **2**, 72

39. Chervenak, F.A., Tortora, M., Moya, F.R. and Hobbins, J.C. (1984). Antenatal sonographic diagnosis of epignathus. *J. Ultrasound Med*, **3**, 235

40. Chervnak, F.A., Isaacson, G., Touloukian, R. *et al.* (1985). The diagnosis and management of fetal teratomas. *Obstet. Gynecol.*, **66**, 666

41. Chudleigh, P., Pearce, J.M. and Campbell, S. (1984). The prenatal diagnosis of transient cysts of the fetal choroid plexus. *Prenat. Diag.*, **4**, 135

42. Nicolaides, K.M., Rodeck, C.G. and Gosden, C.M. (1986). Rapid karyotyping in non-lethal malformations. *Lancet*, **1**, 283

43. Comstock, C.H., Culp, D., Gonzalez, J. *et al.* (1985). Agenesis of the corpus callosum in the fetus: its evolution and significance. *J. Ultrasound Med.*, **4**, 613

44. Comstock, C.H. (1991). Agenesis of the corpus callosum in the fetus: diagnosis and significance. *Female Patient*, in press

45. Chervenak, F.A., Isaacson, G. and Lorber, J. (1988). *Anomalies of the Fetal Head, Neck, and Spine: Ultrasound Diagnosis and Management*, pp.152–210. (Philadelphia: W.B. Saunders)

4 Evaluation of Fetal Skeleton and Diagnosis of Skeletal Dysplasia

V. D'Addario, F. Catizone and A. Ianniruberto

Skeletal dysplasias are a rare and heterogeneous group of anomalies, which are usually genetically determined. Their classification is complicated and controversial, due to their unknown etiopathogenesis, their polymorphic phenotypic expression and finally the lack of uniformity about definition criteria.

The International Nomenclature for Skeletal Dysplasias subdivides the diseases into five different groups[1]:

(1) Osteochondrodysplasias (abnormalities of cartilage or bone growth and development);

(2) Dysostoses (malformations of individual bones singly or in combination);

(3) Idiopathic osteolyses (disorders associated with multifocal reabsorption of bone);

(4) Skeletal disorders associated with chromosomal aberrations; and

(5) Primary metabolic disorders.

A comprehensive description of these diseases is beyond the scope of this chapter. In fact, even though more than 200 skeletal dysplasias are recognizable at birth, only a few of them can be diagnosed *in utero* with ultrasound. Furthermore a specific prenatal diagnosis can be made only in a restricted number of cases. Therefore the attention will be focused on the general aspects of the ultrasonic diagnosis of skeletal dysplasias. Then the ultrasonic findings of the most common skeletal dysplasias will be briefly described.

APPROACH TO THE ULTRASONIC DIAGNOSIS OF SKELETAL DYSPLASIAS

In evaluating a skeletal dysplasia, the ultrasonographer can deal with two different possibilities:

(1) Evaluation of a fetus at risk for a specific familial skeletal dysplasia; or

(2) Occasional recognition of an abnormal skeletal finding during a routine examination of a not at risk patient.

In the former case he will be helped by the knowledge of the anomaly, whose features he will look for, and a specific prenatal diagnosis will be more feasible. In the latter case the routine examination of the fetal skeleton will allow the recognition of a skeletal anomaly, but a specific diagnosis may be

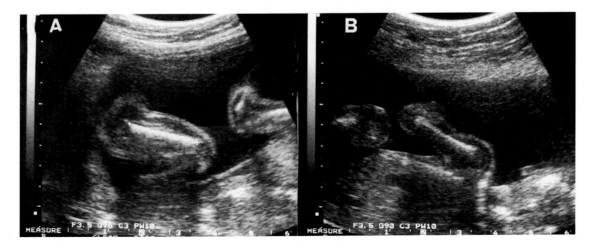

Figure 4.1 Ultrasonic appearance of normal fetal long bones: A = femur; B = humerus. Long bone evaluation includes the assessment of their length, shape and degree of mineralization

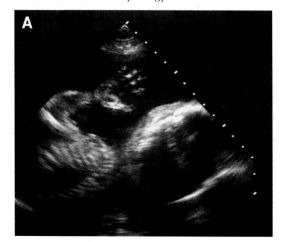
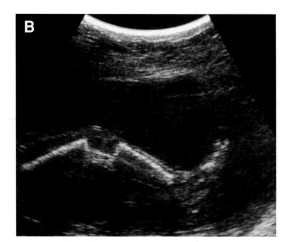

Figure 4.2   Normal appearance of the fetal hand (**A**) and foot (**B**)

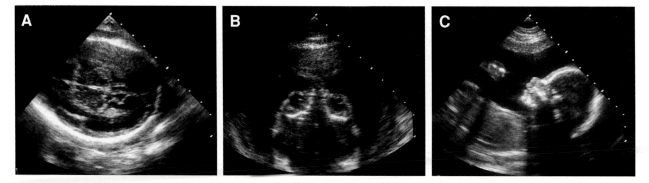

Figure 4.3   Evaluation of the fetal cranium includes the skull size and shape (**A**), the orbits (**B**) and the profile (**C**)

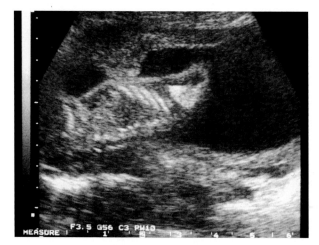
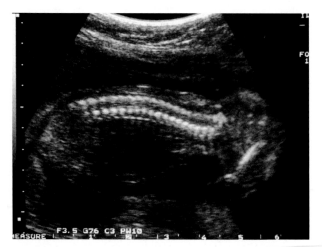

Figure 4.4   Normal appearance of the fetal thorax; the scapula, the ribs and the spine are easily recognized

Figure 4.5   Normal appearance of the fetal spine in longitudinal scan; the spinal canal is clearly identified

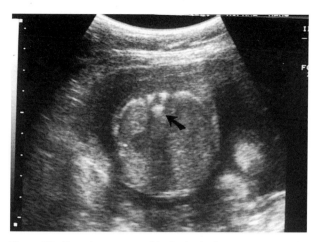

Figure 4.6 Normal appearance of the fetal spine in transverse scan; the ossification centers of the body and of the laminae are clearly identified

difficult or not possible. In both cases a careful examination of the fetal skeleton is necessary, looking for features which can be suggestive of dysplasias[2-4].

The evaluation of the fetal skeleton includes the study of long bones, hands and feet, cranium, spine and chest.

Evaluation of the long bones

Long bone evaluation includes the assessment of their length, shape and degree of mineralization (Figures 4.1A and 4.1B). Long bone biometry refers to the calcified diaphysis and numerous nomograms are available for all fetal long bones. Measurement of long bones allows the recognition of shortening of the extremities. With the exception of heterozygous achondroplasia, bone shortening in affected fetuses is usually dramatic, much lower than the 5th percentile. By comparing the different bone segments, the type of limb shortening can be established:

(1)   Rhizomelic (shortening of the proximal segment);

(2)   Mesomelic (shortening of the intermediate segment);

(3)   Acromelic (shortening of the distal segment); or

(4)   Micromelic (shortening of all limb segments).

In evaluating the shape of a long bone, the degree of its curvature and the possibility of fractures should be considered. Excessive bowing ('campomelia') is characteristic of campomelic dysplasia and osteogenesis imperfecta; fractures are typical of osteogenesis imperfecta and hypophosphatasia.

Finally the degree of mineralization of long bones should be assessed by examining the echogenicity of the bone and its acoustic shadow.

Evaluation of the fetal extremities should include

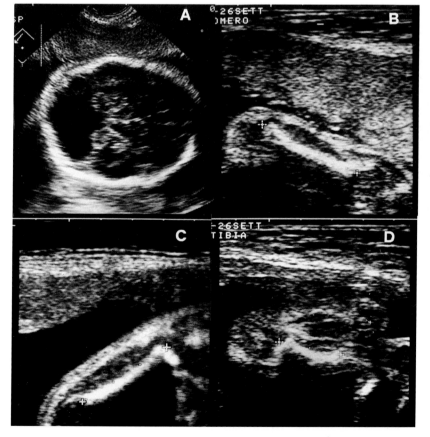

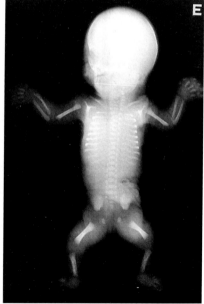

Figure 4.7 Micromelic dwarfism associated with Dandy–Walker malformation. (**A**) shows the absence of the cerebellar vermis and the cyst in the posterior fossa; (**B**), (**C**) and (**D**) show the humerus, the femur and the tibia respectively; (**E**) shows the radiogram of the fetus

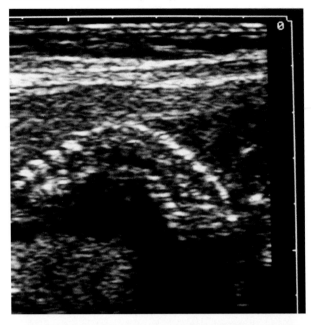

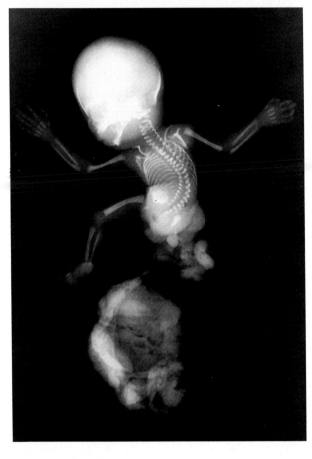

Figure 4.8 Marked angulation of the fetal spine in a fetus with multiple malformations by amniotic band syndrome shown clearly by the scan (**A**) and by the radiogram (**B**)

also the hands and feet (Figures 4.2A and 4.2B), looking for polydactyly or syndactyly, and extreme postural deformities, such as those seen in diastrophic dysplasia.

Evaluation of the cranium

In evaluating the fetal cranium one should consider skull size and shape, orbits and profile (Figures 4.3A–4.3C). Cloverleaf skull deformity is typical of thanatophoric dwarphism. Bone demineralization, typical of congenital hypophosphatasia and osteogenesis imperfecta, produces an impressive ultrasonic visualization of intracranial structures. Furthermore the skull is very thin and can be easily deformed by a slight compression of the ultrasonic probe. Evaluation of the orbits allows the recognition of hypo- and hypertelorism. By observing the fetal profile anomalies such as frontal bossing, depressed nasal bridge, cleft palate and micrognathia can be recognized.

Evaluation of the thorax

Several skeletal dysplasias are associated with hypoplastic thorax (achondrogenesis, thanatophoric dwarphism, asphyxiating thoracic dysplasia, etc.). Chest restriction may lead to pulmonary hypoplasia, a frequent cause of death in these conditions. Thoracic dimensions can be evaluated by measuring the thoracic circumference at the level of the heart. (Figure 4.4).

Evaluation of the spine

Fetal spine should be examined along its whole length, in order to recognize spinal defects or postural abnormalities (Figures 4.5 and 4.6). The degree of mineralization of the spine would also be considered; a highly demineralized spine is typical of achondrogenesis.

Evaluation of associated anomalies

Associated anomalies should be accurately ruled out, since their presence strongly influences the prognosis (Figures 4.7 and 4.8). The severity of most skeletal dysplasias, in fact, mainly depends on three factors: thoracic hypoplasia, bone demineralization and associated anomalies.

Following the general criteria so far described a specific diagnosis or a list of some possible diagnoses can be obtained by comparing the features presented by the single case with the list of anomalies characterized by the same findings, as reported by the following list.

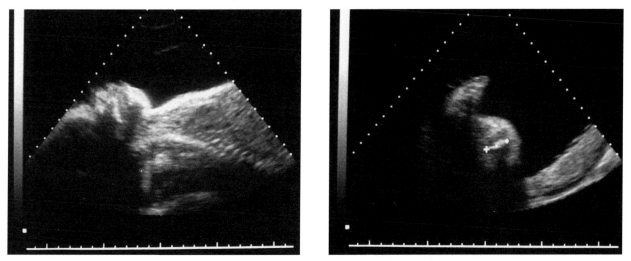

Figure 4.9 Achondrogenesis. Note the severely short femur, the small thorax and the large head; polyhydramnios is associated

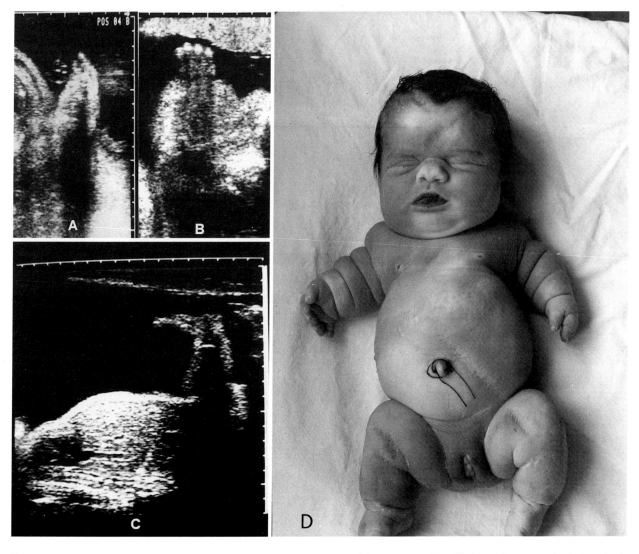

Figure 4.10 Thanatophoric dysplasia. (**A**) and (**B**) show the sonographic appearance of the upper extremities; (**C**) shows a lower extremity, the hypoplastic thorax and the associated polyhydramnios; the newborn is shown in (**D**)

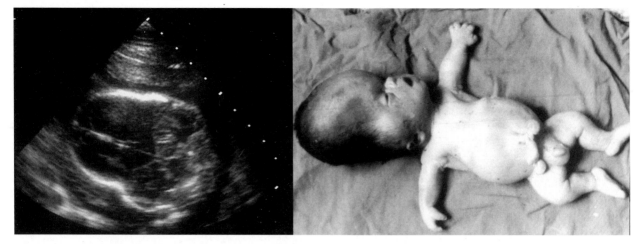

Figure 4.11 Typical cloverleaf skull in a case of thanatophoric dysplasia

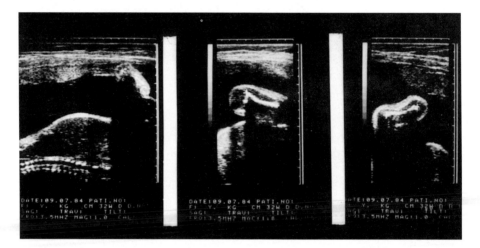

Figure 4.12 Asphyxiating thoracic dysplasia. The thorax is markedly hypoplastic; limb shortening is mild; polyhydramnios is associated

MICROMELIA
  Achondrogenesis
  Thanatophoric dysplasia
  Fibrochondrogenesis
  Short rib–polydactyly syndromes
  Diastrophic dysplasia

RHIZOMELIA
  Thanatophoric dysplasia
  Chondrodysplasia punctata rhizomelic type
  Diastrophic dysplasia
  Congenital short femur

MESOMELIA
  Mesomelic dysplasia
  COVESDEM association (costovertebral
    segmentation defect with mesomelia)

BOWED LONG BONES
  Campomelic dysplasia
  Osteogenesis imperfecta
  Thanatophoric dysplasia
  Hypophosphatasia
  Otopalatodigital syndrome

DEMINERALIZATION
  Achondrogenesis
  Osteogenesis imperfecta
  Hypophosphatasia

BONE FRACTURES
  Osteogenesis imperfecta
  Hypophosphatasia
  Achondrogenesis

HYPOPLASTIC THORAX
  Achondrogenesis
  Thanatophoric dysplasia
  Asphyxiating thoracic dysplasia
  Short rib–polydactyly syndromes
  Chondroectodermal dysplasia
  Fibrochondrogenesis
  Campomelic dysplasia

POLYDACTYLY
  Chondroectodermal dysplasia
  Short rib–polydactyly syndromes

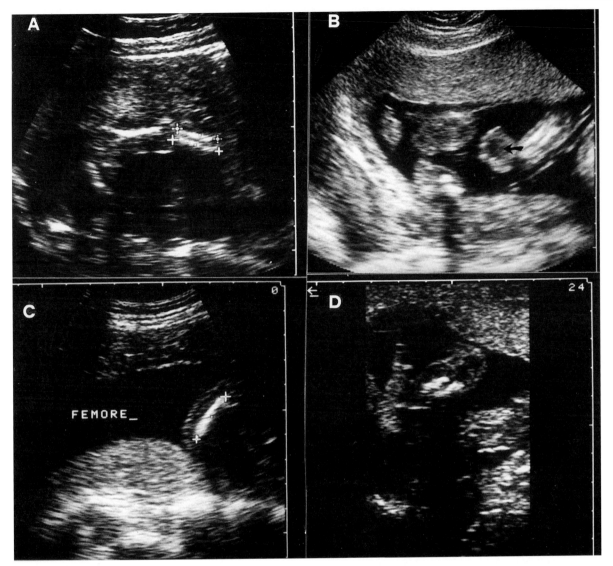

Figure 4.13 Micromelic dwarphism and polydactyly in a case of short limb–polydactyly syndrome. The upper limb is shown in (**A**); polydactyly in (**B**) (arrow); the lower limbs in (**C**) and (**D**)

DEPRESSED NASAL BRIDGE
Atelosteogenesis
Thanatophoric dysplasia
Achondrogenesis
Achondroplasia
Campomelic dysplasia

CLEFT PALATE
Roberts syndrome
Larsen syndrome
Otopalatodigital syndrome
Diastrophic dysplasia
Campomelic dysplasia

MICROGNATHIA
Campomelic dysplasia
Diastrophic dysplasia
Otopalatodigital syndrome
Achondrogenesis
Pena–Shokeir syndrome

HYPERTELORISM
Mesomelic dysplasia
Otopalatodigital syndrome
Larsen syndrome
Roberts syndrome

ULTRASONIC FINDINGS TYPICAL FOR SPECIFIC DYSPLASIAS
Cloverleaf skull (thanatophoric dysplasia)
Hitch-hiker thumbs (diastrophic dysplasia)
Spine demineralization (achondrogenesis)
Hypoplastic scapulae (campomelic dysplasia)
Acromesomelia (chondroectodermal dysplasia)

Looking at the list of skeletal findings it appears evident that only a limited number of skeletal dysplasias are characterized by specific features. In most cases the ultrasonic findings are common to several conditions. However, by combining the different findings, the number of possible diagnoses can be reduced to a short list.

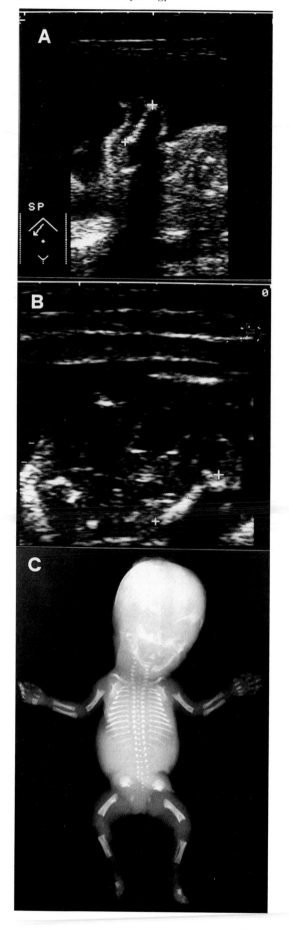

Figure 4.14 Achondroplasia. (**A**) and (**B**) show the humerus and the femur, which are shortened but normally shaped; (**C**) shows the radiogram of the fetus

The ultrasonic findings of the most commonly diagnosed skeletal dysplasias will be now briefly described.

ACHONDROGENESIS

This is characterized by severe micromelic dwarphism, hypoplastic thorax, lack of vertebral ossification and large head (Figure 4.9). Although these findings are quite specific for achondrogenesis the spectrum of the disease is broad[5]. The condition is incompatible with postnatal life.

THANATOPHORIC DYSPLASIA

The sonographic diagnosis can be made in the presence of micromelic dwarphism with bowed femur ('telephone receiver femur'), hypoplastic thorax and cloverleaf skull. This last finding, when present, is specific for the disease[6] (Figures 4.10 and 4.11). The condition is incompatible with postnatal life.

ASPHYXIATING THORACIC DYSPLASIA

The most important diagnostic criterion is the hypoplastic thorax. Limb shortening is frequently associated, but is generally mild. Association with polyhydramnios is common (Figure 4.12). Most of the affected infants die in the neonatal period from respiratory failure.

SHORT RIB–POLYDACTYLY SYNDROMES

These syndromes can be suspected when the following three findings are recognized: micromelic dwarphism, severe hypoplastic thorax with short ribs and polydactyly[8] (Figure 4.13). Anomalies of the heart, of the gastrointestinal tract and the genitourinary tract are frequently associated. The conditions are incompatible with postnatal life.

CAMPOMELIC DYSPLASIA

This is characterized by a marked bowing of the long bones; this finding, however, is not specific for this condition. Craniofacial malformations (macrocephaly, cleft palate and micrognathia) are frequently associated[9]. The condition is lethal in 90% of the cases.

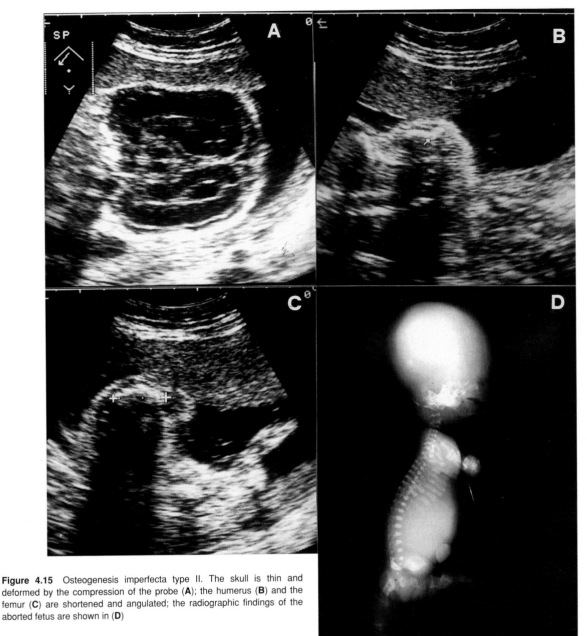

Figure 4.15 Osteogenesis imperfecta type II. The skull is thin and deformed by the compression of the probe (**A**); the humerus (**B**) and the femur (**C**) are shortened and angulated; the radiographic findings of the aborted fetus are shown in (**D**)

CHONDROECTODERMAL DYSPLASIA (ELLIS VAN CREVELD SYNDROME)

This rare condition is characterized by acromesomelic dwarphism, polydactyly and small thorax[10]. Cardiac anomalies are associated in 50% of the cases. The condition is compatible with life but pulmonary failure occurs in 30% of the cases.

ACHONDROPLASIA

The homozygous form is characterized by a severe micromelic dwarphism and can be diagnosed early in pregnancy. In the heterozygous form the alteration in long bone growth may not be observed until the third trimester and, therefore, an early diagnosis is usually impossible. The most useful diagnostic criterion is the ratio of femur length to head circumference, since femur shortening is usually associated with macrocrania. The shape of the long bones is normal[11] (Figure 4.14).

The homozygous achondroplasia is lethal; the heterozygous condition is compatible with a normal life span.

OSTEOGENESIS IMPERFECTA

Among the four types of osteogenesis imperfecta the only one which can be diagnosed *in utero* is type II. The long bones show fractures, angulations,

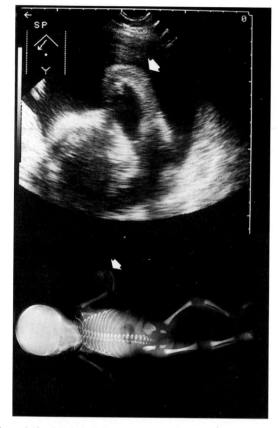

Figure 4.16 Agenesis of the radius: the absence of the radius causes an abnormal posture of the hand

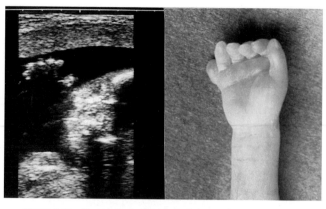

Figure 4.18 Postaxial polydactyly: six digits are clearly identified

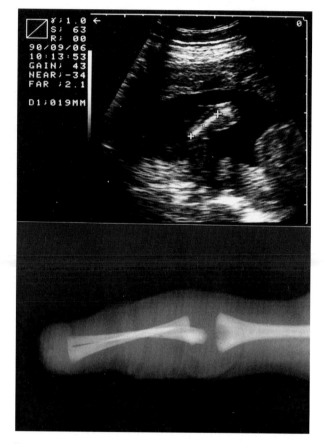

Figure 4.19 Acheiria: the forearm is clearly identified but the hand is absent

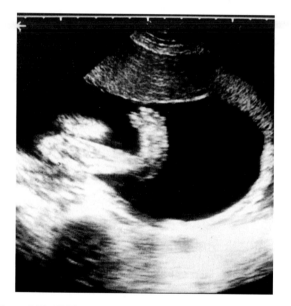

Figure 4.17 Clubfoot: in the same scan the leg bones and both heel and forefoot are shown

shortening, bowing, localized thickening secondary to callous formation and demineralization. This last finding is easily recognized in the skull, which is thinner than normal and easily deformed by the compression of the ultrasonic probe[12] (Figure 4.15).

A precise differential diagnosis with congenital hypophosphatasia may be difficult or impossible[13].

Osteogenesis imperfecta type II is a lethal condition as is hypophosphatasia.

DYSOSTOSES

Dysostoses refer to malformations or absence of individual bones singly or in combination. They can be divided into three groups:

(1) Dysostoses with cranial and facial involvement, such as craniosynostoses;

(2) Dysostoses with predominant axial involvement, such as vertebral segmentation defects;

(3) Dysostoses with predominant involvement of extremities, such as acheira, apodia, emimelia, phocomelia, polydactyly, syndactyly, etc. (Figures 4.16–4.19).

The sonographic diagnosis of the different forms of dysostoses is based on the accurate and systematic evaluation of the fetal skeleton. However, small defects in not at risk patients may be missed even in the hands of experienced operators.

REFERENCES

1. Beighton, P., Cremin, B., Faure, C. *et al.* (1983). International nomenclature of constitutional diseases of bone. *Ann. Radiol.*, **6**, 457

2. Mahony, B.S. (1990). The extremities. In Nyberg, D.A., Mahony, B.S. and Pretorius, D.H. (eds.) *Diagnostic Ultrasound of Fetal Anomalies*, p.492 (Chicago: Year Book Medical Publishers)

3. Romero, R., Pilu, G., Jeanty, P. *et al.* (1988). *Prenatal Diagnosis of Congenital Anomalies*, p.311. (Norwalk: Appleton & Lange)

4. Kurjak, A. (1990). Congenital skeletal abnormalities. In Kurjak, A. (ed.) *Handbook of Ultrasound in Obstetrics and Gynecology*, Vol. I, p.271. (Boca Raton: CRC Press)

5. Mahony, B.S., Filly, R.A. and Cooperberg, P.L. (1984). Antenatal sonographic diagnosis of achondrogenesis. *J. Ultrasound Med.*, **3**, 333

6. Chervenak, F.A., Blakemore, K.J., Isaacson, G. *et al.* (1983). Antenatal sonographic findings of thanatophoric dysplasia with cloverleaf skull. *Am. J. Obstet. Gynecol.*, **146**, 984

7. Schinzel, A., Savoldelli, G., Briner, J. *et al.* (1985). Prenatal sonographic diagnosis of Jeune Syndrome. *Radiology*, **154**, 777

8. Gembruch, U., Hansmann, M. and Fodish, H.J. (1985). Early prenatal diagnosis of short limb-polydactyly (SRP) syndrome type I (Majewski) by ultrasound in a case at risk. *Prenat. Diagn.*, **5**, 357

9. Cordone, M., Lituania, M., Zampetta, C. *et al.* (1989). *In utero* ultrasonographic features of campomelic dysplasia. *Prenat. Diagn.*, **9**, 745

10. Mahoney, M.J. and Hobbins, J.C. (1977). Prenatal diagnosis of chondroectodermal dysplasia (Ellis van Creveld Syndrome) with fetoscopy and ultrasound. *N. Engl. J. Med.*, **297**, 258

11. Kurtz, A.B., Filly, R.A., Wapner, R.J. *et al.* (1986). *In utero* analysis of heterozygous achondroplasia: variable time of onset as detected by femur length measurement. *J. Ultrasound Med.*, **5**, 137

12. Chervenak, F.A., Romero, R., Berkowitz, R.L. *et al.* (1982). Antenatal sonographic findings of osteogenesis imperfecta. *Am. J. Obstet. Gynecol.*, **143**, 228

13. De Lange, M. and Rouse, G.A. (1990). Prenatal diagnosis of hypophosphatasia. *J. Ultrasound Med.*, **9**, 115

5 Prenatal Diagnosis and Management of Fetal Genitourinary Tract Abnormalities

W. Holzgreve, K. Aydinli, M. Evans and P. Miny

INTRODUCTION

Edith L. Potter who worked extensively on fetal renal pathology and provided a very useful classification of these anomalies according to clinical, pathological and genetic aspects summarized her experience in her book on *Normal and abnormal development of the kidney*[1] by writing: 'The more complicated an organ in its development the more subject it is to maldevelopment, and in this respect the kidney outranks most other organs.' This enormous variability in fetal renal pathology ranging from lethal congenital anomalies to slight urinary tract obstructions makes the prenatal diagnosis and management of these disorders a complicated but at the same time fascinating challenge.

With modern real-time ultrasound it has become possible to screen routinely for fetal anomalies, and some countries such as the Federal Republic of Germany (West) have already instituted a general policy of offering two ultrasound examinations to all women during pregnancy[2,3].

Excellent review papers on the prenatal diagnosis and management of fetal urinary tract abnormalities have already been published[4-6] but taking into account the large variability of cystic and obstructive kidney diseases and difficulties with clinical and genetic grouping of these different forms of fetal renal abnormalities there is still a need for a systematic review of the ultrasound findings in accordance with accepted genetic classification criteria[7]. This chapter is based on the analysis of 191 cases with fetal genitourinary tract abnormalities diagnosed in our prenatal diagnosis and therapy center between 1 January, 1982, and 31 December, 1989 (Table 5.1). There was a progressive increase in the number of cases with fetal renal anomalies annually identified in our center during this time period: three in 1982–83; 16 in 1984–85; 68 in 1986–87; and 97 in 1988–89. The minimum follow-up period in this series was 1 year in all cases of children born alive, and of stillbirths and abortions

Table 5.1 Cases with prenatally diagnosed fetal genitourinary tract abnormalities at the University of Münster (January 1982–December 1989)

Diagnosis	n
Bilateral renal agenesis	25
Bilateral polycystic kidney disease	17
Bilateral renal dysmaturity/hypoplasia	8
Unilateral multicystic kidney	21
Unilateral dysplastic kidney with ectopic ureter	6
Unilateral hydronephrosis	37
ureteropelvic or ureterovesical junction	21
duplex system with ectopic ureter/ureterocele	10
transient	6
Bilateral hydronephrosis	59
ureteropelvic or ureterovesical junction	19
megacystis – megaureter	9
posterior urethral valves	18
urethral atresia	7
transient	6
Nephrophthisis	1
Solitary renal cyst	8
Fraser syndrome	1
Hydrometra with bilateral hydronephrosis	1
Ovarian cyst	7
Total	**191**

only those cases were included where autopsy was available after termination or death pre- or postnatally.

Before discussing the pre- and perinatal management in obstructive uropathies, we first present our data with reference to the four types of cystic kidneys as classified by Osathanondh and Potter[8] based on the microdissection technique.

POTTER TYPE I AUTOSOMAL RECESSIVE POLYCYSTIC KIDNEY DISEASE (ARPK)

This form of cystic kidney disease is also often called 'infantile polycystic kidney disease' or 'microcystic kidney disease', but the latter term is more appropriate for congenital nephrotic syndrome[9]. The incidence of ARPK is estimated to be one in 50 000 births[1].

The sonographic picture of large fetal kidneys with hyperechogenic renal structure is very characteristic and easy to recognize once the 'typical pattern' is known to the investigator (Figure 5.1 and 5.2). The kidney involvement in ARPK is invariably bilateral and symmetric and the easily identifiable hyperechogenic structure of the affected kidneys is thought to be due to sound enhancement by the microscopic cystic structure present in the renal parenchyma[10]. Fetuses with Potter type I kidneys also have generalized portal and interlobular fibrosis of the liver accompanied by biliary duct hyperplasia and small distal vein branches, but these hepatic changes are difficult to recognize prenatally.

Blyth and Ockenden[11] have differentiated perinatal, neonatal, infantile and juvenile groups of ARPK corresponding to differences in manifestation and prognosis of survival. Even though this subclassification is not universally accepted, the relatively high intrafamilial constancy may be helpful when counselling after prenatal diagnosis of a recurrent case. In families with a *de novo* diagnosis it is often difficult to know exactly what form of ARPK is present.

In general the recognition of the Potter type I fetal kidneys is not difficult and has been reported frequently[12–16]. Most of the reported cases were diagnosed after the 24th week of pregnancy, but in our series alone nine cases were identified before the 24th week. Severe oligo- and ahydramnios are associated with the so-called 'perinatal' group of Blyth and Ockenden[11] and are associated with a minimal survival period.

In order to define further the individual prognosis prenatally we are also in the process of evaluating the role of pulsed Doppler examinations of the renal artery (Figures 5.3 and 5.4) on the hypothesis that the worst prognosis cases should be associated with a higher resistance index due to renal pathology and disturbance of the microcirculation in the polycystic kidney than, for example, the juvenile forms of ARPK. Even though our preliminary results regarding this additional prognostic marker are encouraging, it is too early to suggest the use of Doppler for this purpose because of the limited follow-up period. Townsend *et al.*[17] pointed out that ARPK can be associated with increased maternal serum and amniotic fluid α-fetoprotein.

POTTER TYPE II (MULTICYSTIC/DYSPLASTIC) KIDNEY DISEASE

This type of fetal cystic kidney disease is usually not inherited. It is characterized by a large variety of pathoanatomic and subsequently also prenatal sonographic findings. A Potter type IIA with enlarged or normal multicystic kidneys often with segmental involvement is differentiated from a type IIB with rudimentary kidneys with few or only small cysts[9]. In cases with bilateral involvement associated anhydramnios is often present[18,19]. The cysts of the kidney may be large and an enlarged Potter type II multicystic kidney can even lead to compression of gastrointestinal organs or of the contralateral urinary tract. The prognosis in general very much depends on the contralateral involvement and even if one side is severely affected, the child will develop normally without problems if the healthy kidney is working properly. Figure 5.5 shows a longitudinal sonogram of a large Potter type IIA kidney in a fetus with a normal contralateral kidney. Even though the child postnatally eventually required a nephrectomy, she is developing normally without any renal or pulmonary functional impairment.

The cross-sectional ultrasound picture of another fetus with unilateral Potter type IIA in Figure 5.6 illustrates the enlarged size of these kidneys. The normal amount of amniotic fluid due to an unimpaired contralateral kidney allowed for an uneventful development of the child pre- and postnatally, whereas in cases with bilateral involvement and severe oligohydramnios (Figure 5.7) the prognosis is extremely poor.

The Potter type IIA fetal kidney in Figure 5.8 composed of multiple, variably sized cysts was so much enlarged that it caused a 'prune belly'-like abdominal distension and displacement of the intestinal tract.

Passarge and Lenz[20] and Grix *et al.*[21] have pointed out that maternal diabetes is associated with an increased risk for the development of fetal Potter type II kidney disease, but in most cases no maternal risk factors can be identified. Although Potter type II kidneys may be present in inherited syndromes such as Zellweger and Fryns syndrome, they are usually not inherited when they are not associated with other malformations.

POTTER TYPE III (AUTOSOMAL DOMINANT POLYCYSTIC) KIDNEY DISEASE (ADPKD)

This type of cystic kidney disease is characterized by the least uniform picture regarding the degree of parenchymal changes and size of the cysts. Although this anomaly normally only shows manifestation in adults between the third and fifth decade, early manifestations have been reported first by Weiß *et al.*[14] and later by Main *et al.*[22] and Fryns *et al.*[23].

We have also diagnosed ADPKD in the second trimester of pregnancy and probably for the first time in one case in the first trimester (Figure 5.9). This very early diagnosis was possible because of the family history and the use of transvaginal sonography which allows visualization of the normal and abnormal fetal urinary tract at an early stage as shown in a series by Bronshtein *et al.*[24] who examined 1940 patients between 10 and 16 weeks of gestation with this method.

In 1985 Reeders *et al.*[25] localized the mutation for ADPKD on the short arm of chromosome 16 by demonstration of a genetic linkage with the α-chain of human hemoglobin, and shortly afterwards the same group reported about the first prenatal diagnosis in a 9-week fetus at risk for the disease by using a highly polymorphic DNA probe genetically linked to the locus of ADPKD[26]. The fetus was diagnosed to have inherited the ADPKD mutation and this was confirmed by microscopic examination of the fetal kidneys at autopsy. The ethical justification for prenatal diagnosis of this frequent disease (1 per 1000) given by the authors of this first prenatal diagnosis report was that 'ADPKD continues to impose a considerable burden on families and the community, accounting for approximately 10% of the total requirement for chronic replacement therapy'.

POTTER TYPE IV KIDNEY DISEASE (CYSTIC KIDNEYS DUE TO URETHRAL OBSTRUCTION)

According to Potter[1], type IV kidney disease only occurs as a result of urethral occlusion, i.e. due to urethral valves. Because of the increase of urine in the fetal urinary tract, the pressure there is exerted against the newly attached nephrons causing their distension and the development of subcapsular cysts[9]. In severe cases the bladder can be profoundly distended (Figure 5.10), often associated with enlarged renal pelvises (Figure 5.11). In cases with

lower urinary tract obstructions due to urethral obstruction the degree of subsequent hydronephrosis can vary profoundly as illustrated by Figures 5.12 and 5.13 of two cases with anatomically similar urethral valves. Since sonography is especially accurate for detecting fluid-filled pathologic lesions, prenatal detection of fetal urinary tract obstruction can easily be achieved[27]. In cases of fetal urethral obstruction the characteristic sonographic finding is the dilatation of both the fetal urinary tract and the proximal urethra (Figure 5.14) resulting in 'key-hole'-like appearance[28,29] usually in a male fetus. Even in cases of urethral or bladder outlet obstruction where one might expect symmetric back-up pressure with uniform degrees of hydronephrosis in both kidneys (Figure 5.15) there is often a considerable asymmetry in the degree of hydronephrosis of both kidneys. (Figure 5.16). With modern gray-scale ultrasonography calyceal dilatation can be identified as illustrated by Figure 5.17 of a fetus with urethral obstruction and only mild hydronephrosis, preserved normal echogenicity of the renal parenchyma and some cortical medullary distinctions still being apparent.

Megacystis and hydronephrosis as the first signs of obstructive uropathy can develop early in pregnancy and they can be associated already late in the first or very early in the second trimester not only with severe oligohydramnios (Figure 5.18), but also with normal amounts of amniotic fluid (Figure 5.19). Wladimiroff *et al.*[30] have pointed out, however, on the basis of a case with weekly ultrasound scans, that slight bilateral hydronephrosis as a first sign of obstructive uropathy due to urethral valves could not be established before 30 weeks of gestation, although anuria developed and bilateral ureterocutaneostomy had to be carried out postnatally. On the other hand, cases of transient *in utero* hydronephrosis have also been reported[31,32] some of which may be due to fetal vesicoureteral reflux resolving in the course of maturation.

Besides urethral obstructions ureteropelvic junction (UPJ) obstruction is the most common cause of hydronephrosis in the neonate and child[33]. These cases can be differentiated prenatally, because hydronephrosis is not associated with megacystis as opposed to urethral obstruction.

It is difficult to quantify prenatally the degree of hydronephrosis. In order to facilitate communication and comparison of results in the literature Grignon *et al.*[34] proposed a morphologic classification of *in utero* urinary tract dilatation. They suggested that grade I dilatation (anteroposterior diameter of the renal pelvis less than 10 mm) should be considered normal, whereas grades II and III with intermediate hydronephrosis require postnatal urologic surgery in nearly half the cases. Grade IV (moderate dilatation of the calyces with easily identified residual renal cortex) and grade V (severe dilatation of the calyces with atrophic cortex) were clearly considered pathologic and would require neonatal corrective surgery. This classification may be helpful for communication, but due to the individual variability of the clinical course of fetal obstructive uropathies any classification scheme is problematic. For practical purposes the systematic evaluation of fetal obstructive uropathies by Filly's group[35,36] provided valuable information, e.g. that cortical cysts had a sensitivity of 44% and specificity of 100% in predicting renal dysplasia, whereas increased echogenicity had a sensitivity of only 57% and a specificity of 89%. The severity of hydronephrosis was least predictive with a sensitivity of 35% and specificity of 78%. Therefore the power of ultrasound to assess the degree of renal residual function after the easy prenatal detection of bilateral hydronephrosis is unfortunately still limited even with the use of the best machines with high resolution. Neither does the degree of dilatation of the ureters correlate well with the degree of renal damage[37] as illustrated by Figures 5.20 and 5.21 which show ureteral dilatation of various degrees in two fetuses with ureteropelvic junction syndrome who both had about the same degree of postnatal renal function. We share, however, the experience of the Fetal Treatment Program in San Francisco[29] that fetal kidneys that are obstructed severely enough to result in rupture of the collecting system and formation of a perinephric urinoma and urinary ascites (Figures 5.22 and 5.23) are unlikely to have adequate residual renal function[38]. It remains to be investigated systematically whether the use of Doppler studies on the renal artery flow which is now greatly aided by the introduction of color-coded Doppler sonography (Figure 5.24) can be helpful for the much needed improvement of prenatal assessment of kidney function in urinary tract obstruction. The hypothesis regarding the Doppler evaluation of the renal artery flow is that an increased resistance index correlates with the degree of parenchymal compression and subsequently with the degree of renal insufficiency.

The four types of cystic kidney diseases according to the classification by Osathanondh and Potter[8] which have been discussed here briefly so far with regard to their prenatal diagnosis are summarized in Table 5.2 following the detailed description of Zerres et al.[9].

PRENATAL ASSESSMENT OF FETAL RENAL FUNCTION *IN UTERO*

Because in cases with sonographically recognized obstructive uropathies ultrasound cannot identify all dysplastic kidneys biochemical studies from fetal urine were performed by the San Francisco Fetal Treatment Group[39]. It is known that fetal urine is produced from the 13th week of gestation onwards and that it is an ultrafiltrate of fetal serum made hypotonic by selective tubular absorption of sodium and chloride. Additionally it has now been determined (U. Nicolini *et al.*, personal communication) that the normal levels of sodium and chloride fall throughout gestation so that a level of 120 mmol/l sodium in fetal urine is still in the normal range at 15 weeks, but clearly pathologic after 20 weeks of gestation. In a retrospective analysis of fetal urine samples in San Francisco it was found that fetuses with hypotonic urine had later been found to have good renal function as opposed to those with isotonic urine who later had poor renal function. Urine osmolarity had a similar predictive value. In summary, the San Francisco retrospective study revealed that urinary sodium levels above 100 mmol/l, chloride above 90 mmol/l and osmolarity above 210 mOsm were associated with insufficient tubular reabsorption capacity and irreversibly damaged renal function at birth.

Lenz et al.[40] showed that – similar to plasma values – concentrations of neutral amino acids in the fetal urine are also predictive of irreversibly destroyed kidneys, because they reflect poor tubular capacity. Later Nicolini et al.[41] pointed out that selection of fetuses for vesicoamniotic shunting can be further improved by serial sampling of each kidney separately. Like others[42,43] however, we found that these useful parameters are not always able to correctly select those cases in which drainage of the obstructed urinary tract might be beneficial. We therefore looked for additional parameters to improve the prenatal prediction about the renal function[44].

In the postnatal as well as in the prenatal period, proteinuria in the course of renal disease is caused either by a pathologic process in the glomeruli and/or by damage in the tubular reabsorption capacity. Because this pathogenetic difference is expressed by the molecular weight of the proteins[45], the site and degree of the underlying lesions in kidneys with pathologic proteinuria can be identified by separating urinary proteins on polyacrylamide gel electrophoresis with sodium dodecyl sulfate as

Table 5.2 Summary of Potter type I–IV cystic kidney diseases

		Potter type I	Potter type II	Potter type III	Potter type IV
1.	*Pathoanatomic findings*	Bilateral symmetrically enlarged kidneys Cysts up to 2 mm in diameter Congenital hepatic fibrosis	Great variety of forms (hypoplastic and hyperplastic 'multicystic') Unilateral or asymmetric finding frequent	Bilateral with considerable renal enlargement Different sized cysts up to several centimetres in diameter	Kidneys often slightly enlarged Often cortical cysts due to urethral obstruction
2.	*Genetics*	Autosomal recessive inheritance	Isolated renal lesion not hereditary Exclusion of a syndrome indispensable	Autosomal dominant inheritance Part of syndromes, e.g. Meckel or tuberous sclerosis	Not hereditary Exclusion of syndromes indispensable
3.	*Clinical features*	Renal insufficiency (childhood) Portal hypertension (adolescence)	Clinically silent to renal non-function syndrome Often some involvement of contralateral urinary tract	Onset usually in adulthood Early manifestations possible	Depending on extent of involvement Megacystis, hydroureter, cortical cysts
4.	*Prenatal diagnosis*	Bilateral enlargement with reniform configuration Increased echogenicity of renal parenchyma In severe cases: oligohydramnios	Multicystic or hypoplastic kidney In severe cases of bilateral involvement: anhydramnios	Only ~ 3 documented cases Early diagnosis by DNA polymorphisms possible	Possible Differentiation from type II by appearance of evident megacystis and peripheral renal cysts

In accordance with ref. 9

detergent (SDS–PAGE). Molecules between 10 and 200 kDa can be separated and stained with amidoblack by this technique. An increase in micromolecular proteins (molecular weight < 70 000) is indicative of an impairment in tubular reabsorption of those proteins which normally pass almost freely through the glomerula[46]. SDS–PAGE not only separates proteins according to their molecular weight, but also allows an estimation of their quantity. In normal pregnancies at 18 weeks hardly any proteins except for some albumin are found in fetal urine (Figure 5.25).

Using this new test we reported a successful case of shunting of a fetus with large megacystis and associated anhydramnios at 19 weeks in which bladder electrolytes and osmolarity (Table 5.3) were compatible with severe renal damage, but the addition of protein analysis by SDS–PAGE was more predictive of the ultimate good outcome after delivery at 36 weeks of gestation[47].

Subsequently we used the SDS–PAGE *in utero* together with the San Francisco profile (modified for gestational age) in a series of 21 cases[3]. We found in this group of patients that the electrolyte and osmolarity evaluations were incorrect in four instances, whereas the SDS–PAGE was in agreement with the ultimate outcome of the pregnancy in all of these cases. We therefore suggest that the SDS–PAGE evaluation should be added to previously described fetal urinary function tests in cases of severe and progressive urinary tract obstructions before decisions about the prenatal management are made.

PRENATAL TREATMENT OF FETAL URINARY TRACT OBSTRUCTIONS

It is well documented experimentally[48] and clinically[49] that severe *in utero* urinary tract obstruction may ultimately lead to delivery of a

Table 5.3 Summary of a case of successful shunting in a fetus of a 28-year-old mother

Gestation (weeks)	Findings
18	Megacystis, key-hole bladder hydronephroses, severe oligohydramnios, karyotype: 46, XY diagnostic bladder puncture, results:

	18 weeks	*19 weeks*
Na⁺	99.8 mmol/l	82 mmol/l
Cl	94 mmol/l	89 mmol/l
Osm.	262	274

19	Double pigtail vesico-amniotic shunt Good filling of amniotic cavity, gradual disappearance of hydronephroses

32	Amniocentesis for lecithin/sphingomyelin ratio, simultaneous bladder puncture, results:

Na⁺	51 mmol/l
Cl	46 mmol/l
Osm.	259

36	Delivery, healthy boy with 'prune belly' appearance, 2820 g, cystogram: dilated posterior urethra, antibiotic treatment

Healthy at 2 years of age

neonate with advanced hydronephrosis and type IV cystic dysplasia incompatible with survival, and the secondary oligohydramnios due to pulmonary hypoplasia leads to skeletal (Figure 5.26) and facial deformities (Potter sequence). Therefore the concept was developed that in some of these cases early *in utero* relief of the obstruction may allow sufficient renal development to support postnatal life and to allow 'catch-up growth' of the lungs.

In 1982 the San Francisco Fetal Treatment Program first reported two different approaches to deal with this problem of decompressing a urinary tract obstruction *in utero*. Golbus *et al.*[50] reported the case of a male fetus who was noted to have ascites at 17 menstrual weeks and during the following 13 weeks developed a dilated and hypertrophied bladder, hydroureters and hydronephrosis. Placement of an indwelling suprapubic catheter *in utero* allowed drainage from the fetal bladder and further prenatal development. The infant was born at 34 weeks and had 'prune belly' syndrome but normal pulmonary and renal function. The transabdominal catheter placement *in utero* (Figure 5.27) and its proper functioning after placement of the vesico-amniotic shunt (Figure 5.28) as well as the postnatal aspect of such a baby (Figure 5.29) are illustrated here

with pictures of cases treated according to the San Francisco technique in our Münster Program.

Because the original vesico-amniotic catheters, however, were difficult to apply and often became obstructed after short time periods (sometimes even were torn out by the fetuses themselves), Harrison *et al.*[51] developed a technique of open fetal surgery with bilateral ureterostomies (Figure 5.30) after extensive experiments in sheep and non-human primates.

Although the experience of the San Francisco Fetal Treatment Program so far has demonstrated clearly the potential applicability of such open fetal treatment, there are potential risks not only for the fetus, but also for the mother including the need for the repeat Caesarean section etc. which have to be balanced against the potential benefits. An improved *in utero* shunt device, originally produced by Rodeck *et al.*[52] (Figure 5.31) for pleuro-amniotic shunting, can now be placed from the inside of a trocar and has better material properties against clotting and dislocation. For this reason it seems debatable what the place for open fetal surgery will be in the future.

Ever since the first reports of *in utero* treatment of obstructive uropathies there has been considerable debate about the need for such procedures[53,54] but it is obvious now that the key to successful management of fetal hydronephrosis is the proper evaluation of renal function *in utero* and prospective, randomized trials would be the best way to evaluate procedures, for example vesico-amniotic shunt placement vs. open fetal surgery.

FLUID INFUSION INTO AMNIOTIC CAVITY IN CASES WITH SEVERE OLIGOHYDRAMNIOS

The incidence of bilateral renal agenesis, a uniformly lethal condition, is about 0.3 of 1000 births[55] with only a few familial cases reported[56]. A reliable prenatal diagnosis is therefore extremely important because it offers the option of elective termination of pregnancy prior to viability or may change the obstetric management later in pregnancy. Failure to identify a fetal bladder is an important diagnostic sign. In doubtful cases the administration of furosemide to the mother has been suggested[30] because it crosses the placenta and is believed to induce fetal diuresis.

Oligohydramnios, however, always obscures the sonographic visibility, and therefore the infusion of fluid into the amniotic cavity to enhance the ultrasound imaging has been suggested[57]. An additional reason for performing this diagnostic test is that with the addition of some dye to the fluid an unnoticed rupture of the membranes may become recognizable. A technical difficulty in needling an amniotic cavity with severe oligohydramnios, however, is the fact that in black and white sonography areas with umbilical cord may look like pockets of amniotic fluid and that an inadvertant injection of large volumes of fluid into the cord may cause complications. The application of color-coded sonography which aids in clearly delineating the blood flow in the umbilical cord can be very helpful in such situations (Figure 5.32).

SPECIAL TYPES OF FETAL URINARY TRACT ABNORMALITIES AND ASSOCIATED ANOMALIES

Cystic changes of fetal kidneys can occur in numerous syndromes[9]. One of the more frequent ones is the autosomal recessive Meckel syndrome (1 in 40 000 births) which is characterized by meningoencephalocele, postaxial hexadactyly and polycystic kidneys similar to a Potter type III aspect[58]. The identification of these major malformations which can then guide the search for minor malformations such as cleft lip or palate or genital malformations is possible now early in the second (Figures 5.33 and 5.34) and even in the first trimester by using vaginal sonography (Figure 5.35).

Another autosomal recessive syndrome with renal involvement is Fraser syndrome, displaying the key symptoms of cryptophthalmos and syndactyly[59].

In our series we also encountered a case of the autosomal recessive Kaufman syndrome[60,61], characterized by hydrometrocolpos, polydactyly, congenital heart disease and sometimes secondary hydronephrosis due to pressure on the ureters from the distended hydrometra like in our case.

Our group first described a syndrome with Potter sequence, persistent buccopharyngeal membrane type II, postaxial polydactyly, cleft palate, cardiac anomalies, intestinal non-fixation and intrauterine retardation[62] which was later also observed by Legius et al.[63] in another case.

In a survey of 80 cases with Potter sequence due to renal or urologic abnormalities Curry et al.[64] found 15 patients with multiple congenital anomalies, four of which had autosomal recessive syndromes and three aneuploidies. Furlong et al.[65] also found a high rate of associated anomalies in fetuses with urinary tract abnormalities.

In our series the most frequent aneuploidy found in cases of sonographically recognized fetal renal anomalies or oligohydramnios was triploidy followed by trisomy 18[66]. In one of the cases with triploidy we found a large pelvic sac-like kidney (Figure 5.36) together with a partial molar degeneration of the placenta[67]. The majority of our cases (eight of 15) with triploidy, however, did not show the typical partial mole picture, but severe oligo- or ahydramnios with growth retardation. In those cases with significantly reduced amniotic fluid volume placental biopsy is the most effective method for rapid karyotyping[68].

There is some confusion in the literature regarding the term 'prune belly' syndrome which is defined as the triad of lax abdominal wall, cryptorchidism and urinary tract anomalies, but the characteristic anterior wall defect can occur secondary to massive bladder dilatation and stretching of the abdominal walls[69,70].

DIFFERENTIAL DIAGNOSIS AND PITFALLS IN PRENATAL DIAGNOSIS

One of the more frequent difficulties after ultrasonic detection of a fetal kidney anomaly is the differential diagnosis between megaureter and primary cysts of the kidney (Figures 5.37 and 5.38). Avni et al.[71] could establish a correct prenatal diagnosis in 43 of 63 cases (70%). They also encountered diagnostic problems in differentiating among multicystic dysplastic kidneys, ureteropelvic junction obstruction and dilatation owing to reflux or obstruction and in lack of visualization of small hypoplastic kidneys. The prenatal ultrasound demonstration of bladder distention and/or hydronephrosis does not always signify true obstruction of the urinary tract which is important to assess before contemplating a prenatal shunting procedure[72,73]. Nor is it always possible in cases with fetal renal pelvises of more than 10 mm to differentiate between an obstructive lesion or exceptional extrarenal pelvises[6]. Figure 5.39 shows an example of a fetal double kidney from our series in which the color-coded Doppler visualization of the renal artery depicts the normal kidney next to the attached hydronephrotic double kidney with adjacent megaureter.

Greenblatt et al.[74] reported the first *in utero* diagnosis of crossed renal ectopia, and Vintzileos et al.[75] presented the sonographic findings in the megacystis-intestinal hypoperistalsis syndrome which has an extremely bad prognosis. The prevalence of ureteral duplication is estimated to range from 0.7 to

1% of the general population and pathological manifestations such as vesicoureteral reflux occur in 20% of these cases[76].

Another important differential diagnosis for a simple urinary tract obstruction is the more complicated common cloaca sequence. We described a case of persistent common cloaca with prune belly and anencephaly (Figure 5.40) detected by sonography in the second trimester of pregnancy[77]. Cloaca malformation again has to be differentiated from a bladder diverticulum which we have visualized early in the second (Figure 5.41) and by vaginal sonography also in the first trimester of pregnancy (Figure 5.42). We encountered an extreme case of a low bladder diverticulum in a fetus with urethral obstruction where the external aspect of the fetus *in utero* was similar to the one seen in cases with cystic sacrococcygeal teratoma (Figure 5.43 and 5.44). In this situation the condition could prenatally be classified as lethal based on the urinary function studies (see above) and the severe degree of pulmonary hypoplasia caused by the upwards pressure of the diaphragm due to the significantly enlarged fetal bladder.

OVARIAN CYSTS

Although it is known from autopsy material of stillbirths and neonatal deaths that small follicular cysts are not unusual in fullterm infants, large cysts are only rarely encountered clinically or by sonography[78]. The diagnosis can be suspected prenatally if a cystic lesion is visualized next to a kidney in a female fetus (Figure 5.45). Prenatally these cysts are usually uncomplicated and often disappear spontaneously postpartum, but sometimes they require surgery because of their size or secondary complications[4,79]. If they are taken out by laparotomy in the neonatal period it is difficult even with microsurgery not to harm the small ovary which is often intimately integrated into the wall of the cyst. It therefore seems prudent either to allow even large cysts to regress spontaneously or to puncture those requiring decompression due to secondary complications.

From our own experience with 11 such cases we know that complications can occur prenatally from torsion of the pedicle and subsequent necrosis or hemorrhage into the cyst. Therefore we recommend prenatal decompression especially if the cyst is large and a 'wandering mass'.

The levels of estradiol, progesterone and testosterone are high in the cyst fluid which confirms the diagnosis after prenatal puncture. The differential diagnosis includes choledochal cysts[80], paranephric, sacrococcygeal, mesenteric and urachal cysts (Figure 5.46). The precise topography aided by color-coded Doppler mapping of the vasculature is helpful in differential diagnosis.

FOLLOW-UP OF CHILDREN WITH PRENATALLY RECOGNIZED URINARY TRACT ABNORMALITIES

Cases with renal agenesis or a complete deficit of renal function are still lethal, because in addition to the pulmonary hypoplasia, which could potentially be prevented by continuous fluid-infusion into the amniotic cavity, it is currently not feasible to transplant kidneys in the newborn period or to apply dialysis directly after birth preceding surgery. Although we have reported about the use of anencephalic donors for kidney transplantation[81] and about 81 such cases are documented in the literature[82] (Figure 5.47) this potential source of organs is also very limited.

With all the current uncertainties about the prenatal assessment of residual renal function it is important to follow up all cases of prenatally diagnosed fetal genitourinary anomalies in order to learn more about prognostic signs and to improve our management protocols. In our follow-up studies we found that 20 of 112 children with prenatally recognized congenital uropathies developed arterial hypertension (Table 5.4). Hypertension in children is a risk factor for progressive renal disease and cardiovascular changes and results in a considerable morbidity and mortality if not recognized early enough and treated accordingly[83]. The main risk

Table 5.4 Incidence of arterial hypertension in newborns with congenital uropathies (20 of 112 newborns investigated at the University of Münster, unpublished results)

Uropathy	n
Unilateral compensated prevesical stenosis	4
Unilateral compensated subpelvic stenosis	3
Urethral valves (bilateral hydronephrosis)	2
Unilateral reflux	2
Bilateral polycystic kidneys	2
Unilateral subpelvic stenosis (after surgery)	2
Bilateral subpelvic stenosis (after surgery)	2
Bilateral subpelvic stenosis and reflux	1
Other	3

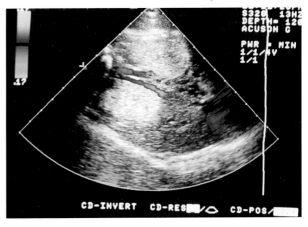

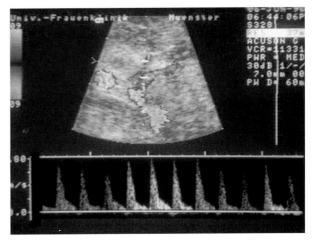

Figure 5.1 Infantile polycystic kidney disease: the typical hyperechogenic renal structure is recognizable

Figure 5.2 Infantile polycystic kidney disease: both large kidneys reach the aorta (clearly outlined by color-coded Doppler sonography)

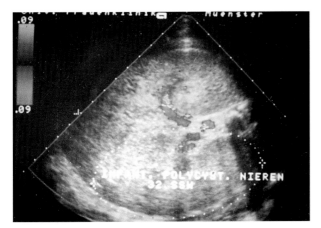

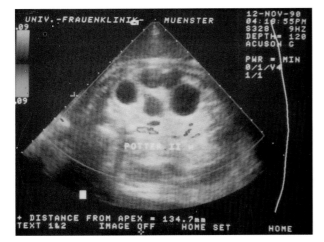

Figure 5.3 Doppler investigations in infantile polycystic kidney disease: the color-coded Doppler sonography outlines renal artery

Figure 5.4 Pulsed Doppler investigation of renal artery in a case of infantile polycystic kidney disease

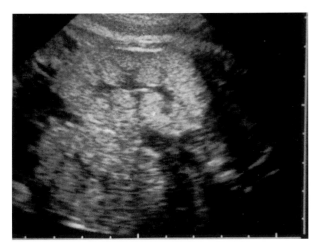

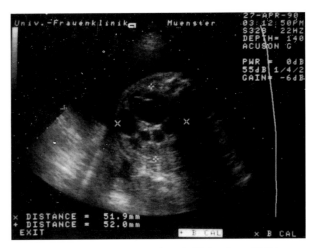

Figure 5.5 Potter IIA unilateral multicystic kidney

Figure 5.6 Cysts of different sizes recognizable in a Potter IIA kidney

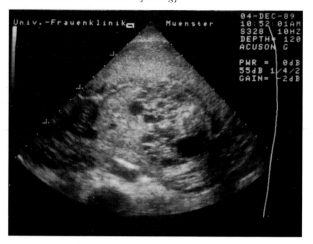

Figure 5.7 Bilateral Potter IIA kidneys

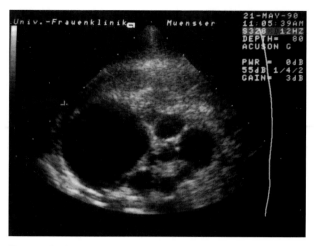

Figure 5.8 Large Potter type IIA kidney which caused abdominal distension

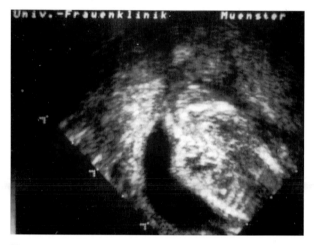

Figure 5.9 First trimester vaginal sonogram of a fetus with autosomal dominant polycystic kidney diease (proven by autopsy and typical family history)

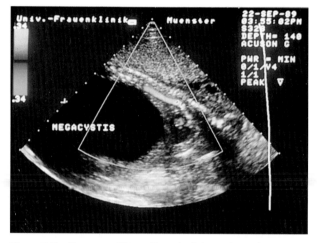

Figure 5.10 Sonogram of fetus with urethral obstruction and megacystis showing grossly distended bladder pushing the diaphragm upwards

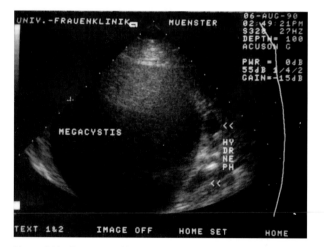

Figure 5.11 Sonogram of fetus with urethral obstruction and megacystis showing bilateral hydronephrosis visible next to the dilated bladder

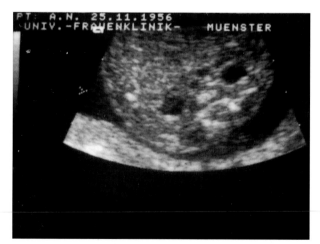

Figure 5.12 Bilateral hydronephrosis in fetus with only mild hydronephrosis

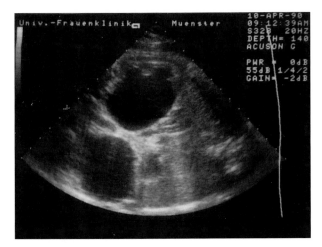

Figure 5.13 Fetus with similar type of urethral valve to the fetus in Figure 5.12 but in this case profound hydronephrosis is present

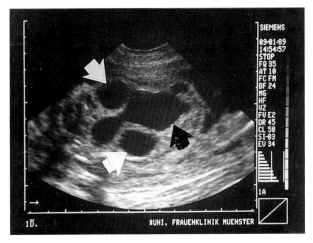

Figure 5.14 Typical key-hole bladder in fetus with urethral obstruction, dilated ureters (white arrows) next to dilated bladder (black arrow)

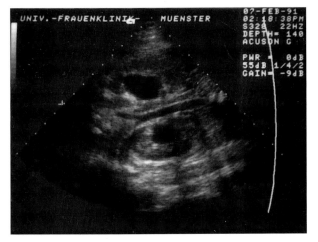

Figure 5.15 Fetus with urethral obstruction and subsequent bilateral symmetric hydronephrosis

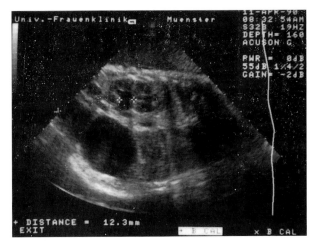

Figure 5.16 Fetus with urethral obstruction and subsequent asymmetric degrees of hydronephrosis

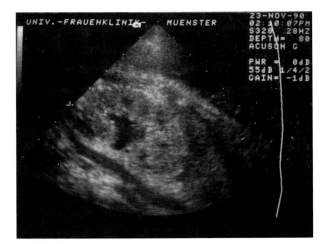

Figure 5.17 Mildly hydronephrotic kidney with preserved echogenicity of the renal parenchyma and cortical medullary distinction in a fetus with urethral valve

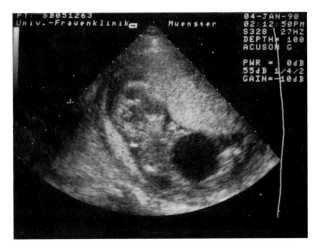

Figure 5.18 Early second trimester fetus with urethral valves with subsequent severe oligohydramnios

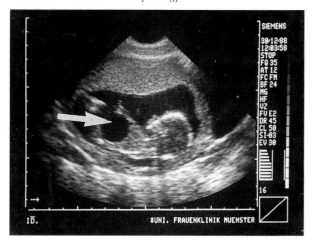

Figure 5.19 Early second trimester fetus with urethral valves associated with almost normal amount of amniotic fluid left (white arrow = megacystis)

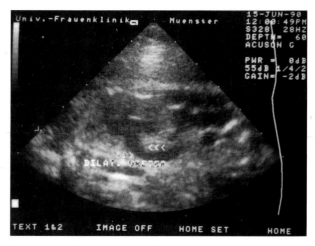

Figure 5.20 Dilated ureters in a fetus with renal insufficiency showing only mild dilatation of the ureter

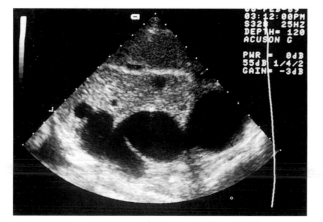

Figure 5.21 Clearly dilated ureters in a fetus with an ultimately similar degree of renal insufficiency to the fetus in Figure 5.20

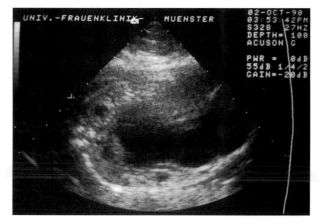

Figure 5.22 Fetus with rupture of the collecting system resulting in urinoma

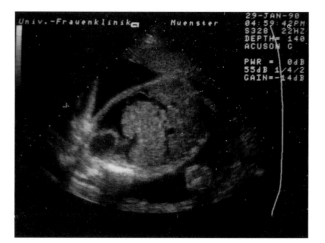

Figure 5.23 Fetus with rupture of the collecting system resulting in urinary ascites

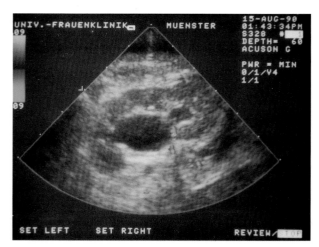

Figure 5.24 Color-coded Doppler sonography outlines the renal artery in a kidney with hydronephrosis

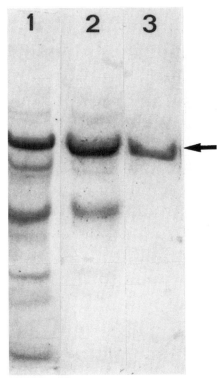

Figure 5.25 SDS-PAGE analysis of fetal urine samples obtained between 18 and 20 weeks of gestation *in utero*. Protein bands are characterized by their mobility in relation to urine albumin (arrow). Severe tubular damage is expressed by the presence of at least six microproteins (molecular weight 10–40 kDa lower half of the gel), exceeding the amount of macroproteins. Lane 1, fetus with irreversibly damaged kidney (Potter type IV dysplasia) due to urethral obstruction; lane 2, fetus with mild tubular damage who subsequently had successful *in utero* placement of vesico-amniotic shunt; and lane 3, normal fetus

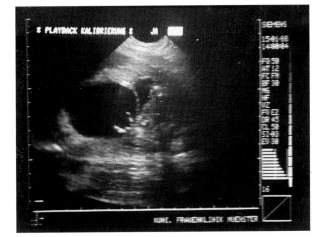

Figure 5.26 Sonographic picture of club foot deformity in a fetus exposed to severe oligohydramnios prior to vesico-amniotic shunt placement

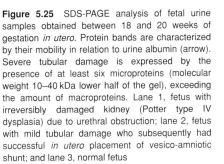

Figure 5.27 Sonographic video reprint at the time of vesico-amniotic catheter placement. The inner coil of the double pigtail shunt can easily be visualized inside the bladder

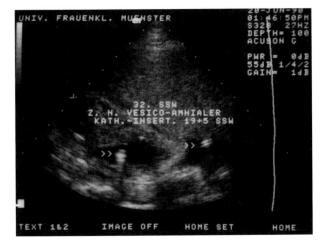

Figure 5.28 Vesico-amniotic shunt (two outer ends marked by arrows) at 32 weeks of pregnancy after catheter placement at 19 weeks 5 days gestation

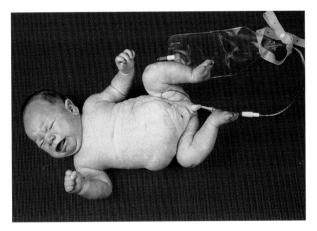

Figure 5.29 Newborn boy with urethral obstruction who had a vesico-amniotic shunt placed at 19 weeks because of severe oligohydramnios at that time. Normal functioning kidneys and lungs now

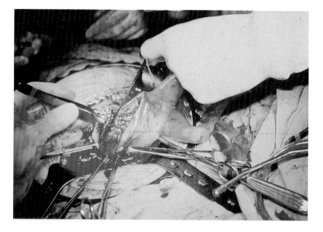

Figure 5.30 Open fetal surgery with ureterostomy because of prenatally recognized fetal urethral obstruction at the San Francisco Fetal Treatment program

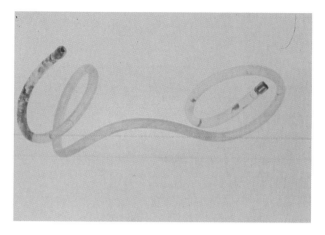

Figure 5.31 New double pigtail indwelling catheter developed by Ch. Rodeck (Rocket of London) which can be pushed through the inside of a trocar

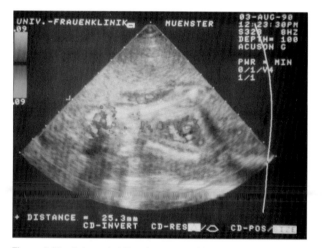

Figure 5.32 Color-coded Doppler sonographic picture of a case with severe oligohydramnios. Those areas which might be confused with pockets of amniotic fluid can easily be identified as areas with coils of umbilical cord

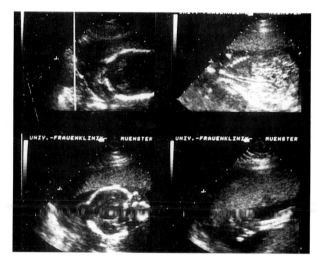

Figure 5.33 Meckel–Gruber syndrome showing ultrasonographic features with encephalocele (left), hexadactyly (lower right) and dysplastic kidneys (upper right)

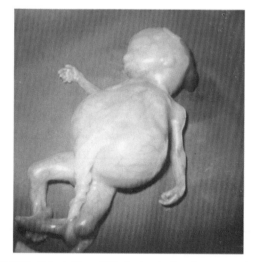

Figure 5.34 Fetus in Figure 5.33 after termination of pregnancy showing encephalocele, hexadactyly and 'prune belly'-like appearance

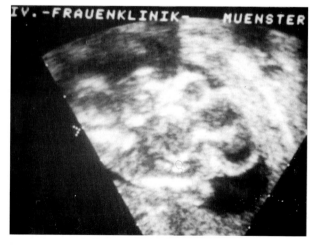

Figure 5.35 First trimester vaginal sonogram of fetus with Meckel syndrome showing encephalocele

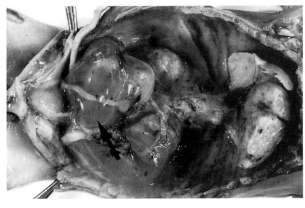

Figure 5.36   Autopsy situs of fetus with triploidy

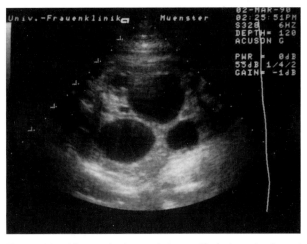

Figure 5.37   Ultrasound picture of fetus with hydronephrosis and megaureters

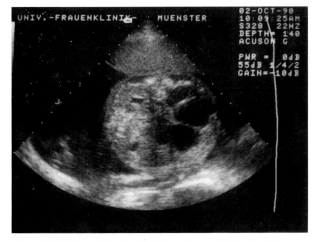

Figure 5.38   Fetus with polycystic kidney disease (Potter type IIA)

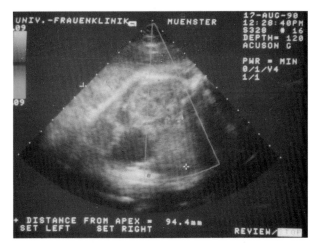

Figure 5.39   Double kidney with normal kidney being depicted by the colour-coded Doppler sonogram of the renal artery next to the smaller hydronephrotic kidneys

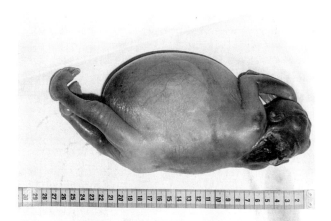

Figure 5.40   Fetus with common cloaca, 'prune belly' aspect and anencephaly

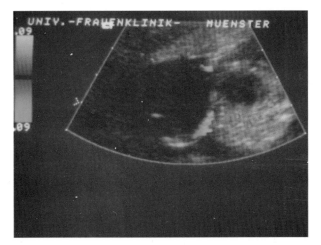

Figure 5.41   Bladder diverticulum in fetus early in the second trimester

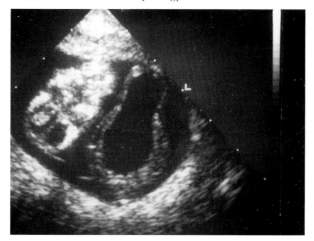

Figure 5.42 Bladder diverticulum in fetus in the first trimester of pregnancy (normal head of co-twin visible next to bladder diverticulum)

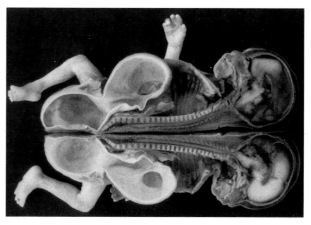

Figure 5.43 Fetus with urethral obstruction and bladder diverticulum, the ureter openings into the distended bladder can be seen

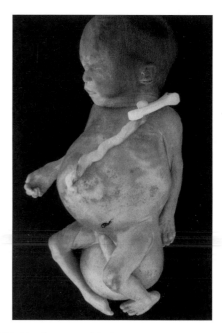

Figure 5.44 Exterior aspect of the fetus in Figure 5.43 looks similar to a fetus with sacrococcygeal teratoma

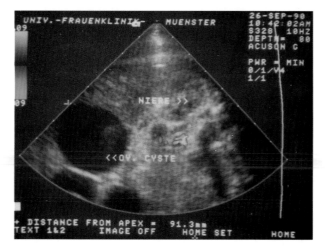

Figure 5.45 Sonogram of a fetus with ovarian cyst next to a normal kidney

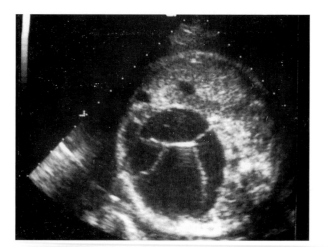

Figure 5.46 Urachal cyst (fluid-filled with septations) in a fetus medially and cranially to the urinary tract towards the anterior abdominal wall

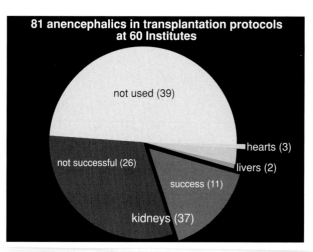

Figure 5.47 Current experience with the use of anencephalic donors for kidney transplantation (taken from ref. 82)

factor for the development of arterial hypertension is pyelonephritis due to vesicorenal reflux, obstructive uropathy and fistulation of the renal pelvis, which can develop even after successful surgery.

In summary, although some congenital renal anomalies cannot be recognized prenatally, e.g. non-Finnish nephrotic syndrome without amniotic fluid α-fetoprotein increase[84], most urogenital fetal anomalies can be detected now by modern gray-scale ultrasound screening[85].

The prenatal recognition offers the chance to prevent postnatal complications more easily, e.g. pyelonephritis from unrecognized hydronephrosis, or to make prognostic statements about the treatability of these conditions, but the development of the most appropriate pre- and perinatal management protocols requires further studies including careful postnatal follow-up investigations.

REFERENCES

1. Potter, E.L. (1972). *Normal and Abnormal Development of the Kidney.* (Chicago: Year Book Medical Publishers)
2. Hansmann, M., Hackelöer, B.J. and Staudach, A. (1985). *Ultraschalldiagnostik in Geburtshilfe und Gynäkologie.* (Berlin-Heidelberg-New York-Tokyo: Springer)
3. Holzgreve, W., Lison, A., Bulla, M. *et al.* (1991). Protein analysis to determine fetal kidney function (Abstr.). *Am. J. Obstet. Gynecol.*, **164** (suppl.), 336
4. Kurjak, A., Latin, V., Mandruzzato, G. *et al.* (1984). Ultrasound diagnosis and perinatal management of fetal genito-urinary abnormalities. *J. Perinat. Med.*, **12**, 291–312
5. D'Ottavio, G., Bogatti, P., Rustico, M.A. *et al.* (1989). Anatomic correlates of ultrasound in prenatal diagnosis of urinary tract abnormalities. *Eur. J. Obstet. Gynecol. Reprod. Biol.*, **32**, 79–87
6. Arger, P.H., Coleman, B.G. and Mintz, M.C. (1985). Routine fetal genitourinary tract screening. *Radiology*, **156**, 485–9
7. Zerres, K. (1987). Genetics of cystic kidney disease. Criteria for classification and genetic counselling. *Pediatr. Nephrol.*, **1**, 397–404
8. Osathanondh, V. and Potter, E.L. (1964). Pathogenesis of polycystic kidneys. *Arch. Pathol.*, **77**, 459–65
9. Zerres, K., Völpel, M.C. and Weiß, H. (1984). Cystic kidneys. *Hum. Genet.*, **68**, 104–35
10. Romero, R., Cullen, M., Jeanty, P. *et al.* (1984). The diagnosis of congenital renal anomalies with ultrasound. II. Infantile polycystic kidney disease. *Am. J. Obstet. Gynecol.*, **150**, 259–62
11. Blyth, H. and Ockenden, B.G. (1971). Polycystic disease of kidneys and liver presenting in childhood. *J. Med. Genet*, **8**, 257–84
12. Hobbins, J.C., Grannum, P.A.T., Berkowitz, R.L. *et al.* (1979). Ultrasound in the diagnosis of congenital anomalies. *Am. J. Obstet. Gynecol.*, **134**, 331
13. Main, D., Mennuti, M.T., Cornfeld, D. and Coleman, B. (1983). Prenatal diagnosis of adult polycystic kidney disease. *Lancet*, **2**, 337–8
14. Weiß, H., Zerres, K. and Hansmann, M. (1981). Pränatale Diagnose zystischer Nierenveränderungen mit Hilfe der Ultraschalltechnik. *Ultraschall*, **2**, 244–8
15. Simpson, J.L., Sabbagha, R.E., Elias, S. *et al.* (1982). Failure to detect polycystic kidneys *in utero* by second trimester ultrasonography. *Hum. Genet.*, **60**, 295
16. Habif, D.V., Berdon, W.E. and Yeh, M.N. (1982). Infantile polycystic kidney disease: *in utero* sonographic diagnosis. *Radiology*, **142**, 475
17. Townsend, R.R., Goldstein, R.B., Filly, R.A. *et al.* (1988). Sonographic identification of autosomal recessive polycystic kidney disease associated with increased maternal serum/amniotic fluid alpha-fetoprotein. *Obstet. Gynecol*, **71**, 1008–12
18. Garrett, W.J., Grunwald, G. and Robinson, D.E. (1970). Prenatal diagnosis of fetal polycystic kidney by ultrasound. *Aust. N.Z. J. Obstet. Gynaecol.*, **10**, 7–9
19. Venn, H.J., Weiss, H., Zerres, K. *et al.* (1983). Sonographische Differentialdiagnose cystischer Veränderungen der fetalen Niere. In Otto, R.C. and Jann, F.X. (eds.) *Ultraschalldiagnostik 82*, pp.156–9. (Stuttgart: Thieme Verlag)
20. Passarge, E. and Lenz, W. (1966). Syndrome of caudal regression in infants of diabetic mothers: observations of further cases. *Pediatrics*, **37**, 672–75
21. Grix, A., Curry, C. and Hall, B.D. (1982). Patterns of multiple malformations in infants of diabetic mothers. *Birth Defects*, **18**, 3A, 55–77
22. Main, D., Mennuti, M.T., Cornfeld, D. *et al.* (1983). Prenatal diagnosis of adult polycystic kidney disease. *Lancet*, **2**, 337–8
23. Fryns, J.P., Vandenberghe, K. and Moerman, F. (1986). Mid-trimester ultrasonographic diagnosis of early manifesting 'adult' form of polycystic kidney disease. *Hum. Genet.*, **74**, 461
24. Bronshtein, M., Yoffe, N., Brandes, M. *et al.* (1990). First and early second-trimester diagnosis of fetal urinary tract anomalies using transvaginal sonography. *Prenat. Diagn.*, **10**, 653–66
25. Reeders, S.T., Breuning, M.H., Davies, K.E. *et al.* (1985). A highly polymorphic DNA marker linked to adult polycystic kidney disease on chromosome 16. *Nature*, **317**, 542–4
26. Reeders, S.T., Zerres, K. and Gal, A. (1986). Prenatal diagnosis of autosomal dominant polycystic kidney disease with a DNA probe. *Lancet*, **2**, 6–8
27. Hobbins, J.C., Romero, R., Grannum, P. *et al.* (1984). Antenatal diagnosis of renal anomalies with

ultrasound. I. Obstructive uropathy. *Am. J. Obstet. Gynecol.*, **148**, 868–77

28. Garrett, W.J., Kossow, G. and Osborn, R.A. (1975). The diagnosis of fetal hydronephrosis, megaureter and urethral obstruction by ultrasonic echography. *Br. J. Obstet. Gynaecol.*, **82**, 115–20

29. Harrison, M.R. and Filly, R.A. (1990). The fetus with obstructive uropathy: pathophysiology, natural history, selection, and treatment. In Harrison, M.R., Golbus, M.J. and Filly, R.A. (eds.) *The Unborn Patient*, pp. 328–98. (Philadelphia: Saunders)

30. Wladimiroff, J.W., Beemer, F.A., Scholtmeyer, R.J. *et al.* (1985). Failure to detect fetal obstructive uropathy by second trimester ultrasound. *Prenat. Diagn.*, **5**, 41–6

31. Sanders, R. and Graham, D. (1982). Twelve cases of hydronephrosis *in utero* diagnosed by ultrasonography. *J. Ultrasound Med.*, **1**, 341

32. Baker, M.E., Rosenberg, E.R., Bowie, J.D. *et al.* (1985). Transient *in utero* hydronephrosis. *J. Ultrasound Med.*, **4**, 51–3

33. Flake, A.W., Harrison, M.R., Sauer, L. *et al.* (1986). Ureteropelvic junction obstruction in the fetus. *J. Pediatr. Surg.*, **21**, 1058–63

34. Grignon, A., Filion, R., Filiatrault, D. *et al.* (1986). Urinary tract dilatation *in utero*: classification and clinical applications. *Radiology*, **160**, 645–7

35. Mahony, B.S., Filly, R.A., Callen, P.W. *et al.* (1984). Sonographic evaluation of renal dysplasia. *Radiology*, **152**, 143

36. Appelman, Z. and Golbus, M.S. (1986). The management of fetal urinary tract obstruction. *Clin. Obstet. Gynecol.*, **29**, 483–9

37. Golbus, M.S., Filly, R.A., Callen, P.W. *et al.* (1985). Fetal urinary tract obstruction: management and selection for treatment. *Semin. Perinatol.*, **9**, 91–7

38. Holzgreve, W. (1990). The fetus with nonimmune hydrops. In Harrison, M.R. *et al.* (eds.) *The Unborn Patient*, pp.228–45. (Philadelphia: Saunders)

39. Appelman, Z. and Golbus, M.S. (1990). The mangement of fetal urinary tract obstruction. *Clin. Obstet. Gynecol.*, **29**, 483–9

40. Lenz, S., Lund-Hansen, T., Bang, J. *et al.* (1985). A possible prenatal evaluation of renal function by amino acid analysis on fetal urine. *Prenat. Diagn.*, **5**, 259–67

41. Nicolini, U., Rodeck, C.H. and Fisk, N.M. (1987). Shunt treatment for fetal obstructive uropathy. *Lancet*, **2**, 1338–9

42. Wilkins, I.A., Chitkara, U., Lynch, L. *et al.* (1987). The nonpredictive value of fetal urinary electrolytes: preliminary report of outcomes and correlations with pathologic diagnosis. *Am. J. Obstet. Gynecol.*, **157**, 694–8

43. Reuss, A., Wladimiroff, J.W., Pijpers, L. *et al.* (1987). Fetal urinary electrolytes in bladder outlet obstruction. *Fetal Ther.*, **2**, 148–53

44. Holzgreve, W., von Bassewitz, D.B., Ullrich, K. *et al.* (1986). Pränatale Funktionsdiagnostik bei obstruktiven Uropathien des Feten. In Hansmann, M. *et al.* (eds.) *Ultraschalldiagnostik 86*, pp. 391–6. (Berlin: Springer Verlag)

45. Peterson, P.A., Errin, P.E. and Berggard, (1969). Differentiation of glomerular, tubular and normal proteinuria: determinations of urinary excretion of β_2-microglobulin, albumin and total protein. *J. Clin. Invest.*, **48**, 1189–96

46. Pesce, A.J., Boreisha, I. and Pollak, V.E. (1972). Rapid differentiation of glomerular and tubular proteinuria by sodium dodecyl sulfate polyacrylamide gel electrophoresis. *Clin. Chim. Acta*, **40**, 27–34

47. Holzgreve, W., Lison, A. and Bulla, M. (1989). SDS–PAGE as an additional test to determine fetal kidney function prior to intrauterine diversion of urinary tract obstruction. *Fetal Ther.*, **4**, 93–6

48. Adzick, N.S., Harrison, M.R., Glick, P.L. *et al.* (1985). Fetal urinary tract obstruction: experimental pathophysiology. *Semin. Perinatol.*, **9**, 79–90

49. Golbus, M.S., Harrison, M.R. and Filly, R.A. (1983). Prenatal diagnosis and treatment of fetal hydronephrosis. *Semin. Perinatol.*, **7**, 102–7

50. Golbus, M.S., Harrison, M.R., Filly, R.A. *et al.* (1982). *In utero* treatment of urinary tract obstruction. *Am. J. Obstet. Gynecol.*, **142**, 383–8

51. Harrison, M.R., Golbus, M.S., Filly, R.A. *et al.* (1982). Fetal surgery for congenital hydronephrosis. *N. Engl. J. Med.*, **306**, 591–3

52. Rodeck, C.H., Fisk, N.M., Fraser, D.I. *et al.* (1988). Long-term *in utero* drainage of fetal hydrothorax. *N. Engl. J. Med.*, **319**, 1135–8

53. Berkowitz, R.L., Glickman, M.G., Smith, G.J.W. *et al.* (1982). Fetal urinary tract obstruction: what is the role of surgical intervention *in utero*? *Am. J. Obstet. Gynecol.*, **144**, 367–75

54. Elder, J.S., Duckett, J.W. and Snyder, H.M. (1987). Intervention for fetal obstructive uropathy: has it been effective? *Lancet*, **2**, 1007–10

55. Romero, R., Cullen, M., Grannum, P. *et al.* (1985). Antenatal diagnosis of renal anomalies with ultrasound. III. Bilateral renal agenesis. *Am. J. Obstet. Gynecol.*, **151**, 38–43

56. Wilson, R.D. and Hayden, M.R. (1985). Bilateral renal agenesis in twins. *Am. J. Med. Genet.*, **21**, 147–52

57. Hansmann, M. (1985). Ultraschallkontrollierte Therapie des Feten. *Arch. Gynecol.*, **238**, 169–84

58. Duval, J.M., Milon, J., Coadou, Y. *et al.* (1986). Ultrasonographic anatomy and diagnosis of fetal uropathies affecting the upper urinary tract. *Surg. Radiol. Anat.*, **8**, 131–45

59. Ramsing, M., Rehder, H., Holzgreve, W. *et al.* (1990). Fraser syndrome (cryptophthalmos with syndactyly) in the fetus and newborn. *Clin. Genet.*, **37**, 84–96

60. Knowles, J.C., Brandt, I.K. and Bull, M.J. (1981).

Kaufman syndrome (hydrometrocolpos, polydactyly, and congenital heart disease) with pituitary dysplasia, choanal atresia, and vertebral anomalies. *Am. J. Med. Genet.*, **8**, 389–93

61. Haspeslagh, M., Fryns, J.P., Van den Berghe, K. *et al.* (1981). Hydrometrocolpos–polydactyly syndrome in a macerated female fetus. *Eur. J. Pediatr.*, **136**, 307–9

62. Holzgreve, W., Wagner, H. and Rehder, H. (1984). Bilateral renal agenesis with Potter phenotype, cleft palate, anomalies of the cardiovascular system, skeletal anomalies including hexadactyly and bifid metacarpal. A new syndrome? *Am. J. Med. Genet.*, **18**, 177–82

63. Legius, E., Moerman, P., Fryns, J.P. *et al.* (1988). Holzgreve–Wagner–Rehder syndrome: Potter sequence associated with persistent buccopharyngeal membrane. A second observation. *Am. J. Med. Genet.*, **31**, 269–72

64. Curry, C.J.R., Jensen, K., Holland, J. *et al.* (1984). The Potter sequence: a clinical analysis of 80 cases. *Am. J. Med. Genet.*, **19**, 679–702

65. Furlong, L.A., Williamson, R.A., Bonsib, S. *et al.* (1986). Pregnancy outcome following ultrasound diagnosis of fetal urinary tract anomalies and/or oligohydramnios. *Fetal Ther.*, **1**, 134–45

66. Holzgreve, W. and Miny, P. (1989). Genetic aspects of fetal disease. *Semin. Perinatol.*, **13**, 260–77

67. Holzgreve, W., Miny, P., Holzgreve, A. and Rehder, H. (1986). Ultraschall-Befund als Hinweiszeichen auf eine fetale Triploidie. *Ultraschall*, **7**, 169–71

68. Holzgreve, W., Miny, P., Gerlach, B. *et al.* (1990). Benefits of placental biopsies for rapid karyotyping in the second and third trimesters (late chorionic villus sampling) in high-risk pregnancies. *Am. J. Obstet. Gynecol.*, **162**, 188–92

69. Bovicelli, L., Rizzo, N., Orsini, L.F. *et al.* (1980). Prenatal diagnosis of the prune belly syndrome. *Clin. Genet.*, **18**, 79–82

70. Burton, B.K. and Dillard, R.G. (1984). Prune belly syndrome: observations supporting the hypothesis of abdominal overdistension. *Am. J. Med. Genet.*, **17**, 669–72

71. Avni, E.F., Rodesch, F. and Schulman, C.C. (1985). Fetal uropathies: diagnostic pitfalls and management. *J. Urol.*, **134**, 921–5

72. Gruenewald, S.M., Crocker, E.F., Walker, A.G. *et al.* (1984). Antenatal diagnosis of urinary tract abnormalities: correlation of ultrasound appearance with postnatal diagnosis. *Am. J. Obstet. Gynecol.*, **148**, 278–83

73. Dunn, V. and Glasier, C.M. (1985). Ultrasonographic antenatal demonstration of primary megaureters. *J. Ultrasound Med.*, **4**, 101–3

74. Greenblatt, A.M., Beretsky, I., Lankin, D.H. *et al.* (1985). *In utero* diagnosis of crossed renal ectopia using high-resolution real-time ultrasound. *J. Ultrasound Med.*, **4**, 105–7

75. Vintzileos, A.M., Eisenfeld, L.I., Herson, V.C. *et al.* (1986). Megacystis–microcolon–intestinal hypo-peristalsis syndrome. Prenatal sonographic findings and review of the literature. *Am. J. Perinat.*, **3**, 297–302

76. Duval, J.M., Milon, J., Coadou, Y. *et al.* (1985). Ultrasonographic anatomy and diagnosis of fetal uropathies affecting the upper urinary tract. *Anat. Clin.*, **7**, 301–32

77. Holzgreve, W. (1985). Prenatal diagnosis of persistent common cloaca with prune belly and anencephaly in the second trimester. *Am. J. Med. Genet.*, **20**, 729–32

78. Kirkinen, P. and Jouppila, P. (1985). Perinatal aspects of pregnancy complicated by fetal ovarian cyst. *J. Perinat. Med.*, **13**, 245–51

79. Jouppila, P., Kirkinen, P. and Tuononen, S. (1982). Ultrasonic detection of bilateral ovarian cysts in the fetus. *Eur. J. Obstet. Gynecol. Reprod. Biol.*, **13**, 87–92

80. Dewbury, K.C., Aluwihare, A.P.R., Birch, S.J. *et al.* (1980). Prenatal ultrasound demonstration of a choledochal cyst. *Br. J. Radiol.*, **53**, 906–7

81. Holzgreve, W., Beller, F.K., Buchholz, B. *et al.* (1989). Kidney transplantation from anencephalic donors. *N. Engl. J. Med.*, **316**, 1069–70

82. Medical Task Force on Anencephaly (1990). *N. Engl. J. Med.*, **322**, 669–74

83. Mendoza, S.A. (1990). Hypertension in infants and children. *Nephron*, **54**, 289–95

84. Bulla, M., Kuwertz-Bröking, E., Helmchen, U. *et al.* (1990). Idiopathisches Congenitales Nephrotisches Syndrome (CNS) unter dem histologischen Bild einer intra- und extrakapillären Glomerulonephritis – Kasuistik einer türkischen Familie. *Monatsschr. Kinderheilkd.*, **138**, 526

85. Holzgreve, W. (1990). Sonographic screening for anatomic defects. *Semin. Perinatol.*, **14**, 504–13

6 Normal Anatomy and Malformation of the Fetal Cardiovascular System

P.A. Stewart

NORMAL FETAL CARDIAC ULTRASOUND ANATOMY

The four-chamber view

Approximately 70–80% of congenital heart abnormalities can be excluded from a normal four-chamber view[1,2]. It is the easiest view to obtain and recognize and is achieved by a direct transverse plane across the fetal thorax. It is the easiest plane to use in routine scanning as it lies between that for measuring the biparietal diameter and that for measuring the abdominal circumference. The fetal stomach and the apex of the heart should be visualized on the left side of the fetus. The fetal position is not important as the position of the spine is always used for orientation. The 'rule of thumb' for orientation is given by first checking the position of the spine. The descending aorta lies on the spine and the left atrium lies on the aorta while the sternum lies opposite the spine and the right ventricle lies beneath the sternum (Figure 6.1).

On ultrasound the four-chamber view is presented as follows (Figures 6.2 and 6.3):

(1) The heart fills approximately one-third of the fetal thorax;

(2) The right and left atria are approximately equal in size;

(3) The right and left ventricular cavities are more or less equal in size at the level of the valves;

(4) The right ventricle is closest to the sternum, the left atrium closest to the spine (Figure 6.2);

(5) Mitral and tricuspid valves open with each cardiac cycle;

(6) Ventricular walls and interventricular septum are more or less equal in thickness;

(7) The tricuspid valve inserts more apically than the mitral valve;

(8) The right ventricular apex has a 'triangular' shape due to increased trabeculations and the moderator band;

(9) The foramen ovale flap is seen with movement into the left atrium;

(10) The pulmonary veins insert into the left atrium – seen on either side of the spinal crest; and

(11) The ventricular septum appears intact.

Left heart connections

From the four-chamber position (orientation unimportant, spine as landmark), cranial angulation of the transducer produces the 'five-chamber view' or the four-chamber aortic root view (Figures 6.4–6.6). Turning the transducer lengthwise will produce a left ventricular long axis view. Continuity between the anterior wall of the aorta and interventricular septum, and the posterior wall of the aorta and anterior mitral valve leaflet should be identified. Still turning the transducer longitudinally shows the aortic arch with innominate, carotid and subclavian arteries to the head and neck. The ascending aorta lies to the right of the main pulmonary artery and angles out to the right.

Right heart connections

The pulmonary artery is closer to the chest wall and runs straight towards the spine (Figure 6.7). Orientating the transducer along the length of the right ventricular outflow tract shows the pulmonary valve. Scanning the base of the heart lengthwise brings the inferior and superior vena caval connections into view (Figure 6.8). Further angulation in a horizontal direction visualizes the main pulmonary artery, right and left pulmonary arteries and/or the ductus arteriosus (Figures 6.9 and 6.10). A parasternal short axis view shows both

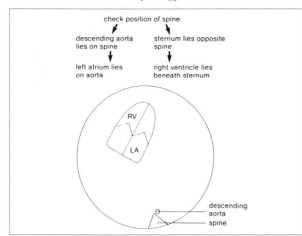

Figure 6.1 Diagram to show orientation for obtaining a four-chamber view

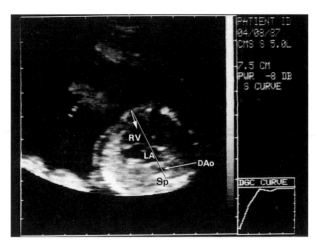

Figure 6.2 Fetal four-chamber view; if an imaginary line is drawn from the spine (Sp) to the sternum, the first structure under the sternum will be the right ventricle (RV) and the structure closest to the descending aorta (DAo) will be the left atrium (LA)

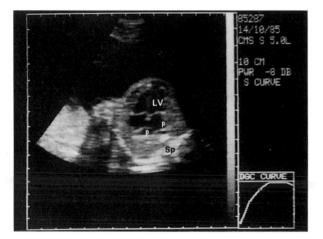

Figure 6.3 Fetal four-chamber view; LV = left ventricle, p = pulmonary vein, Sp = spine

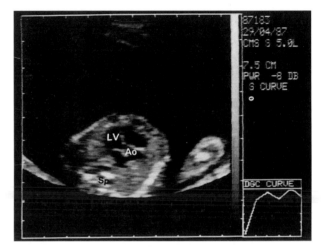

Figure 6.4 Fetal 'five'-chamber view; Ao = aortic root, LV = left ventricle, Sp = spine

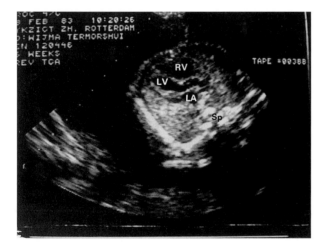

Figure 6.5 Fetal left ventricular long-axis view; LV = left ventricle, RV = right ventricle, LA = left atrium, Sp = spine

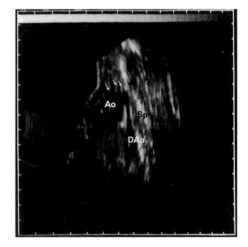

Figure 6.6 Fetal aortic arch view; the head and neck vessels are seen vertically from this orientation (arrows); DAo = descending aorta, Ao = aorta, Sp = spine

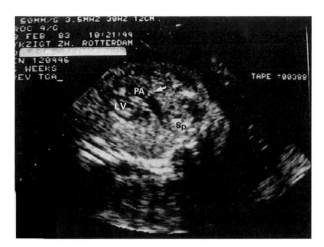

Figure 6.7 Fetal right ventricular outflow tract; PA = pulmonary artery, LV = left ventricle, Sp = spine, arrow indicates closed pulmonary valve

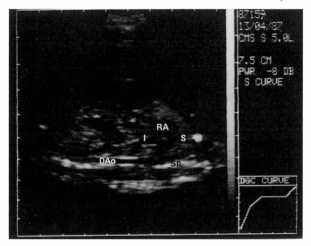

Figure 6.8 Fetal inferior (I) and superior (S) vena caval connections to the right atrium (RA); DAo = descending aorta, Sp = spine

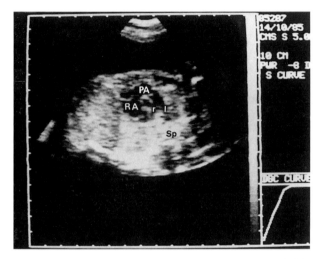

Figure 6.9 Fetal parasternal short axis pulmonary artery view with right (r) and left (l) pulmonary arteries; RV = right ventricle, LV = left ventricle, Sp = spine

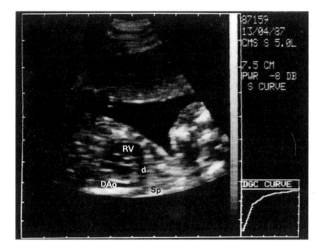

Figure 6.10 Fetal ductus arteriosus (d) connecting the right ventricle (RV) and the descending aorta (DAo); Sp = spine

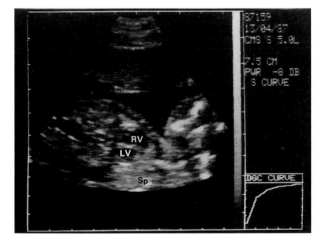

Figure 6.11 Fetal parasternal short axis view; LV = left ventricle, RV = right ventricle, Sp = spine

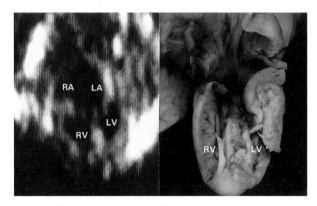

Figure 6.12 Case 1 – 17 weeks. Ultrasound: complete atrioventricular septum defect; Pathology: complete atrioventricular septum defect; RA = right atrium, LA = left atrium, RV = right ventricle, LV = left ventricle

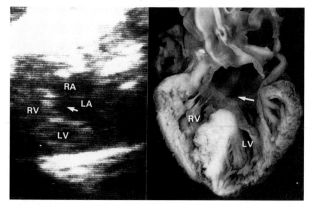

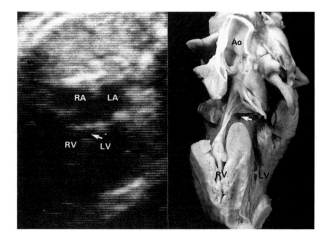

Figure 6.13 Case 2 – 27 weeks. Ultrasound: complete atrioventricular septum defect; Pathology: complete atrioventricular septum defect and hypoplastic aortic isthmus; RA = right atrium, LA = left atrium, RV = right ventricle, LV = left ventricle

Figure 6.14 Case 3 – 30 weeks. Ultrasound: complete atrioventricular septum defect and over-riding aorta (Ao); Pathology: complete atrioventricular septum defect, aorta probably normal – appeared displaced due to septal architecture; RA = right atrium, LA = left atrium, RV = right ventricle, LV = left ventricle

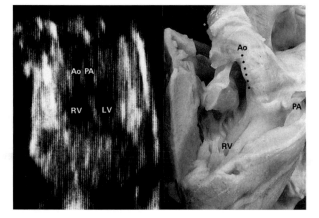

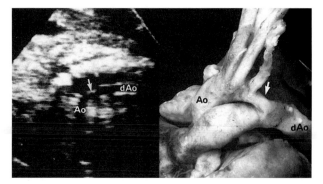

Figure 6.15 Case 4 – 25 weeks. Ultrasound: ventricular septal defect and double outlet right ventricle; Pathology: ventricular septal defect, double outlet right ventricle and dysplastic tricuspid valve; RA = right atrium, LA = left atrium, RV = right ventricle, LV = left ventricle, Ao = aorta, PA = pulmonary artery

Figure 6.16 Case 5 – 28 weeks. Ultrasound: hypoplastic aortic isthmus; Pathology: hypoplastic aortic isthmus; Ao = aorta, DAo = descending aorta

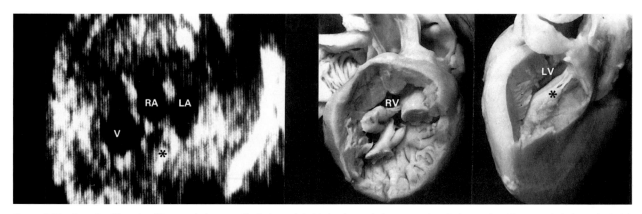

Figure 6.17 Case 6 – 31 weeks. Ultrasound: dextrocardia, ? absent left-sided atrioventricular connection, ? abnormal papillary muscle in hypoplastic left ventricle and double outlet right ventricle; RA = right atrium, LA = left atrium, V = ventricle; Pathology: dextrocardia, hypoplasia left heart, parachute mitral valve, and double outlet right ventricle (RV) with pulmonary outflow tract stenosis and preductal coarctation; LV = left ventricle

ventricles, the right rather elongated and the left seen as a circle, 'sitting' on the diaphragm (Figure 6.11).

Outflow tracts

The pulmonary valve is anterior and cranial to the aortic valve. The pulmonary artery is connected to the anterior (right) ventricle and gives rise to the right and left pulmonary arteries and the ductus arteriosus (Figures 6.6, 6.9 and 6.10). The origins of the pulmonary artery and aorta are at 90° to each other.

The aorta arises from the posterior (left) ventricle, is in the center of the chest and continues into the aortic arch. The arch gives rise to the innominate, carotid and subclavian arteries (Figures 6.4–6.6).

SUMMARY

The morphologic characteristics and connections of the fetal heart should be sequentially identified. Using both transverse and longitudinal planes the *venous–atrial junctions* are identified by visualizing the venae cavae to the right atrium and pulmonary veins to the left atrium.

To visualize the *atrioventricular junction* the transverse plane should be used to identify the four-chamber view.

The *ventriculoarterial connections* are identified using transverse and longitudinal planes to visualize the pulmonary artery and branches to the right, and aorta and branches, to the left.

FETAL CARDIAC PATHOLOGY: ULTRASOUND AND PATHOLOGY CORRELATES

Where possible an attempt was made to correlate the prenatal ultrasound findings with the postmortem specimens. This is mandatory, to confirm the prenatal diagnosis and to understand how errors (misclassifications, false-positive diagnoses etc.) in interpretation may have occurred.

Sequential segmental analysis of cardiac morphology was performed during both ultrasound and postmortem examinations[3,4]. When feasible specimens were opened, and photographed in planes as close as possible to the appropriate ultrasound images to aid comparison (Figures 6.12–6.21). Close correlation may be achieved (case 8; Figure 6.19) even when the specimen is very small.

Concomitant defects such as aortic arch anomalies, dysplasia of the valve leaflets (Figures 6.15 and 6.18) and outflow tract stenoses (Figure 6.17) may be missed by prenatal ultrasound. In some cases this may be caused by inability to visualize all structures completely, especially later in gestation or when multiple defects are present. Certain types of defect may not be identifiable by ultrasound. In yet other cases (cases 9 and 10; Figures 6.20 and 6.21) rare anatomic variants may confuse the issue, leading to erroneous interpretation.

Given the above it is obvious that, whenever possible, careful postmortem examination should be performed.

FETAL COLOR-CODED DOPPLER FLOW MAPPING

The most recent advance has been the introduction of color-coded Doppler flow mapping techniques whereby the Doppler shift is displayed in color during the real-time examination[5–7]. Doppler color flow mapping displays the Doppler shift in three ways:

(1) Red color indicates a Doppler shift towards the transducer;

(2) Blue color indicates a Doppler shift away from the transducer; and

(3) Mosaic color (red/orange or blue/green) indicates multiple Doppler shifts suggestive of turbulent flow.

The power output (SPTA, spatial-peak temporal average) required for fetal real-time color-coded Doppler flow mapping is considered to be acceptable at less than 100 mW/cm^2[8,9].

The advantages of this method are:

(1) Rapid visualization of fetal cardiovascular blood flow in normal hearts;

(2) Easy identification of significant valvular regurgitation (and stenoses);

(3) Visualization of abnormal shunting across interatrial and interventricular structures;

(4) Adjunctive information to be obtained in complex lesions; and

(5) The possibility to study extracardiac blood flow directions and profiles.

Currently color-coded Doppler flow mapping offers most benefit for fetal cardiovascular

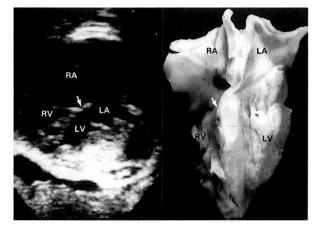

Figure 6.18 Case 7 – 35 weeks. Ultrasound: severe RA dilatation, and ? Ebstein anomaly or obstructed foramen ovale (no echographic evidence of valve displacement – arrow indicates septal leaflet insertion); Pathology: severe RA dilatation, and tricuspid dysplasia with 'knobbly' tissue. No septal leaflet displacement; RA = right atrium, LA = left atrium, RV = right ventricle, LV = left ventricle

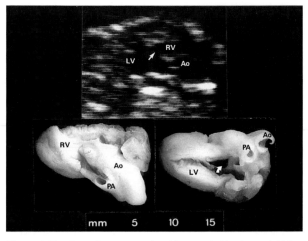

Figure 6.19 Case 8 – 16 weeks. Ultrasound: Tetralogy of Fallot; Pathology: Tetralogy of Fallot; LV = left ventricle, RV = right ventricle, Ao = aorta, PA = pulmonary artery, arrow indicates ventricular septal defect

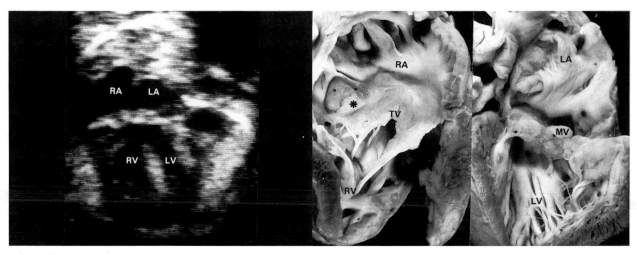

Figure 6.20 Case 9 – 34 weeks. Ultrasound: complete atrioventricular septum defect, and Tetralogy of Fallot; RA = right atrium, LA = left atrium, RV = right ventricle; LV = left ventricle; Pathology: deficiency of the muscular atrioventricular septum (replaced by membranous septum*), dysplastic tricuspid (TV) and mitral (MV) valves – MV with no papillary muscles, and Tetralogy of Fallot; RA = right atrium, LA = left atrium, RV = right ventricle, LV = left ventricle

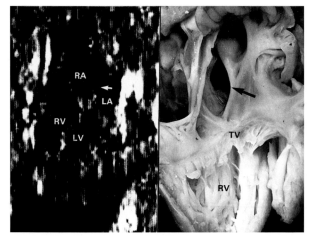

Figure 6.21 Case 10 – 29 weeks. Ultrasound: secundum atrial septal defect; Pathology: anatomic variant, superior and inferior limbus met in central fibrous body; RA = right atrium, LA = left atrium, RV = right ventricle, LV = left ventricle, TV = tricuspid valve

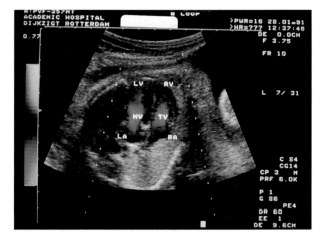

Figure 6.22 Fetal color four-chamber view showing normal forward flow through the mitral (MV) and tricuspid (TV) valves; LV = left ventricle, RV = right ventricle, LA = left atrium, RA = right atrium

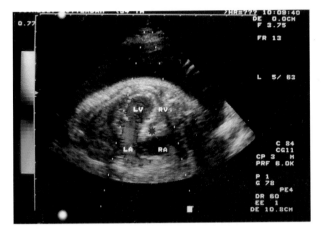

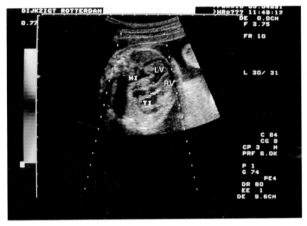

Figure 6.23 Fetal color four-chamber view showing normal forward flow through left atrium (LA) and left ventricle (LV) and no detectable flow through right atrium (RA) and right ventricle (RV) due to tricuspid valve atresia (*)

Figure 6.24 Fetal color four-chamber view showing mitral (MI) and tricuspid (TI) insufficiency related to fetal hydrops in a case of twin–twin transfusion; LV = left ventricle, RV = right ventricle

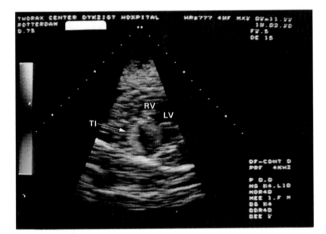

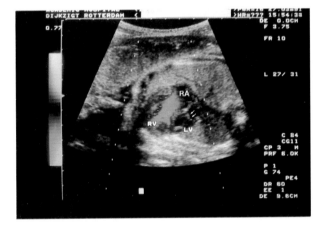

Figure 6.25 Fetal color four-chamber view in a case with Ebstein anomaly showing severe tricuspid insufficiency (TI) (coded in blue) and normal forward flow (coded in red) during diastole; RV = right ventricle, LV = left ventricle

Figure 6.26 Fetal color four-chamber view showing normal flow through the right atrium (RA) and ventricle (RV) and no detectable flow through the left side of the heart due to mitral atresia (arrows); LV = left ventricle

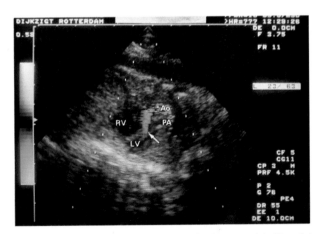

Figure 6.27 Fetal color-modified long-axis view in a case of double outlet right ventricle with anterior aorta (Ao). Blood flow from left ventricle (LV) shunts through a ventricular septal defect (arrow) across the right ventricle (RV) and is coded in red. Aortic arch blood flow is coded in blue. No flow was detected through the narrowed pulmonary artery (PA)

examination and is a valuable adjunct to the other ultrasound techniques already described (Figures 6.22–6.27). Ultrasound examination time may be reduced, especially for hemodynamic evaluation, as interfacing the color-coded information allows more rapid identification of the areas to be interrogated, especially when abnormal flow patterns are expected.

Expected technological advances will further improve the usefulness of this technique as enhanced processing of information will allow evaluation of smaller structures more accurately than is presently feasible.

REFERENCES

1. Allan, L.D., Crawford, D.C., Chita, S.K. and Tynan, M.J. (1986). Prenatal screening for congenital heart disease. *Br. Med. J.*, **292**, 1717–19
2. Copel, J.A., Pilu, G., Green, J., Hobbins, J.C. and Kleinman, C.S. (1987). Fetal echocardiographic screening for congenital heart disease: the importance of the four-chamber view. *Am. J. Obstet. Gynecol.*, **157**, 648–55
3. Becker, A.E. and Anderson, R.H. (1981). *Pathology of Congenital Heart Disease*, pp.3–27. (London: Butterworth)
4. Gussenhoven, W.J. and Becker, A.E. (1983). *Congenital Heart Disease: Morphologic Echocardiographic Correlations.* (Edinburgh: Churchill Livingstone)
5. Maulik, D., Nanda, N.C. and Hsiung, M.C. (1986). Doppler color flow mapping of the fetal heart. *Angiology*, **37**, 628–32
6. Kurjak, A., Breyer, B., Jurkovic, D., Alfirevic, Z. and Miljan, M. (1987). Colour flow mapping in obstetrics. *J. Perinat. Med.*, **15**, 271–81
7. Devore, G.R., Hovenstein, J., Siassi, B. and Platt, L.D. (1987). Doppler color flow mapping: a new technique for the diagnosis of congenital heart disease. *Am. J. Obstet. Gynecol.*, **156**, 1054–64
8. Centers for Disease Control (1985). Temporal trends in the incidence of malformation in the United States, selected years, 1970–71, 1982–83. *MMWR*, **34**, 1SS–3SS
9. Health Council of the Netherlands (1986). The safety of ultrasound in clinical diagnostic examinations. In *Ultrasound in Medicine. Recommendations on the Subject of Ultrasound*, vol.13, pp.33–49. (The Hague: Health Council)

7 Normal and Abnormal Anatomy of the Respiratory System

J. Zmijanac and A. Kurjak

The upper respiratory system can be partially seen by ultrasound (Figure 7.1). Portions of the pharynx and hypopharynx are commonly visible because of the presence of fluid (Figure 7.2). Details of laryngeal anatomy are not particularly evident but the larynx itself can be easily recognized as a superior constriction of the tracheal fluid column. The trachea can be easily visualized due to the fact that it is consistently filled with fluid. Mainstem bronchi are usually invisible.

The fetal chest can be easily recognized by using the fetal heart as a landmark. The thoracic circumference is derived on the plain of section used for the four-chamber view of the heart. Displacement of the fetal heart or mediastinum indicates the presence of intrathoracic space-occupying lesions, like an intrathoracic mass or fluid collection.

The right and left pulmonary arteries and several pulmonary veins are visible in a large percentage of cases. They are usually examined during fetal heart examination.

The lung tissue can be seen from late first trimester onward (Figure 7.3). The structures that surround it include ribs, heart and liver. Sonography routinely visualizes the fetal lungs by the mid-second trimester (Figure 7.4). They appear as two moderately and homogeneously echogenic areas on either side of the heart[1]. On longitudinal section the diaphragm can be recognized between the lungs and the liver as a relatively transonic line moving during respiratory excursions (Figure 7.5). Lung echogenicity increases after 35–36 weeks, approaching that of the liver. It has been suggested that fetal pulmonic maturity has been achieved when lung echogenicity is equal to, or greater than liver echogenicity.

Impaired maturation of fetal lungs frequently results in postnatal respiratory distress or death. Derangements of the intrauterine environment, thorax, or extrathoracic organ systems profoundly affect the prenatal development of the lungs. Pulmonary hypoplasia detected prenatally usually occurs in prolonged and severe oligohydramnios or primary thoracic abnormalities[2,3]. In the case of an abnormal thoracic mass or pleural fluid collection, evaluation of the size may assist in prediction of associated pulmonary hypoplasia. The severity of pulmonary hypoplasia depends upon the gestational age and onset, duration of the inciting conditions and severity of the insult. Since the fetal thorax normally grows at a regular rate from 16 to 40 weeks, comparison of the measured thoracic size with the predicted size at different gestational ages may assist in the prediction of small lungs indicative of pulmonary hypoplasia. An absolute thoracic circumference measurement less than the 5th percentile for expected values or a declining thoracic circumference to abdominal circumference ratio has been suggested as evidence for pulmonary hypoplasia.

Hydrothorax is abnormal fetal pleural fluid collection developed from various etiologies (Figure 7.6)[4]. Excluding hydrops, the most common cause of fluid accumulation in the fetal thorax is chylothorax. Chylothorax is particularly likely when the pleural effusion is unilateral. The right side is affected more often than the left, and males twice as often as females. Congenital chylothorax probably results from a malformation of the fetal thoracic duct. The specific diagnosis is made postnatally, because prior to oral milk feeding the fluid appears clear.

Hydrothorax produces an anechoic space located on the periphery of the thoracic cavity (Figure 7.7). Anechoic pleural fluid collection displaces the lungs away from the chest wall and compresses the lungs. The partially collapsed lungs usually retain their normal shape (Figures 7.8 and 7.9).

Cystic adenomatoid malformation of the lung (CAML) is a lung hamartoma with overgrowth of the mesenchymal elements[5]. Type I contains one or several large cysts ranging from 2 to 10 cm in diameter, and small cysts along the periphery of the hemithorax (Figures 7.10–7.12). These cysts can involve the entire lobe. Type II has multiple small cysts measuring less than 1 cm in diameter. On ultrasound scan, type II creates a mass with numerous

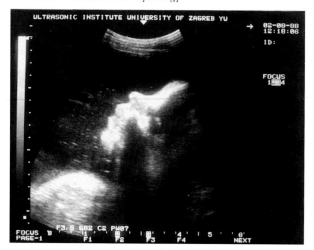

Figure 7.1 The upper respiratory system: fetal nose and mouth are clearly visualized on fetal profile

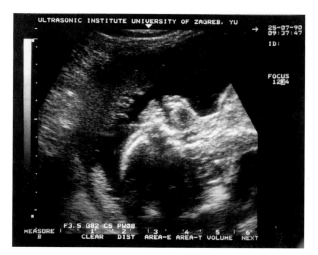

Figure 7.2 Fetal hydropharynx and larynx are filled with fluid and therefore visible

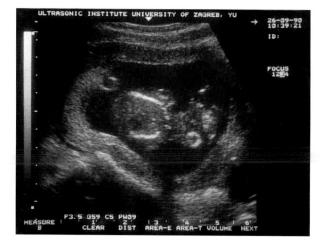

Figure 7.3 Early pregnancy: fetal lung tissue is defined more from structures that surround it, like fetal ribs

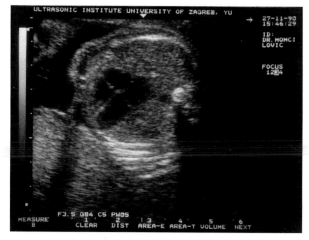

Figure 7.4 Second trimester: fetal lungs create homogeneous, midrange echoes that surround fetal heart

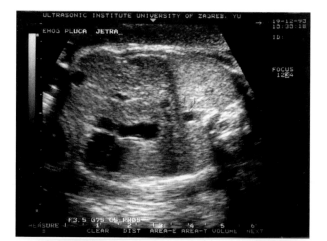

Figure 7.5 Different echogenicity of fetal lungs and fetal liver. The diaphragm appears as a hypoechoic line between lungs and liver

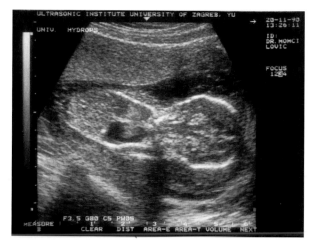

Figure 7.6 Fetal hydrothorax detected at 20 weeks of pregnancy

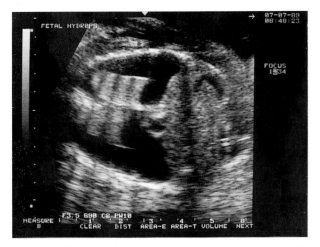

Figure 7.7 Hydrothorax can be visualized as an anechoic space within the thoracic cavity

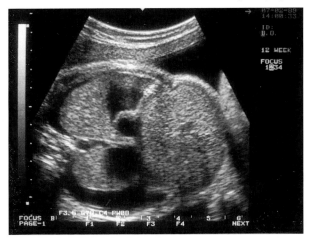

Figure 7.8 The partially collapsed lungs retain their normal shape, although the anechoic pleural fluid displaces them away from the chest wall

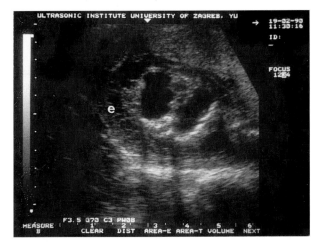

Figure 7.9 Transverse section through the fetal thorax. Lungs are totally collapsed or hypoplastic and compressed to the mediastinum. Thoracic cavity is completely filled with fluid. There is severe soft tissue edema (e)

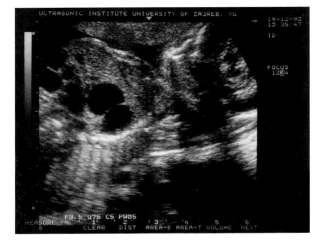

Figure 7.10 Cystic adenomatoid malformation of the lungs. Multiple large cysts are seen in the fetal thorax

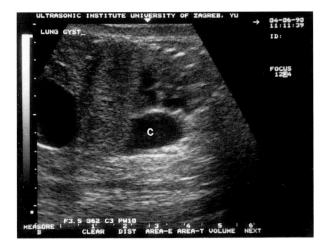

Figure 7.11 Longitudinal scan of the fetus with a solitary cystic mass (c) in the left hemithorax

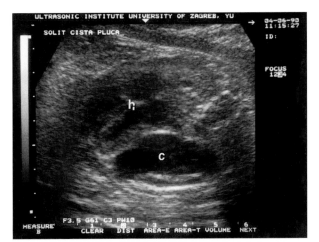

Figure 7.12 Transverse scan of the fetus with huge solitary cystic mass (c) in the left hemithorax. The heart (h) and mediastinum are shifted to the right side of the chest

small cysts. Type III creates a large solid mass involving the entire lobe. It produces a homogeneous echogenic mass without individual cysts.

Lung sequestration is a malformation in which a part of the bronchopulmonary tissue is separated from the normal bronchial system[6]. It is a rare anomaly, classified as extra- and intralobar sequestration, depending on the extent of pleural covering. A sequestration produces a well defined homogeneous echogenic mass usually in the inferior part of the hemithorax or upper abdomen.

Bronchogenic cysts result from abnormal budding of the foregut diverticulum, and can occur within the mediastinum, within the lung or below the diaphragm[7]. They do not communicate with the tracheobronchal tree. Ultrasonographically, they appear as small, well defined, unilocular intrathoracic cystic lesions adjacent to the mediastinum. They do not impair fetal development, although infants may occasionally present with dysphagia or pneumonia during childhood[8].

REFERENCES

1. Fried, A.M., Loh, F.K., Umer, M.A. *et al.* (1985). Echogenicity of fetal lungs: relation to fetal age and maturity. *Am. J. Radiol.*, **145**, 591–4

2. Castillo, R.A., Devoe, L.D., Falls, G. *et al.* (1987). Pleural effusions and pulmonary hypoplasia. *Am. J. Obstet. Gynecol.*, **157**, 1252–5

3. Nimrod, C., Nicholson, S., Davies, D. *et al.* (1988). Pulmonary hypoplasia testing in clinical obstetrics. *Am. J. Obstet. Gynecol.*, **158**, 277–80

4. Rodeck, C.H., Fisk, N.M., Fraser, D.I. *et al.* (1988). Long term *in utero* drainage of fetal hydrothorax. *N. Engl. J. Med.*, **319**, 1135–8

5. Fine, C., Adzick, N.A. and Doubilet, P.M. (1988). Decreasing size of a congenital adenomatoid malformation *in utero*. *J. Ultrasound Med.*, **7**, 405–8

6. Davies, R.P., Ford, W.D.A., Lequesne, G.W. *et al.* (1989). Ultrasonic detection of subdiaphragmatic pulmonary sequestration *in utero* and postnatal diagnosis by fine needle aspiration biopsy. *J. Ultrasound Med.*, **8**, 47–9

7. Albright, E.B., Crane, J.P. and Shackelford, G.D. (1988). Prenatal diagnosis of a bronchogenic cyst. *J. Ultrasound Med.*, **7**, 91–5

8. Nyberg, D.A., Mahony, B.S. and Pretorius, D.H. (1990). *Diagnostic Ultrasound of Fetal Anomalies. Text and Atlas.* (Chicago: Year Book Medical Publishers)

8 Normal Anatomy and Malformations of Fetal Gastrointestinal System

A. Kurjak and J. Zmijanac

Intra-abdominal anomalies present a particular challenge to the obstetric sonographer since they can arise from a variety of different organs and anatomic sites.

Potential sites of gastrointestinal abnormalities include esophagus, stomach, duodenum, jejunoileum and colon, liver, spleen, gallbladder, pancreas and mesentery or peritoneal cavity. Despite the diversity, diagnosis can usually be made after carefully considering the location and sonographic appearance of the abnormality[1].

NORMAL SONOGRAPHIC APPEARANCE

The upper portion of the fetal abdomen is occupied by liver which has a homogeneous echogenicity higher than that of the lungs. At any gestational age, the liver comprises most of the upper abdomen in the fetus (Figure 8.1). The most commonly obtained section through the fetal abdomen is the transverse section through the liver at the level of the intrahepatic portion of the umbilical vein (Figure 8.2). The umbilical vein can be followed from its entrance into the fetal abdomen until the portal sinus (Figures 8.3 and 8.4). A smaller part of the umbilical vein blood is directed through the ductus venosus directly into the inferior vena cava. Ductus venosus can be visualized intrahepatically in the oblique scan.

The gallbladder is normally visualized as an ovoid or pear-shaped fluid-filled structure to the right and inferior to the intrahepatic portion of the umbilical vein (Figure 8.5). It can be mistaken for the umbilical vein unless the characteristic course of the vein or its intrahepatic branches is visualized.

The fetal stomach becomes visible at the age of 11 menstrual weeks[2]. By 16 weeks, the stomach should be demonstrated in nearly all normal fetuses in the left upper quadrant of the abdomen (Figures 8.6 and 8.7). It appears as a fluid-filled structure the size and shape of which vary according to the ingestion of amniotic fluid and active peristaltic movements.

Fetal spleen is visualized on a transverse plane just posterior and to the left of the fetal stomach. It appears as a semilunar, hypoechoic structure.

Fluid-filled bowel loops are often seen in the second and third trimester (Figures 8.8 and 8.9). Distinguishing large bowel from small bowel is possible after 20 menstrual weeks and this distinction becomes more obvious with advancing gestational age. Characteristically, the large bowel appears as a continuous tubular structure located in the periphery of the abdomen that is filled with hypoechoic meconium. The small bowel is located centrally and remains more echogenic in appearance until the late third trimester. The small bowel undergoes peristalsis that can be observed during the third trimester.

GASTROINTESTINAL ANOMALIES

The normal appearance of fetal bowel can be altered by a number of pathological processes[3]. Most commonly bowel obstruction results in proximal bowel dilatation that is characteristically recognized as one or more tubular or cystic structures within the fetal abdomen. Fetal bowel obstruction may be secondary to a congenital malformation such as intestinal atresia, duplication of the bowel, volvulus, or meconium ileus.

Atresias are the most commonly encountered type of digestive system obstructions.

Esophageal atresia can sometimes be visualized with careful real-time scanning alternating filling and emptying of a large proximal esophagus. The presence of swallowing and regurgitation during an ultrasound examination is further presumptive evidence for esophageal atresia. In cases without tracheoesophageal fistula the fetal stomach is not visualized. Esophageal atresia alone would also be expected to cause polyhydramnios. However, demonstration of fluid in the stomach does not necessarily exclude esophageal atresia, since enough fluid may be excreted by the gastric mucosa to make

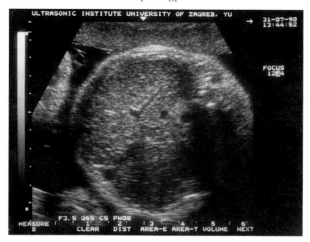

Figure 8.1   Transverse scan of fetal abdomen showing the liver which has a homogeneous echogenicity and occupies most of the upper abdomen in the fetus

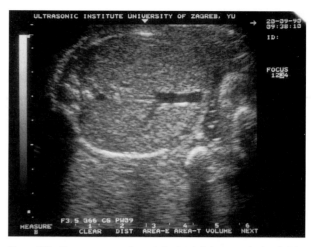

Figure 8.2   Transverse scan through the fetal abdomen at the level of the umbilical vein

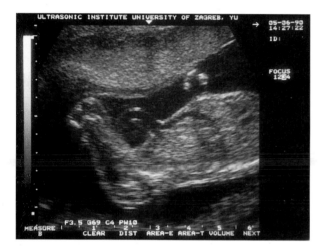

Figure 8.3   Longitudinal scan of the fetus showing the entrance of umbilical cord into the fetal abdomen and its course in the fetal liver

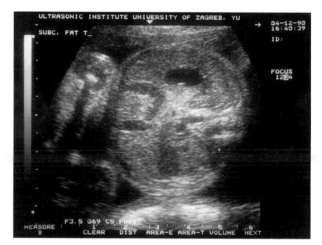

Figure 8.4   Transverse section through the fetal abdomen at the level of the portal sinus. Fetal stomach and gallbladder are also displayed

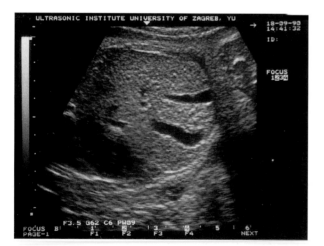

Figure 8.5   Gallbladder can be visualized on the right side of the umbilical vein. The umbilical vein is a tubular structure, while the gallbladder can be recognized by its typical pear-shaped appearance

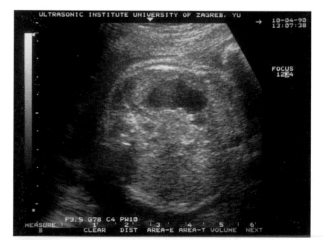

Figure 8.6   Fetal stomach can be visualized in the left upper quadrant of the abdomen. The size and the shape of fetal stomach vary according to the amount of ingested amniotic fluid

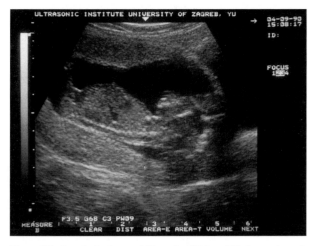

Figure 8.7 Longitudinal scan of 16-week-old fetus. At that age, stomach should be demonstrated in nearly all normal fetuses

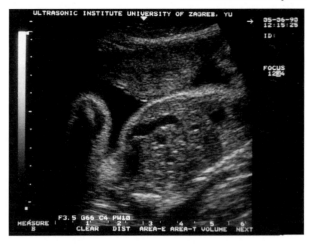

Figure 8.8 Beneath the umbilical vein, multiple small bowel loops can be demonstrated as small anechoic structures in the abdomen

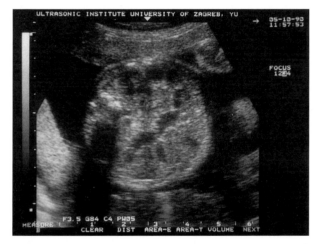

Figure 8.9 Fetal colon transversum is visualized as a predominantly anechoic tubular structure coursing across the abdomen

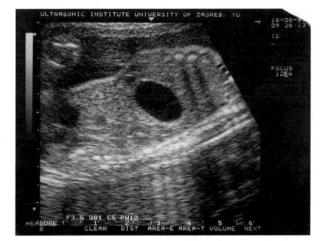

Figure 8.10 Dilated fetal stomach: the finding is highly indicative of pyloric atresia, but the size of the stomach should be checked on subsequent examinations

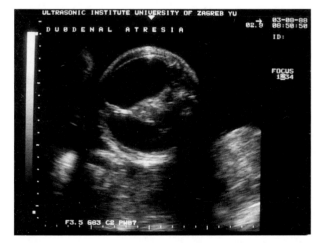

Figure 8.11 Duodenal atresia: the transverse scan through the fetal abdomen illustrates the typical 'double-bubble' sign. The upper cyst represents the dilated stomach and is usually larger than the lower cyst representing the dilated duodenum

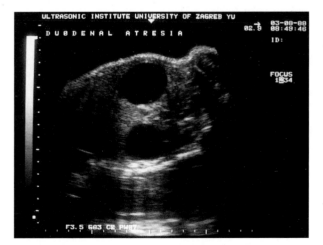

Figure 8.12 Double-bubble sign on a longitudinal sonogram

it visible. If the stomach is not visualized, particularly in the presence of polyhydramnios, other congenital anomalies such as diaphragmatic hernia, situs inversus, facial cleft and central nervous system anomalies should also be suspected.

Pyloric atresia is a rare anomaly accounting for approximately 1% of all intestinal atresias (Figure 8.10). Ultrasound visualization of a dilated, fluid-filled stomach associated with polyhydramnios is highly suggestive of this anomaly.

Duodenal atresia has frequently been detected on prenatal sonography (Figures 8.11 and 8.12)[4]. It affects 1 in 5000 pregnancies, and approximately 30% of these are associated with trisomy 21. A characteristic finding is the so-called 'double-bubble' sign, representing the fluid-filled stomach and duodenum. Two round-shaped cystic structures are ultrasonically visualized in the upper abdomen of the affected fetus. The left cyst represents the dilated stomach and the right one is duodenum. Continuity with the stomach should be demonstrated to distinguish a distended duodenum from other cystic masses in the right upper quadrant, such as choledochal cysts and hepatic cysts. Other causes that could produce 'double-bubble' sign include annular pancreas, obstructing bands, volvulus or intestinal duplications.

Normal stomach with prominent incisura angularis should not be mistaken for duodenal atresia (Figure 8.13). This potential pitfall can be avoided by scanning in a transverse plane.

Polyhydramnios develops in most cases of duodenal atresia, presumably because at a variable gestational age the volume of amniotic fluid swallowed by the fetus exceeds the resorptive capacity of the stomach and proximal duodenum.

Intestinal atresia is characterized by several cystic structures in the upper abdomen representing dilated bowel loops (Figures 8.14 and 8.15). Polyhydramnios is seen less frequently. When dilated small bowel is demonstrated, meconium ileus should be considered (Figures 8.16 and 8.17) as well as jejunoileal atresia and volvulus. Care should be taken to distinguish dilated bowel from hydroureter or other intra-abdominal cystic masses.

More distal obstructions include colonic and anorectal atresias. In distal obstruction there is sufficient length of the proximal bowel for complete resorption of swallowed fluid and polyhydramnios does not occur. Nevertheless, anorectal atresia can sometimes be recognized as dilated colon in the lower abdomen or pelvis (Figures 8.18 and 8.19)[5]. Calcified intraluminal meconium is another possible manifestation of anorectal atresia. Colonic atresia is

an isolated anomaly and is extremely rare. Anal atresia is associated with anomalies of other systems (genitourinary or skeletal) in more than half of cases (Figure 8.20).

Congenital megacolon (Hirschsprung's disease) is the most common cause of colonic obstruction[6]. It is due to the congenital absence of ganglion cells in the distal intestine. Characteristically, only the rectum and sigmoid colon are involved. Sonographically, severely distended small bowel loops proximally from the site of obstruction and polyhydramnios can be detected.

A variety of cystic masses can be observed in the fetal abdomen (Figure 8.21). Cystic masses arising from the digestive system, excluding dilated bowel are hepatic cysts and tumors, choledochal cyst, enteric duplication cyst, and mesenteric cyst. The prevalence, location and sonographic appearance of cystic malformation can help in making a diagnosis.

Congenital anomalies of the liver are quite rare. Solitary hepatic cysts can be described as an intrahepatic cystic structure, multilocular in 10% of cases. Solitary cysts are derived from the developmental interruption of the intrahepatic biliary tree. They are most frequently located at the inferior margin of the right lobe. Less likely considerations for a cystic mass located in liver include cystic hepatoblastoma, hemangioma or hamartoma.

Choledochal cyst most frequently results from cystic dilatation of the common duct. Other types of choledochal cysts are derived from multiple intrahepatic and extrahepatic cysts, diverticula of the common bile duct and choledochoceles. Choledochal cysts are rare and can be identified as a simple cystic mass in the upper abdomen or right upper quadrant.

Enteric duplication cysts may occur at any level along the gastrointestinal tract. The stomach is involved less frequently than other regions. On prenatal sonography, duplication cysts are reported as cystic intra-abdominal masses that should be distinguished from mesenteric or omental cysts, urachal cyst, ovarian cyst or hepatic cyst.

The sonographic findings of mesenteric, omental and retroperitoneal cysts are variable. They can be unilocular or multiseptate and of various sizes. Usually sonolucent, they may appear solid when hemorrhagic. They are usually located in mid-abdomen. Mesenteric (Figure 8.22) and omental cysts are characteristically mobile.

Although ovarian cysts do not belong to the gastrointestinal system, they should be considered in the differential diagnosis of cystic structures in the fetal abdomen. Ovarian cysts are usually unilateral

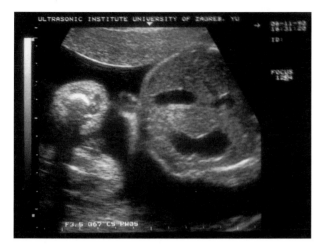

Figure 8.13 Normal stomach with prominent incisura angularis

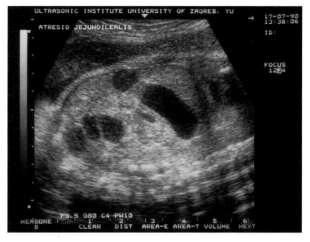

Figure 8.14 Small bowel obstruction: the stomach is dilated and several cystic structures are present in the fetal abdomen

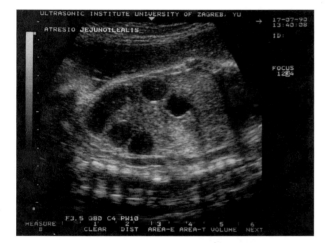

Figure 8.15 Longitudinal scan through the fetus with small bowel obstruction. Note the presence of several cysts representing dilated bowel loops

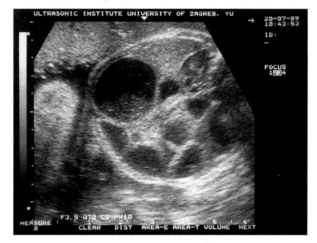

Figure 8.16 Meconium ileus: multiple distended bowel loops are seen inside the fetal abdomen. Presence of solid matter inside the cysts reveals the diagnosis of meconium ileus

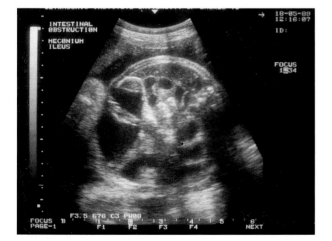

Figure 8.17 Meconium ileus with signs of meconium peritonitis. Note the hyperechogenic areas of calcifications surrounded by the distended bowel loops

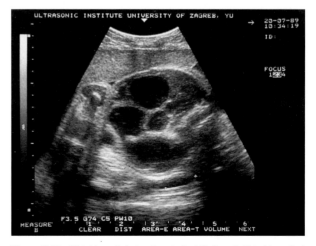

Figure 8.18 Distal bowel obstruction: typical finding of dilated intestinal loops in the lower parts of the fetal abdomen is illustrated

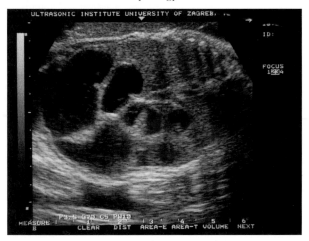

Figure 8.19 Longitudinal scan of the fetus with distal bowel obstruction. Dilated, fluid-filled bowel loops are located caudally in the fetal abdomen

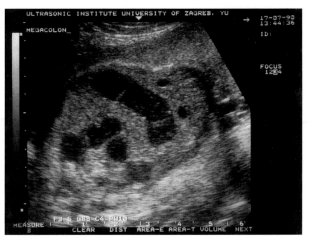

Figure 8.20 Marked dilatation of the colon transversum at 37 weeks. The clinical significance of such a finding can be evaluated only after delivery

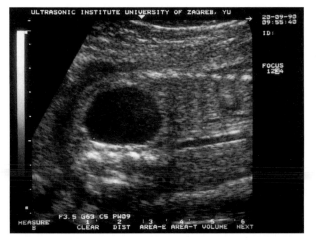

Figure 8.21 Cystic structure in the lower abdomen. Identification of fetal sex is important in such cases and helps in the differential diagnosis

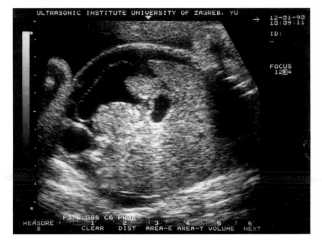

Figure 8.22 Mesenteric cyst (lymphangioma) is clearly visible due to associated ascites

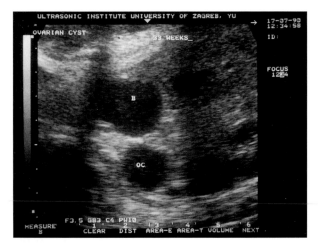

Figure 8.23 Fetal ovarian cyst (OC) in 33-week-old female fetus. Urinary bladder (B) is also displayed

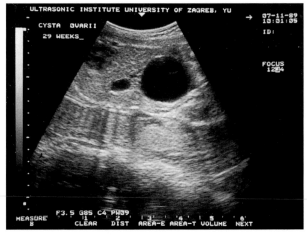

Figure 8.24 Fetal ovarian cyst

and unilocular (Figures 8.23 and 8.24)[7]. They vary in size from small cysts to structures filling the entire abdomen[8]. An ovarian cyst should be suspected when a cystic intra-abdominal mass is found in a female fetus. The cyst should be separate from the organs of the urinary and gastrointestinal systems. Extremely large cysts may impair fetal lung development and should therefore be treated by puncture under ultrasonic guidance.

REFERENCES

1.   Hill, L.H. (1988). Sonographic detection of fetal gastrointestinal anomalies. *Ultrasound Q.*, **6**, 35–67

2.   Pretorius, D.H., Gosink, B.B., Clautice-Engle, T. *et al.* (1988). Sonographic evaluation of the fetal stomach: significance of non-visualization. *Am. J. Radiol.*, **151**, 987–9

3.   Kurjak, A. (1990). Congenital and perinatal anomalies of the gastrointestinal tract. In Kurjak, A. (ed.) *Handbook of Ultrasound in Obstetrics and Gynecology*, pp.229–50. (Boca Raton: CRC Press)

4.   Romero, J., Jeanty, P., Pilu, G. *et al.* (1988). The prenatal diagnosis of duodenal atresia. Does it make any difference? *Obstet. Gynecol.*, **71**, 739–41

5.   Harris, R.D., Nyberg, D.A., Mack, L.A. *et al.* (1987). Anorectal atresia: prenatal sonographic diagnosis. *Am. J. Radiol.*, **149**, 395–400

6.   Vermish, M., Mayden, K.L., Confino, E. *et al.* (1986). Prenatal sonographic diagnosis of Hirschsprung's disease. *J. Ultrasound Med.*, **5**, 37–9

7.   Rizzo, N., Gabrielli, S., Perolo, A. *et al.* (1989). Prenatal diagnosis and management of fetal ovarian cysts. *Prenat. Diagn.*, **9**, 97–104

8.   Romero, R., Pilu, G., Jeanty, P. *et al.* (1988). *Prenatal Diagnosis of Congenital Anomalies.* (Norwalk: Appleton & Lange)

9 Normal Anatomy and Malformations of Fetal Abdominal Wall

A. Kurjak and J. Zmijanac

Abdominal wall defects occur early in embryologic development[1-5]. Routine views of the anterior abdominal wall and umbilical cord insertion site are recommended (Figures 9.1–9.3). A false-positive diagnosis of abdominal wall defect is possible between 6 and 12 weeks when the rapidly elongating midgut normally herniates into the base of the body stalk. Because of this embryologic process, a reliable diagnosis of gastroschisis or omphalocele may not be possible before 12 weeks.

OMPHALOCELE

This is defined as a herniation of a variable amount of abdominal viscera into the base of the umbilical cord. It results from a failure of the intestines to return to the abdomen or from a failure of four embryonic disc folds to fuse into the primitive pleuroperitoneal cavity. The result of fusion failure is a midline abdominal wall defect. The viscera are covered with a membranous sac of peritoneum and amnion. The umbilical cord inserts into the sac with it vessels spreading within the sac wall. The herniated sac contains, according to the degree of the defect, the intestines, liver, stomach and spleen. If the sac ruptures prenatally, an omphalocele could be mistaken for gastroschisis. Regardless of the size of the defect in the fetal skin, the underlying rectus muscles are intact.

Sonographically, omphalocele may demonstrate a variable appearance depending on the size of the abdominal wall defect, type of eviscerated organs, presence of ascites and associated anomalies. The primary diagnostic feature of omphalocele is the central location of the abdominal wall defect at the base of the umbilical cord insertion site (Figure 9.4). The presence of a limiting membrane is another essential feature of omphalocele. However, the membrane itself may be difficult to visualize as a discrete structure when not outlined by ascites. The existence of the membrane is inferred by showing that extracorporeal structures appear contained rather than floating freely in the amniotic fluid (Figures 9.5–9.8). The liver in an omphalocele can be identified by its homogeneous appearance and the presence of intrahepatic vessels. The bowel in the sac is more echogenic and irregular in appearance.

Omphalocele involves a high degree of association with other abnormalities. Cardiovascular and gastrointestinal malformations are most frequent (Figure 9.9). Chromosome abnormalities have been reported in 10–40% of neonates with omphalocele, mostly trisomies 18 and 13. In view of all this, the prenatal work-up should include a complete ultrasound evaluation of the affected fetus. An irregular abdominal shape in transverse section is usually caused by limb compression (Figure 9.10). Misinterpretation of this finding as omphalocele must be avoided and the continuity of the skin layer should be verified.

GASTROSCHISIS

This is an abdominal wall defect mainly located in the right paraumbilical region. The defect involves all layers of the abdominal wall and is usually 2–5 cm in size. It has been suggested that gastroschisis results from abnormal involution of the right umbilical vein or from the disruption of the omphalomesenteric artery. Gastroschisis is sporadic, and no genetic association or recurrence risks have been described. The ultrasonic finding of bowel loops floating in the amniotic fluid outside the fetal abdomen is characteristic (Figures 9.11–9.13). As the defect is located paraumbilically, the umbilical cord is inserted normally. The sonographic diagnosis of gastroschisis is highly reliable when:

(1)   The full-thickness abdominal wall defect is located just to the right of a normal umbilical cord insertion site;

(2)   A variable amount of bowel protrudes through the defect and floats freely in the amniotic fluid

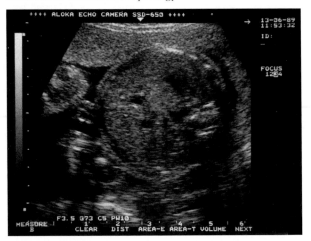

Figure 9.1 Normal round-shaped section through the fetal abdomen. The umbilical cord insertion site is visible between the fetal legs

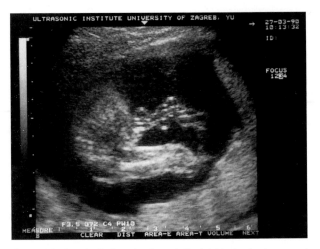

Figure 9.2 Longitudinal section through the fetal body showing normal umbilical cord insertion site

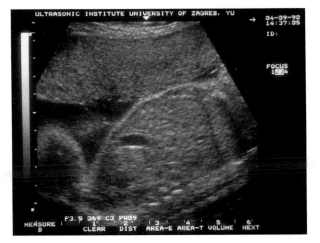

Figure 9.3 Longitudinal scan through the fetal body showing continuity of abdominal wall. The different echogenicity of fetal liver and lungs can be seen with a diaphragm between those organs. The diaphragm is displayed as a thin hypoechogenic line

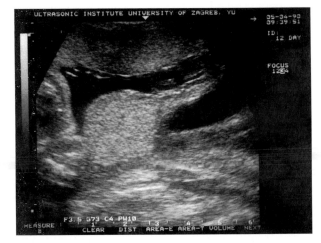

Figure 9.4 Typical ultrasonic finding of a solid sac attached to the fetal abdomen, in case of omphalocele. The insertion of the umbilical cord to the sac wall is clearly visible

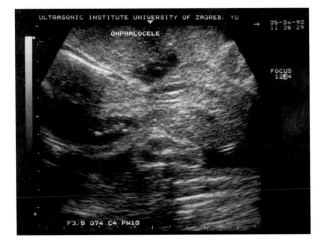

Figure 9.5 Omphalocele: herniated viscera and umbilical vein are visible within the sac

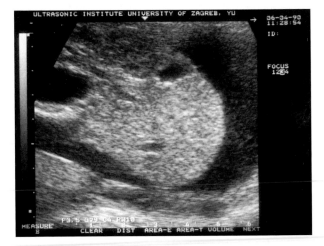

Figure 9.6 Omphalocele: a closer look at the sac

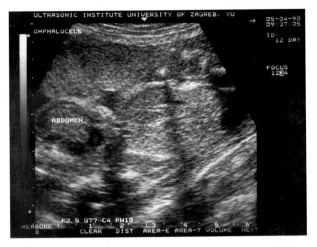

Figure 9.7 Sac containing herniated viscera appears very large compared to the abdomen

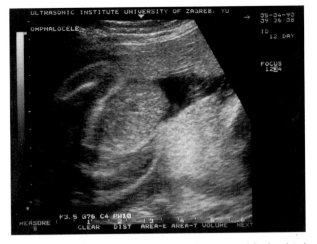

Figure 9.8 Typical appearance of omphalocele: sac containing herniated viscera is seen between fetal legs

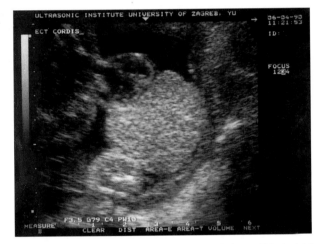

Figure 9.9 Omphalocele associated with ectopic heart. Ectopic fetal heart is clearly seen in the amniotic fluid above the omphalocele

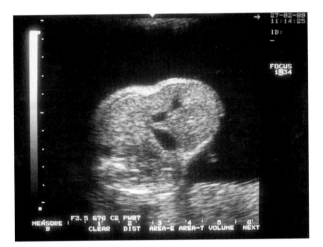

Figure 9.10 'Pseudosac': irregular abdominal shape on the transverse section usually caused by limb compression. Note the continuous skin layer. Misinterpretation of this finding as omphalocele has to be avoided

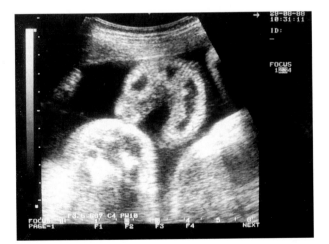

Figure 9.11 Gastroschisis: typical finding of intestinal loops floating freely in the amniotic fluid

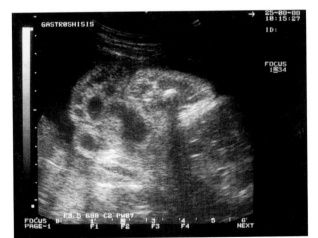

Figure 9.12 Gastroschisis: the fetal trunk and fluid-filled intestinal loops protruding from the fetal abdomen are visible

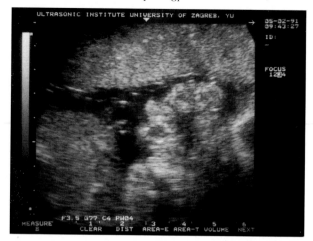

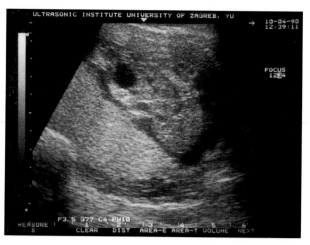

Figure 9.13   Free floating loop of intestine is visible between fetal trunk and placenta. In this case loops are of a more solid appearance

Figure 9.14   A case of evisceration: most of the fetal abdominal organs are found in the amniotic fluid

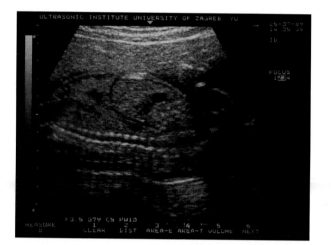

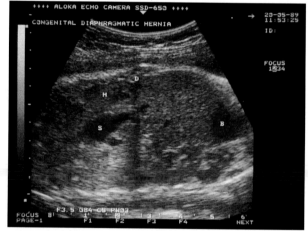

Figure 9.15   Longitudinal scan of a normal fetus showing fetal thorax and abdomen separated by a thin anechoic line representing fetal diaphragm

Figure 9.16   A case of congenital diaphragmatic hernia: diaphragm (D) is seen between thorax and abdomen, but fetal heart (H) and stomach (S) are lying next to each other in the thoracic cavity; the urinary bladder (B) is also displayed

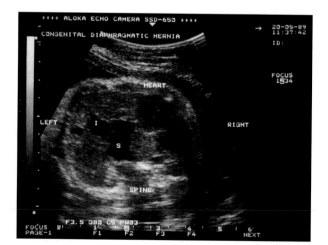

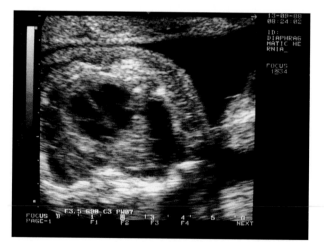

Figure 9.17   Transverse scan of the fetus with congenital diaphragmatic hernia. Heart, stomach (S) and intestine (I) are in the same level in the thoracic cavity

Figure 9.18   A diagnosis of congenital diaphragmatic hernia is certain when abdominal organs (the stomach in this case) are displayed at the same level as a four-chamber view of the heart

and may appear disproportionately large to the small wall defect; and

(3) There is no covering membrane.

The abdominal cavity may be reduced in size, depending on the amount of eviscerated bowel (Figure 9.14). Near term, eviscerated bowel appears slightly thickened probably due to chemical peritonitis induced by prolonged exposure of bowel to the amniotic fluid.

CONGENITAL DIAPHRAGMATIC HERNIA

This is another very important malformation involving both abdomen and thorax. Ultrasound diagnosis of diaphragmatic hernia is based upon three characteristic signs: polyhydramnios, mediastinal shift and inability to visualize stomach in its normal place in the upper abdomen (Figures 9.15 and 9.16). As most hernias contain the small bowel, bowel loops can be seen in the thoracic cavity (Figure 9.17). The fluid-filled stomach and small bowel contrast to the more echogenic fetal lung especially in the left-sided hernias. Polyhydramnios is a non-specific sign and it seems that impaired fetal swallowing due to compression of the esophagus plays a role in its etiology. Displacement of the fetal mediastinum is predominantly lateral and it can be easily identified on the transverse section taken at the level of the fetal heart. It can be stated that when abdominal organs are at the level of the four-chamber view, they lie within the fetal thorax and congenital diaphragmatic hernia is present (Figure 9.18).

CLOACAL AND BLADDER EXTROPHY

These share a common embryologic origin in abnormal cloacal development. Bladder extrophy is characterized by a defect in the lower abdominal wall and anterior wall of the urinary bladder. Cloacal extrophy results in extrophy of the bladder, in which there are two hemibladders separated by intestinal mucosa. Other malformations include abdominal and pelvic defects, anorectal atresia and spinal abnormalities.

The primary finding in cases of bladder extrophy is failure to visualize the normal urinary bladder although the amount of amniotic fluid is normal. The abdominal wall defect may be difficult to visualize due to its small size. Abnormal genitalia and hydronephrosis can also be identified.

Anterior abdominal wall defect may be the primary sonographic finding in cloacal extrophy. Cloacal extrophy should be considered whenever an atypical abdominal wall defect is identified. The diagnosis can be made by failure to demonstrate a urinary bladder together with the presence of low abdominal wall defect, soft tissue abdominal mass and splaying of the pubic rami.

REFERENCES

1. Langer, J.C. and Harrison, M.R. (1990). The fetus with an abdominal wall defect. In Harrison, M.R., Golbus, M.S. and Filly, R.A. (eds.) *The Unborn Patient*, 2nd edn. (Philadelphia: WB Saunders Co)

2. Hill, L.M. (1988). Sonographic detection of fetal gastrointestinal anomalies. *Ultrasound Q.*, **6**, 35–67

3. Romero, R., Pilu, G., Jeanty, P., Ghidini, A. and Hobbins, J.C. (1988). *Prenatal Diagnosis of Congenital Anomalies.* (Norwalk: Appleton & Lange)

4. Winter, R.M., Knowles, S.A.S., Bieber, F.R. and Baraitser, M. (1988). *The Malformed Fetus and Stillbirth. A Diagnostic Approach.* (Chichester: John Wiley & Sons)

5. Kurjak, A. (1990). *Handbook of Ultrasound in Obstetrics and Gynecology.* (Boca Raton: CRC Press)

10 Normal and Abnormal Multiple Gestation

A. Kurjak and J. Zmijanac

The antenatal diagnosis of twins is best made by ultrasound examination. In early gestation ultrasound is helpful in confirming gestational age and fetal number and in evaluating fetal growth and placentation (Figures 10.1–10.5).

However, an assessment of amnionicity and chorionicity constitutes the initial step in the prenatal sonographic evaluation of a twin pregnancy. This can be accomplished by visualization of a separating membrane, two separate placentae, and fetal sex. Visualization of separate placental masses or opposite-sexed twins is consistent with a diagnosis of dichorionic placentation. However, the presence of a single placenta may represent a fused dichorionic placenta or a single monochorionic placenta, and thus is not definitive in differentiating chorionic types. Visualization of a separating membrane indicates a diamniotic pregnancy (Figures 10.6–10.8). Nevertheless, non-visualization of a separating membrane is not sufficient evidence for a monoamniotic gestation (Figures 10.9 and 10.10). In diamniotic–dichorionic gestation, the separating membrane is comprised of two amnions and two chorions and is therefore thicker than in a diamniotic–monochorionic gestation (Figure 10.11). In the latter, it is composed of only two layers – two amnions (Figure 10.12). The thick membrane is easily seen in the first trimester, while a thin membrane is often not visible until the second trimester.

Intrauterine growth retardation is seen in increased frequency in twins. Individual twin growth curves are similar to those of singletons up until the early third trimester. As the third trimester progresses, increasing differences in birth weight are found between twins and singletons. Intrauterine growth in multiple gestations should be evaluated differently from in a singleton gestation. The growth status of each twin should be evaluated individually using the same sonographic parameters as for singletons: biparietal diameter, abdominal circumference, femur length and amniotic fluid volume. These findings then should be compared with prior sonograms of the same twin to assess the appropriateness of interval growth. Moreover, fetal size should be regarded as a comparison between the twins rather than to normalized standards and growth charts.

Discordant growth in twin pregnancy can be caused by fetal growth retardation of one fetus or by twin-to-twin transfusion syndrome. Birth weight discordancy is calculated as the birth weight difference divided by the weight of the heavier twin. A commonly used definition describes discordancy as a birth weight difference of greater than 20% between twins.

Twin transfusion syndrome occurs only in monozygotic twins and is caused by placental vascular anastomoses in the monochorionic placenta. Through the anastomoses, blood shunts from one twin (the donor) to the other (the recipient). This sequence results in one anemic twin and a fluid overloaded cotwin (Figures 10.13 and 10.14). The clinical presentation of twin transfusion syndrome depends on the quantity of blood transferred. The sonographic criteria suggesting the diagnosis of twin transfusion syndrome include significant disparity in size between fetuses of the same sex, especially if one twin shows evidence for asymmetric growth retardation and the other is macrosomic, disparity in size between two amniotic sacs, a single placenta, and evidence of hydrops in one fetus or congestive cardiac failure. Twin transfusion usually occurs in the second trimester. When twin transfusion syndrome is suspected, diagnosis may be confirmed by showing a hemoglobin difference of 5 mg/ml or more between blood samples from each twin.

Acardiac twin probably represents the most extreme manifestation of the twin transfusion syndrome in most cases. The acardiac twin has no direct vascular connections with the placenta. He is present without a well defined cardiac structure and is kept alive through umbilical vascular anastomoses by the viable fetus. Acardiac monsters can range in appearance from an unrecognizable mass of tissue to a fairly complete and well formed fetus. If the

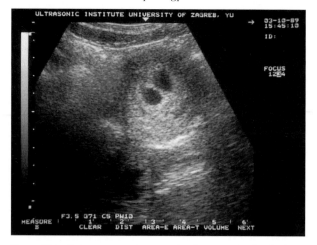

Figure 10.1 Twin pregnancy: two gestational sacs can be visualized at 6 weeks of pregnancy

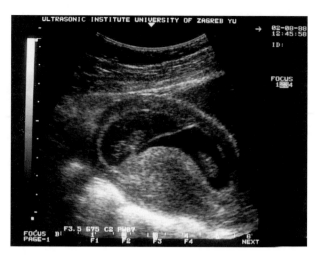

Figure 10.2 Two living embryos at 8 weeks of pregnancy

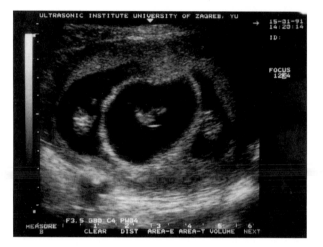

Figure 10.3 Three gestational sacs are clearly seen with three living embryos: triplets at 7 weeks of gestation

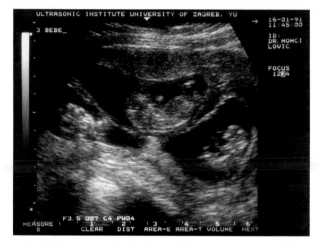

Figure 10.4 Triplets at 10 weeks of gestation: each embryo has its own gestational sac and is separated from the others by a thick membrane

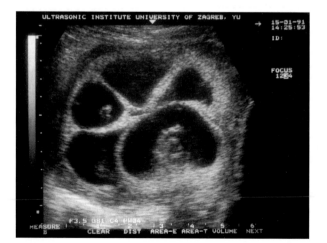

Figure 10.5 A rare case of quintuplets: five gestational sacs are displayed on this scan

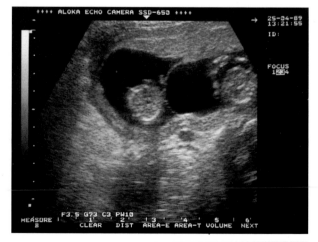

Figure 10.6 Twins at 13 menstrual weeks: fetuses are separated by a thin membrane

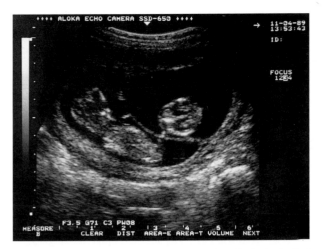

Figure 10.7 Thirteen-week-old twins: one is displayed in the longitudinal section, while the head of the other is in transverse section

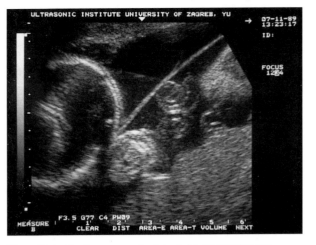

Figure 10.8 Membrane separating twins in the second trimester

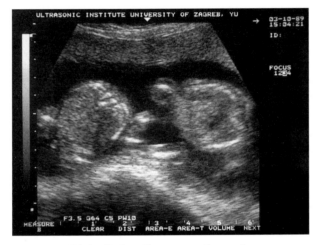

Figure 10.9 Two fetal bodies without a separating membrane

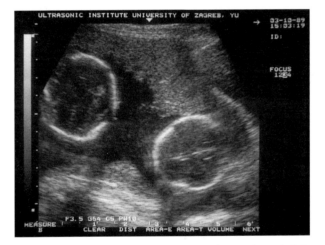

Figure 10.10 Two fetal heads without a separating membrane. In both Figures 10.9 and 10.10 there remains a risk of monoamnionicity

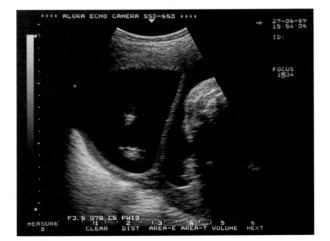

Figure 10.11 Thick membrane indicates diamniotic–dichorionic gestation

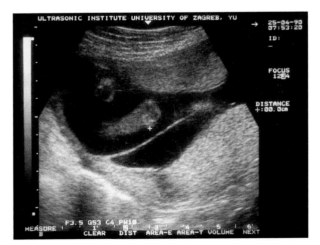

Figure 10.12 Thin membrane indicates diamniotic–monochorionic gestation

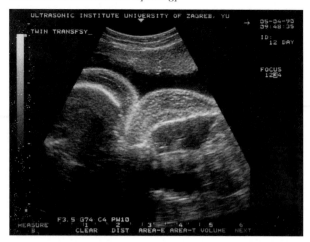

Figure 10.13 Twin transfusion syndrome: hydropic twin with scalp edema and hydrothorax

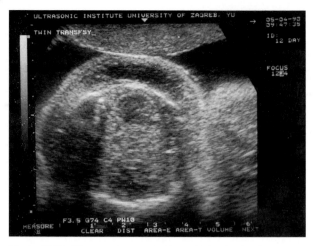

Figure 10.14 The same fetus as in Figure 10.13 showing the extreme scalp edema

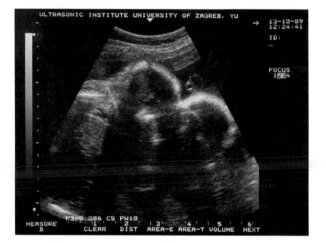

Figure 10.15 Conjoined twins: two fetal heads are abnormally close. The fetuses were fused in the thoracic region

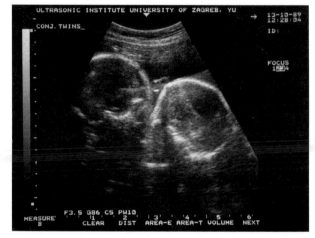

Figure 10.16 The abnormal position of the fetal heads seen in Figure 10.15 did not change on subsequent examinations. It was not possible to demonstrate separate fetal bodies

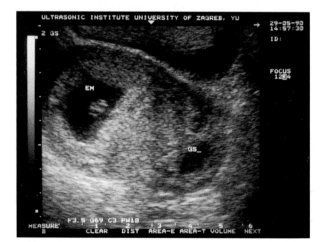

Figure 10.17 Two gestational sacs at the age of 7 menstrual weeks. One gestation sac contains a living embryo (EM), but the other is empty (GS–). The empty sac is already resolving

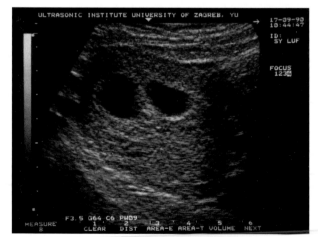

Figure 10.18 Twin blighted ova: no embryonic echo is seen in either of the sacs

vascular connection to the acardiac twin is insufficient, early in pregnancy the acardiac embryo can reabsorb. Demise later in pregnancy results in fetus papyraceus. Sonographically, an acardiac twin can be visualized as an amorphous mass of tissue with recognizable fetal parts, or as an anomalous twin who moves independently but has no heart action. Other findings include polyhydramnios, two-vessel umbilical cord, structural anomalies in the acardiac twin and evidence of cardiac failure in the normal twin.

Arrest of separation in monozygotic twins results in the development of conjoined twins (Figures 10.15 and 10.16). Although the site and extent of fusion vary markedly, conjoined twins are most commonly joined at the chest and/or abdomen and less commonly at the sacrum, ischium or head and face. Sonographic evaluation of twins must always attempt to determine whether the twins are conjoined. Visualization of a separating membrane excludes conjoined twinning. The sonographic criterion that verifies the presence of conjoined twins is a demonstration of continuous external skin contour of both monoamniotic twins. Demonstration of shared fetal organs also provides definitive evidence for conjoined twins. Other findings suggestive of conjoined twinning are constant fetal positions and unusual positioning, with hyperextension of the spine or unusual extremity posture.

Another potential complication of twin pregnancies is *in utero* demise of one of the fetuses. Twin pregnancies suffer from a high rate of single fetal loss resulting in the delivery of only one viable child. This loss is most commonly seen early in the pregnancy (Figures 10.17 and 10.18), but can occur at any time in gestation. Cotwin demise in early pregnancy results in the 'vanishing twin' phenomenon. This carries no significant risk for the surviving twin. Sonographic detection of two gestational sacs in early pregnancy with two living embryos is usually the only evidence of multiple pregnancy, since the vanished twin is usually not detected at the time of delivery.

Cotwin demise that occurs in the second trimester results in fetus papyraceus. The dead fetus has undergone flattening, atrophy and sometimes mummification. Sonographically it can be detected as a small, non-living fetus within a smaller gestational sac near the uterine wall. The surviving twin should be carefully examined for presence of anomalies that can occur secondary to embolization following death of a cotwin.

Numerous reports indicate that twins have an increased prevalence of congenital anomalies, especially monozygotic twins. Thromboembolic insults resulting from vascular anastomoses have been postulated to cause a great majority of detected anomalies. However, monozygotic twins are also at greater risk for congenital anomalies due to abnormal embryologic development. Twins are also more likely to have defects related to anomalous positioning within the uterus.

Because of the increased risk present, women with multiple pregnancies should be seen at more frequent intervals by the ultrasonographer. With the goal of improved pregnancy outcome, sonography helps to evaluate these pregnancies, improves antenatal care and helps in the choice of the optimal route of delivery.

READING LIST

1. Blickstein, I., Shoham-Schwartz, Z. and Lancet, M. (1988). Growth discordancy inappropriate for gestational age term twins. *Obstet. Gynecol.*, **72**, 582–4

2. Bronsteen, R.A., and Evans, M.I. (1989). Multiple gestation. In Evans, M.I., Fletcher, J.C., Dixler, A.O. and Schulman, J.D. (eds.) *Fetal Diagnosis and Therapy*, pp.242–65. (Philadelphia: J.B. Lippincot Co.)

3. Jaunieaux, E., Elkazen, N. and Leroy, F. (1988). Clinical and morphologic aspects of the vanishing twin phenomenon. *Obstet. Gynecol.*, **72**, 577–81

4. Kurjak, A. (1990). Abnormalities in multiple pregnancies. In Kurjak, A. (ed.) *Handbook of Ultrasound in Obstetrics and Gynecology*, pp.291–301. (Boca Raton: CRC Press)

5. Little, J. and Bryan, E. (1986). Congenital anomalies in twins. *Semin. Perinatol.*, **10**, 50

6. Sekiya, S. and Hafez, E. (1977). Physiomorphology of twin transfusion syndrome: a review of 86 twin gestations. *Obstet. Gynecol.*, **50**, 288–92

7. Townsend, R. and Filly, R.A. (1988). Sonography of nonconjoined monoamniotic twin pregnancies. *J. Ultrasound Med.*, **7**, 665–70

8. Townsend, R., Simpson, G. and Filly, R. (1988). Membrane thickness in ultrasound prediction of chorionicity of twin gestations. *J. Ultrasound Med.*, **7**, 327–32

11 Normal Anatomy and Malformations of the Placenta and Umbilical Cord

A. Kurjak and J. Zmijanac

THE UMBILICAL CORD

The umbilical cord normally contains three vessels: two arteries and one vein, surrounded by a connective tissue known as Wharton's jelly (Figures 11.1 and 11.2). Floating in the amniotic fluid, the umbilical cord can be visualized as early as 8 menstrual weeks. Initially, it is small, but it grows in diameter and length during pregnancy. At 28 weeks, it has attained its final length of 50–60 cm.

Coiling is a characteristic of the umbilical cord that is established by 9 menstrual weeks (Figures 11.3 and 11.4). More twists are present near the fetal insertion site (Figures 11.5 and 11.6).

On sonography, the intracorporeal umbilical vein can be seen to deviate from the umbilical arteries after entry through the umbilicus. On entering the liver, the umbilical vein becomes the umbilical portion of the left portal vein which turns posteriorly and is continuous with the main portal vein.

The most common anomaly of the umbilical cord is a single umbilical artery. The normal umbilical cord contains two arteries and one vein visible in transverse or longitudinal sections (Figure 11.2). A single umbilical artery can be seen in transverse sections by identifying a cord with only two vessels. The single umbilical artery is larger than normal, and can be as large as the umbilical vein. Identification of this anomaly can be difficult before the third trimester because of the small size of the umbilical cord. A false-positive diagnosis can be made when the umbilical cord is examined near the placental insertion site, since the two umbilical arteries may normally fuse at a variable distance from the placenta. Infants with a single umbilical artery are at risk for intrauterine growth retardation and have a higher prevalence of congenital anomalies. Thus, the detection of a single umbilical artery should prompt a search for associated anomalies.

Umbilical cord presentation is defined as a cord lying between the presenting part and the lower pole of the intact membranes. This situation may result in cord compression and fetal distress. The sonographic diagnosis is easily made by demonstrating loops of umbilical cord in the lower segment below the presenting part.

Nuchal cord can occasionally be demonstrated by sonography, by visualization of one or more loops of cord encircling the fetal neck (Figure 11.7).

Umbilical cord cysts can originate from remnants of either the omphalomesenteric or allantoic ductal systems. Omphalomesenteric cysts are usually small and are observed near the fetal insertion site. Allantoid cysts are also located close to the fetus. Differential diagnosis is not possible. Other umbilical anomalies that can appear cystic on sonography are focal accumulation of Wharton's jelly, resolving hematoma, dilatation of umbilical vessels, hemangiomas and angiomyxomas (Figure 11.8).

Umbilical cord hematomas usually result from needle puncture. They can appear as a hypoechogenic septated mass or an echogenic mass conforming to the umbilical cord. Hematomas may be more irregular than other cystic lesions.

Hemangioma of a cord is a tumor arising from the endothelial cells of the vessels of the umbilical cord. It appears as a hyperechogenic mass. Localized edema of the umbilical cord can also be present.

THE PLACENTA

The chorion frondosum can be identified on sonography as early as 8 menstrual weeks (Figure 11.9). Between 8 and 20 weeks the placenta appears homogeneous and uniform in thickness, measuring 2–3 cm. After 20 weeks, intraplacental echo-free areas and placental calcifications may begin to appear.

Differential growth of the lower uterine segment is responsible for the impression of placental ascension during pregnancy. Many low-lying placentas or suspected partial previas improve due to this process.

Between placenta and myometrium lies a subplacental venous complex that can sometimes

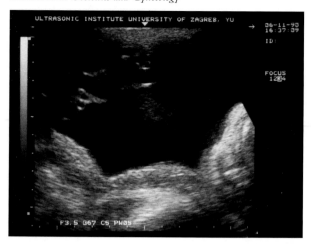

Figure 11.1 Scan of the umbilical cord displaying two arteries and one vein

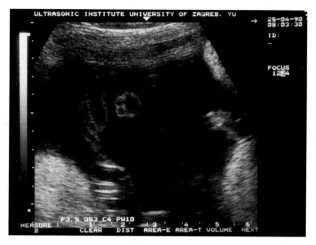

Figure 11.2 Transverse scan of umbilical cord on the right side shows two arteries and one vein. On the left side the umbilical cord is displayed in the longitudinal section

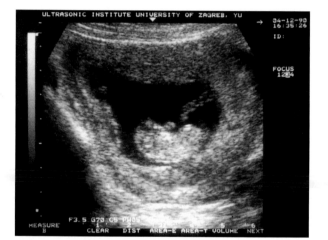

Figure 11.3 Scan at 9 menstrual weeks shows the umbilical cord attaching the embryo with the developing placenta or chorion frondosum

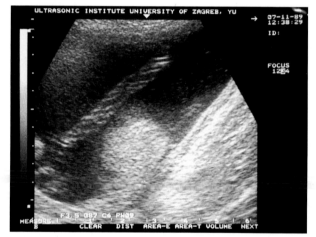

Figure 11.4 Umbilical cord at 20 weeks showing typical spiral pattern of umbilical vessels

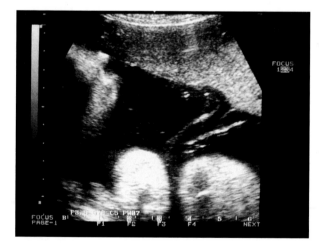

Figure 11.5 Placental cord insertion in a case of anterior placenta

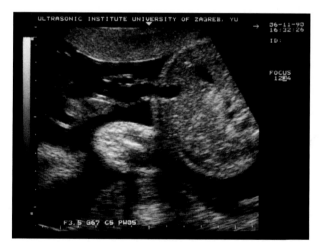

Figure 11.6 Cord insertion showing vessels traced into the fetal abdomen

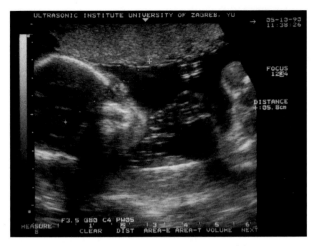

Figure 11.7 Nuchal cord: umbilical cord loop is encircling fetal neck

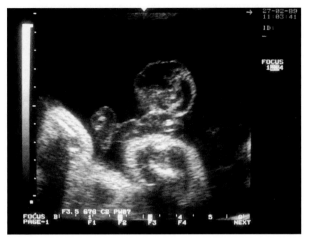

Figure 11.8 Angiomyxoma of the umbilical cord

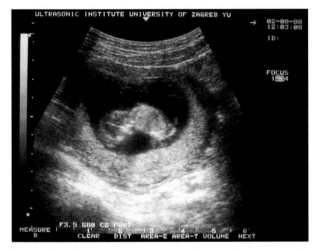

Figure 11.9 Placenta at the end of the first trimester of pregnancy. At this stage, it appears as an echogenic, falciform, soft tissue mass occupying a large part of the uterine wall. In this case, it is situated on the posterior uterine wall

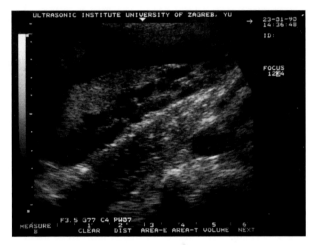

Figure 11.10 Prominent subplacental venous complex in posterior placenta

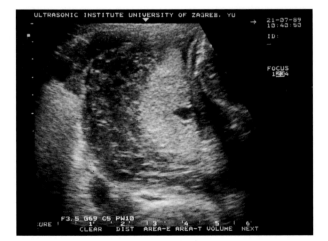

Figure 11.11 Another example of prominent subplacental venous complex. In this case the placenta is lateral, and the venous complex should not be mistaken for retroplacental or marginal hemorrhage

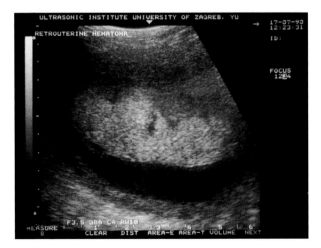

Figure 11.12 Retroplacental hematoma: large extramembranous clot is occupying most of the posterior uterine wall

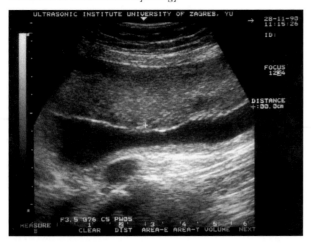

Figure 11.13 Homogeneous placenta with no densities within the placental substance. The chorionic plate is straight and well defined: Grannum grade 0

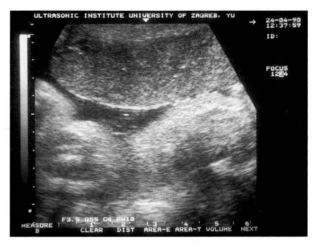

Figure 11.14 Anterior placenta with small areas of echogenic densities randomly dispersed in the placental tissue: Grannum grade I

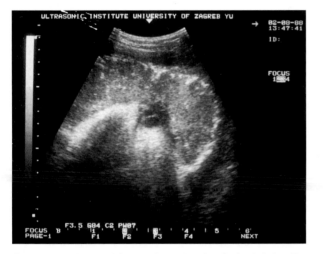

Figure 11.15 Anterior placenta with prominent basal echogenic densities and comma-like densities extending from the chorionic plate: Grannum grade II

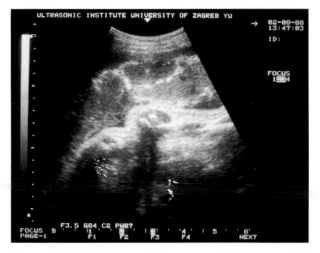

Figure 11.16 Calcified intercotyledonary septa in Grannum grade III placenta

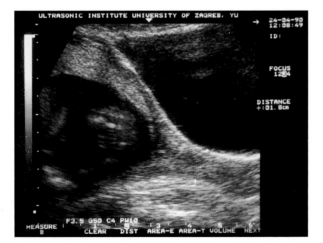

Figure 11.17 Marginal placenta previa: the lower placental margin extends to the internal cervical os

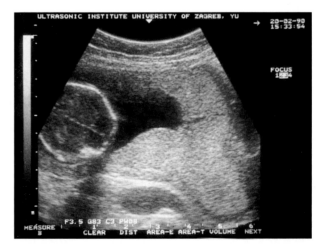

Figure 11.18 Total (complete) placenta previa: the placenta covers the entire internal os

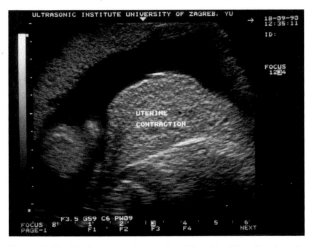

Figure 11.19 Uterine contraction can be distinguished from the placenta because of its different shape and echogenicity

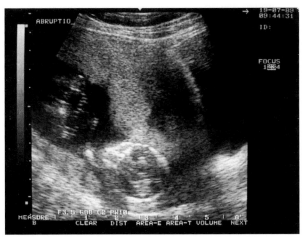

Figure 11.20 Abruptio placentae with a hematoma appearing as an anechoic area on the anterior uterine wall

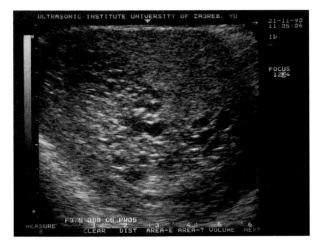

Figure 11.21 Hydatidiform mole: characteristic vesicular changes can be demonstrated throughout the placenta

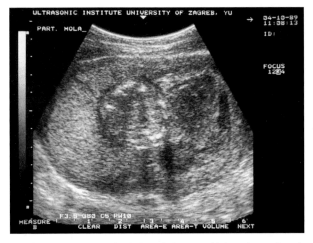

Figure 11.22 Partial mole: thickened placenta with intraplacental cystic areas and calcifications

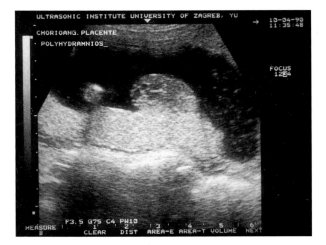

Figure 11.23 Chorioangioma placentae appears as a cystic or solid tumor arising from placental tissue. It is accompanied by polyhydramnios

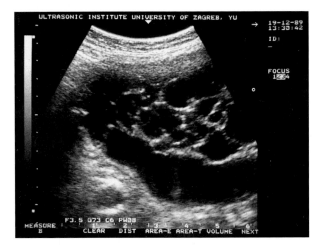

Figure 11.24 Large, predominantly cystic chorioangioma placentae

become quite prominent (Figures 11.10 and 11.11). These prominent veins should not be mistaken for retroplacental (Figure 11.12) or marginal hemorrhage.

Placental maturation can be divided into grades based on the pattern of calcification. According to Granum *et al.*, grade 0 is a homogeneous placenta (Figure 11.13); grade I shows small intraplacental calcifications (Figure 11.14); grade II shows calcifications of the basilar plate (Figure 11.15); and grade III shows compartmentalization of the placenta from the chorionic plate to the basal layer (Figure 11.16). Grade 0 is most common in the first trimester, Grade I may appear as early as 14 weeks and is most common until 34 weeks and grade II usually appears after 30 weeks and peaks at 36 weeks. Grade III is usually seen after 35 weeks.

Abnormally thickened placenta (placentomegaly) may be associated with maternal diabetes, anemia, Rhesus sensitization, chronic intrauterine infections, twin transfusion syndrome, or congenital neoplasms. An abnormally small placenta may be associated with intrauterine growth retardation, infection or chromosome abnormalities.

Placenta previa can be total (placental tissue completely covering the internal cervical os) or marginal (Figures 11.17 and 11.18). Partial (marginal) previa is suggested when the lower placental margin appears to extend to, but not across the internal cervical os. An overly distended urinary bladder and focal uterine contractions are the two most common technical factors responsible for false-positive diagnoses of placenta previa (Figure 11.19). Rescanning after partial voiding or after a 30-min delay will usually resolve normal anatomic relationships.

Succenturiate placenta can be suspected when a discrete lobe separate from the body of the placenta is demonstrated by ultrasound. Occasionally a vascular band connecting the lobes can be seen within the amniotic fluid.

Placental abruption can be demonstrated by visualization of a hemorrhage produced by the placental detachment (Figure 11.20). Sonographic appearance of periplacental hemorrhage depends on the time at which the ultrasound examination is performed. Acute hemorrhage is hyperechoic to the placenta, whereas older hemorrhage (more than 2 weeks) is almost sonolucent. Occasionally, a retroplacental abruption can be seen as a well-defined hematoma located between the placenta and uterus. Marginal hemorrhage is the most common site of placental abruption. The hematoma can mimic other mass lesions like myoma, succenturiate lobe, chorioangioma, or molar pregnancy.

Trophoblastic disease can be manifested as complete mole, partial mole, or coexistent mole and fetus. Invasive mole and metastatic trophoblastic disease can be regarded as subgroups of complete mole. Simple hydropic degeneration should be distinguished from trophoblastic disease.

The sonographic appearance of complete mole varies with gestational age. In the first trimester, it can be mistaken for an incomplete abortion. After that period, characteristic vesicular changes can be demonstrated (Figure 11.21).

Partial mole may be visualized as thickened placenta with intraplacental cystic areas, accompanied by oligohydramnios (Figure 11.22). A living fetus may be present.

A coexisting mole is more likely when more than one placenta is identified, whereas partial mole is more likely with fetal demise, or fetal anomalies. Sonographic findings include an enlarged, hyperechoic placenta with multiple small cysts, and a coexisting living embryo.

Chorioangioma is the most common tumor of the placenta (Figures 11.23 and 11.24). Other tumors, such as teratomas or metastatic neoplasms are exceedingly rare. Sonographically, they are seen as solid, hyperechoic or hypoechoic, circumscribed masses that often protrude from the fetal surface of the placenta. Polyhydramnios is present in one-third of cases. Fetal hydrops can also be associated with large tumors involving the placenta or umbilical cord.

READING LIST

1. Brown, H.L., Miller, J.M., Khawli, O. *et al.* (1988). Premature placental calcifications in maternal cigarette smokers. *Obstet. Gynecol.*, **71**, 914–17

2. Fortune, D.W. and Ostor, A.G. (1980). Angiomyxomas of the umbilical cord. *Obstet. Gynecol.*, **55**, 375–81

3. Gallagher, P., Fagan, C.J., Bedi, D.G. *et al.* (1987). Potential placenta previa: definition, frequency and significance. *Am. J. Radiol.*, **149**, 1013–15

4. Herrman, U.J. and Sidropoulos, D. (1988). Single umbilical artery: prenatal findings. *Prenat. Diagn.*, **8**, 275–80

5. Hertzberg, B.J., Bowie, J.D., Bradford, W.D. *et al.* (1988). False knot of the umbilical cord: sonographic appearance and differential diagnosis. *J. Clin. Ultrasound*, **16**, 599–602

6. Hill, L.M., Kislak, S. and Runco, C. (1987). An ultrasonic view of the umbilical cord. *Obstet. Gynecol. Surv.*, **42**, 82–8

7. Nyberg, D.A. and Finberg, H.J. (1990). The

placenta, placental membranes and umbilical cord. In Nyberg, D.A., Mahony, B.S. and Pretorius, D.H. (eds.) *Diagnostic Ultrasound of Fetal Anomalies. Text and Atlas*, pp.623–75. (Chicago: Year Book Medical Publishers Inc.)

8. Nyberg, D.A., Mack, L.A., Benedetti, T.J. *et al.* (1987). Placental abruption and placental hemorrhage: correlation of sonographic findings with fetal outcome. *Radiology*, **164**, 357–61

9. Rempen, A. (1989). Sonographic first trimester diagnosis of umbilical cord cyst. *J. Clin. Ultrasound*, **17**, 53–5

10. Romero, R., Pilu, G., Jeanty, P., Ghidini, A. and Hobbins, J.C. (1988). *Prenatal Diagnosis of Congenital Anomalies*. (Norwalk: Appleton & Lange)

12 Ultrasound Investigations of Placental and Cord Morphology

E. Jauniaux, D. Jurković, A. Kurjak and S. Campbell

INTRODUCTION

The improvement of ultrasound equipment and the advent of color imaging enable us to explore the placenta and the cord morphology in detail before delivery. The correlation of *in vivo* and *in vitro* features is a fundamental step for a better comprehension of the pathophysiology of the different placental and cord abnormalities. The sonographic diagnosis of these abnormalities is reviewed in this chapter as well as their possible clinical significance.

NORMAL PLACENTAL DEVELOPMENT

The placental size and its echogenicity increase progressively as pregnancy advances.

Placental maturation and grading

Grannum *et al.*[1] have proposed a sonographic classification system for grading placentas *in utero* according to maturational changes. The placentas were graded from 0 to III on the basis of compound B-scan changes in the placental structures (Figure 12.1A–12.1D). The sonographic features were correlated with fetal pulmonary maturity evaluated by amniotic fluid lecithin to sphingomyelin (L/S) ratios and mature L/S ratios were found in 100% of Grade III placentas. Several authors did not confirm these findings and subsequent reports have shown that a grade III placenta was associated with an immature L/S ratio in 8–42% of the cases and this method was therefore not accurate enough to replace amniocentesis in predicting fetal pulmonary maturity[2].

The grading system may be useful as a predictive indicator of potential perinatal problems later in pregnancy. A very well conducted, randomized, controlled trial has demonstrated that pregnant women presenting with mature placental sonographic features (grade III) between 34 and 36 weeks' gestation have an increased risk of problems during labor and their babies have an increased risk of low birth weight, intrapartum distress and perinatal death[3].

Placental size

Determination of the placental size is part of the overall assessment of the intrauterine environment. Placental growth can be estimated by measuring the placental thickness or by estimation of the placental volume.

The placental thickness is not diagnostic of any particular condition but can contribute to the management of a fetus at risk[4]. Thick placentas (> 4 cm) can be an early sign of developing fetal hydrops (Figure 12.2A and 12.2B) and can also be found in pregnancies with elevated midtrimester maternal serum α-fetoprotein and an anatomically normal fetus (Figures 12.3A–12.3F).

Sonographic methods for determination of the placental volume are usually complex and time consuming in routine. The development of new computerized systems, integrated within ultrasound equipment such as three-dimensional sonography, may open new perspectives in this particular field of placental investigation.

Doppler ultrasound investigation of placental circulations

The use of color Doppler ultrasound techniques combined with high-resolution sonography offers a novel approach for the investigation of human placental circulations very early in pregnancy[5–7]. It is now possible to image and to investigate small vessels within placental tissue from 16 weeks of gestation (Figures 12.4 and 12.5). Small branches of both uterine and umbilical arteries are clearly visualized with the color mode and identification of terminal

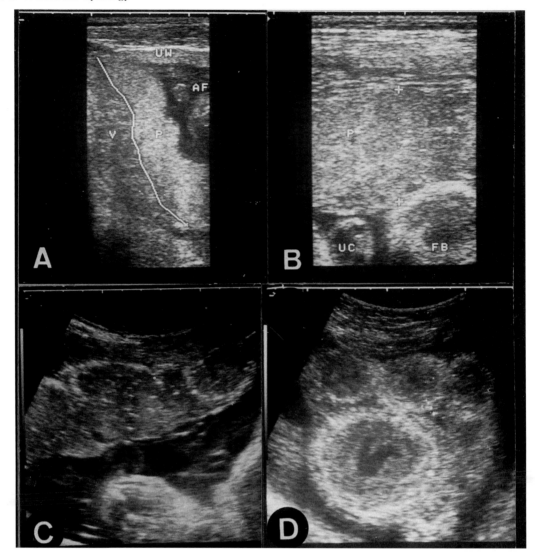

Figure 12.1 Composite compound scan of the four placental grades. (**A**) grade 0 at 14 weeks of gestation; V, vessels (uteroplacental); UW, uterine wall; P, placenta; AF, amniotic fluid; (**B**) grade I at 30 weeks of gestation; P, placenta; UC, umbilical cord; FB, fetal body; (**C**) grade II, partially grade III at 38 weeks of gestation; and (**D**) premature grade III at 32 weeks in a pregnancy complicated by chronic hypertension

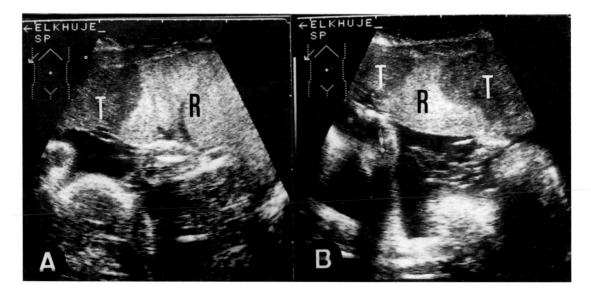

Figure 12.2 Transverse and longitudinal scans of the placenta in a monochorionic–diamniotic twin pregnancy at 30 weeks, complicated by a twin-transfusion syndrome. The hemiplacenta corresponding to the recipient (R) or perfused twin is thicker and hyperechoic compared to the edematous placental area corresponding to the transfuser (T) or donor

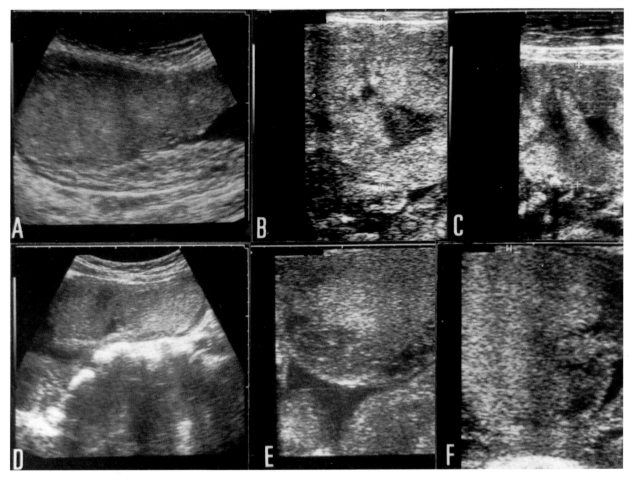

Figure 12.3   Sonograms at 20 weeks of gestation showing large placentas 'jelly-like placentas' in pregnancies complicated by increased levels of maternal serum α-fetoprotein without associated fetal anomalies. The placentas are > 4 cm in thickness, present with patchy decreased echogenicity (**A,D**) and large sonolucent spaces (**B,E**) containing turbulent blood flows (**C,F**)

branches of the uteroplacental vessels (Figure 12.6), intervillous blood flow (Figure 12.7), chorionic vessels (Figure 12.8) and intraplacental fetal arterioles (Figure 12.9) can be easily performed[5,6].

The overall structure of placental vasculature as shown *in vivo* with color imaging and spectral analysis correlates well with the classical anatomic features[8]. The waveforms obtained from both fetal and maternal sides of the placental circulation show a significant decrease in flow resistance towards the placental mass[6] which has been suggested by different mathematical models[9].

MAJOR PLACENTAL ABNORMALITIES

Many inaccurate and misleading expressions have been used by ultrasonographers to describe placental lesions. This is probably due to the fact that little attempt has been made to compare ultrasound and pathologic findings. Until a better terminology can

be proposed we will refer to the classical pathologic terminology[8] to categorize these lesions. Table 12.1 summarizes the dynamic sonographic features and the perinatal complications associated with the main placental abnormalities. More details are available in pathologic textbooks and in recent literature reviews.

We have recently proposed a classification of the different placental sonographic features (Table 12.2 and Figures 12.10–12.15) and we would like to highlight the following points.

(1)   Depending on the delay between the development of a lesion *in utero* and delivery, both the sonographic and the pathologic findings can be very different. The ultrasound features of most placental vascular lesions may undergo major changes within a few days. When a placental abnormality which could be associated with perinatal complications is suspected, serial sonographic examinations should be performed[2].

Table 12.1 Pathologic classification and sonographic features of the principal placental abnormalities

Pathologic classification	Sonographic features	Location	Associated complications ★
Vascular lesions			
Thrombosis	Sonolucent → Hyperechoic turbulent blood flow	Intervillous or subchorial	Materno–fetal blood incompatibility
Infarcts irregular shape	Hyperechoic → Isoechoic	Maternal plate	Chronic hypertension and/or PIH and/or IUGR
Hematomas	Hyperechoic → Hypoechoic → sonolucent	Subamniotic, retroplacental	PIH
Fibrin	Hyperechoic	Diffuse	IUGR
Non-trophoblastic tumors			
Chorioangioma	Hypoechoic → Hyperechoic, round and encapsulated	Fetal plate or intraplacental	Polyhydramnios and/or NIHF-IUGR
Mesenchymal hyperplasia	Multiple small hypoechoic spaces often containing blood flow	Diffuse	Giant placenta
Trophoblastic tumors			
Classical mole	Snowstorm appearance no fetus	Diffuse	Vaginal bleeding and/or severe vomiting and/or PIH and/or ovarian cyst
Triploidy	Swiss cheese appearance	Diffuse	IUGR and/or poly- or oligo-hydramnios, fetus abnormal, PIH, vaginal bleeding
Abnormalities of placentation			
Placenta circumvallate	Mammelonnated fetal plate marginal hematoma	Placental margin	PROM and/or premature labor Vaginal bleeding
Placenta accreta	No placental–uterine interface	Maternal plate	Post or antepartum bleeding Uterine rupture
Placenta membranacea	Uterine cavity covered with placental tissue	Continuous placental mass always previa	Vaginal bleeding Premature labor

★ IUGR, intrauterine growth retardation; PROM, premature rupture of membranes; PIH, pregnancy-induced hypertension; and NIHF, non-immune hydrops fetalis

(2) Placental sonographic examination must be combined with other prenatal investigations some of which may help in the differential diagnosis. For example, elevated maternal serum levels of human chorionic gonadotropin are suggestive of trophoblastic disorders while elevated α-fetoprotein levels are less specific of a typical placental lesion, but indicate a breakdown of the maternal barrier such as may occur in infarcts or thromboses[2,4,10]. Indeed, a large range of placental and also cord abnormalities are associated with elevated maternal serum α-fetoprotein and are potentially diagnosable by routine sonographic examination at the time of α-fetoprotein screening[4].

(3) Knowledge of the expected fetal or placental waveform characteristics may help the differential diagnosis between placental and other intrauterine abnormalities[6,10,11]. For

Table 12.2 Differential diagnosis of the principle placental sonographic features (reproduced from ref. 2 with permission)

Location	Sonographic features	Pathologic classification
Fetal plate	Multiple sonolucent areas limited to the placental periphery (Figure 12.10A)	Circumvallate placentas Circummarginate placentas
	Single sonolucent or hypoechoic area surrounded by a thin membrane	Subamniotic cysts Old subamniotic hematomas
(Figures 12.10C and 12.10F)	Single hyperechoic area surrounded by a thin membrane (Figure 12.10E)	Recent subamniotic hematoma
	Heterogeneous mass protruding into the amniotic cavity (Figure 12.11A)	Chorioangiomas
Placental tissue	Small sonolucent area in the center of the cotyledon (Figure 12.12A)	Centrocotyledonary cavity
	Large sonolucent area (Figures 12.12A and 12.13)	Large avillous zone (cavern) Septal cysts Early stage of thrombosis formation
	Large hyperechoic area (Figures 12.12C and 12.12E)	Old thrombosis Infarcts
	Multiple sonolucent areas of various sizes and shapes (Figure 12.14)	Hydatidiform transformations
Maternal plate	Large hyperechoic area	Recent retroplacental hematoma
	Large hypoechoic area (Figure 12.15)	Old retroplacental hematoma

Table 12.3 Comparison of the prenatal sonographic features and the postnatal findings in a series of 80 cases of single umbilical artery (modified from ref. 13)

	Prenatal sonographic findings		Postnatal findings	
Number of fetuses with associated malformation(s)	21	(26.6%)	34	(42.5%)
Total IUGR★	28.3%		36.4%	
Isolated IUGR	15%		20%	
Distribution of the different associated fetal malformations				
Musculoskeletal system	15	(28.8%)	32	(32%)
Urogenital system	11	(21.1%)	20	(20%)
Gastrointestinal system	3	(5.8%)	11	(11%)
Central nervous system	12	(23.1%)	11	(11%)
Integument	3	(5.8%)	9	(9%)
Cardiovascular system	4	(7.7%)	8	(8%)
Respiratory system	4	(7.7%)	6	(6%)
Miscellaneous	0	(0%)	3	(3%)
Total	52	(100%)	100	(100%)

★ IUGR, intrauterine growth retardation

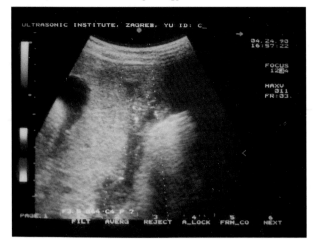

Figure 12.4 Color flow mapping of the placental bed at 18 weeks gestation

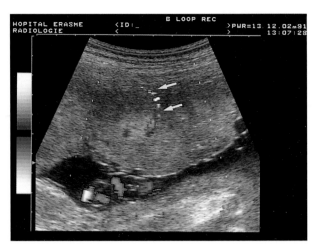

Figure 12.5 Color flow mapping of the placenta and umbilical cord at 32 weeks gestation showing the terminal part of a uteroplacental vessel (arrows)

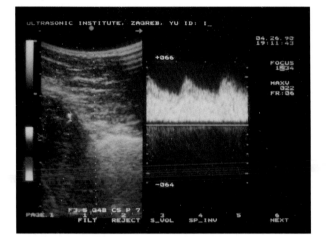

Figure 12.6 Color flow mapping and flow velocity waveforms of a radial artery at 28 weeks gestation

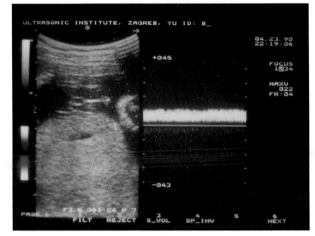

Figure 12.7 Color flow mapping and flow velocity waveforms obtained from the intervillous circulation under the fetal plate at 24 weeks gestation

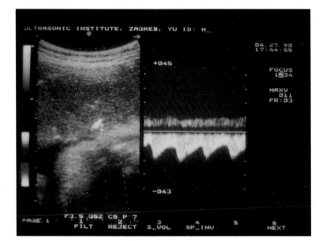

Figure 12.8 Color flow mapping and flow velocity waveforms of a chorionic artery at 36 weeks gestation

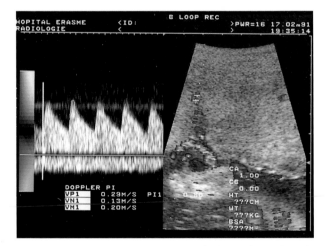

Figure 12.9 Color flow mapping and flow velocity waveforms of a main (stem) villous artery at 29 weeks' gestation

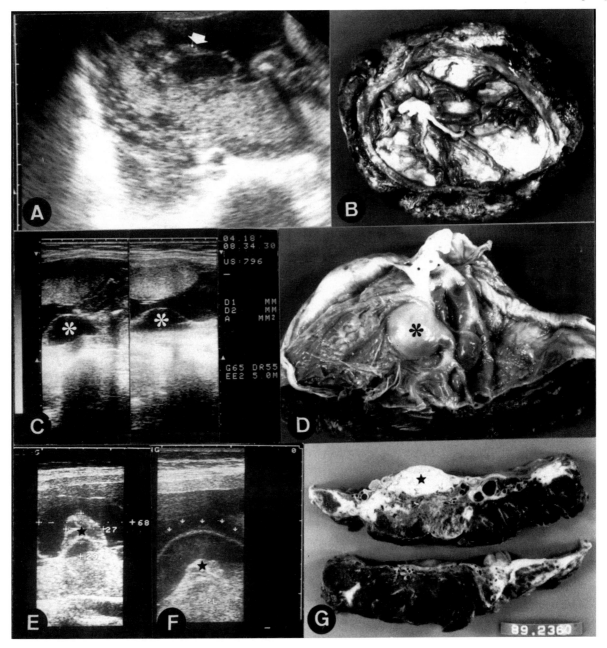

Figure 12.10 (**A**) Transverse scan at 20 weeks of gestation of the marginal zone of the placenta, showing sonolucent areas over the fetal plate (arrows). These abnormalities were found only near the placental edge. (**B**) Pathologic examination demonstrated a circumvallate placenta. (**C**) Transverse and longitudinal scans of a single sonolucent subamniotic area (*) at 32 weeks corresponding to (**D**) a subamniotic cyst (*). (**E**) and (**F**) Longitudinal sonograms at 24 and 32 weeks, respectively, showing hyperechogenic placental lesions on the top of the fetal plate (stars), surrounded by a thin membrane (arrows). The lesion becomes less echogenic as the clot resolves. Pathologic examination revealed an old subamniotic hematoma (star). (Reproduced from ref. 2 with permission)

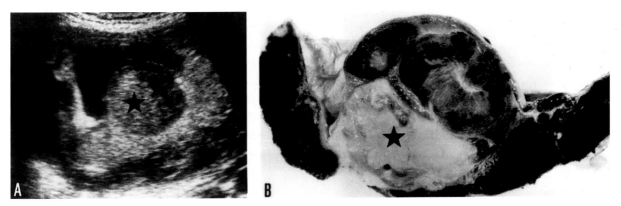

Figure 12.11 (**A**) Heterogeneous placental mass at 30 weeks, protruding from the fetal plate near the cord insertion. Half of the lesion was more echogenic (star). (**B**) At delivery the lesion corresponded to a large chorioangioma partly grooved by bands of fibrous tissue (star)

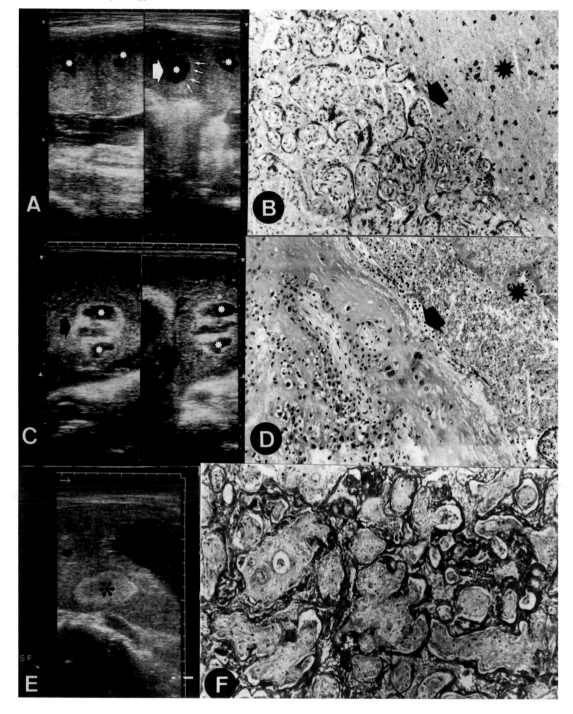

Figure 12.12 (**A**) Sonograms at 35 weeks, showing small and large placental sonolucent spaces (*), containing turbulent blood flow. Note the increased echogenicity of the surrounding villi (small arrows). (**B**) Histological section (H&E x 50) at the level of the large arrow showing a recent intervillous thrombosis (*) and normal villi (arrow). The villi surrounding the lesion at the level of the small arrows were compressed and infarcted. (**C**) Sonograms at 39 weeks showing a large placental lesion (*) corresponding, (**D**) to an organized intervillous thrombosis (*) with extensive fibrin desposition (large arrows) in periphery (H&E x 50). (**E**) Large placental hyperechoic area (*) located near the basal plate at 32 weeks of gestation corresponding, (**F**) to a chronic infarct (H&E x 50). (Reproduced from ref. 2 with permission)

example, in cases of undetermined placental mass, demonstration of fetal waveforms strongly suggests chorioangioma, whereas maternal waveforms favor the diagnosis of uterine myoma[6]. Furthermore, the association of abnormal placental features with abnormal Doppler indices will clarify the hemodynamic changes occurring in these cases[12].

MAJOR CORD ABNORMALITIES

In transverse sonographic sections the arteries and umbilical vein appear as three separately circular lucencies while in longitudinal sections, a portion of the cord will be seen as a series of parallel lines or as a central vein with the two arteries looping around it (Figures 12.16 and 12.17).

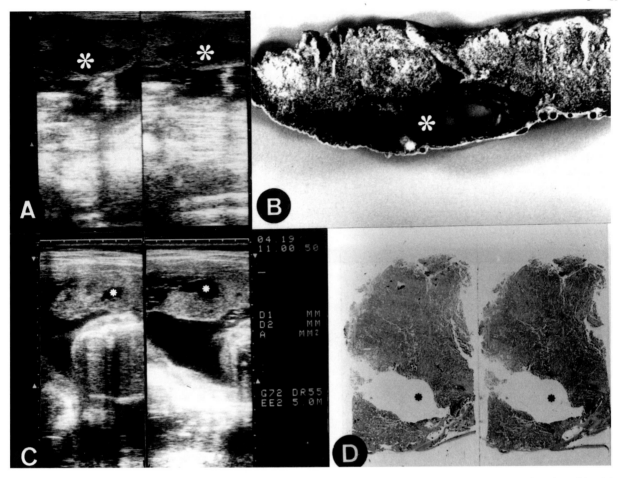

Figure 12.13 (A) Longitudinal sonograms at 27 weeks of gestation of a large sonolucent space (*). The shape of the lesion and the echogenicity of the surrounding placental tissue remain unchanged until delivery. (B) Macroscopic view of the lesion (*) at term. Transverse sonograms of a large sonolucent space (*) at 37 weeks of gestation. (C) Histological sections of the lesion showing a large avillous area (*) surrounded by normal placental tissue

The umbilical cord anatomy can often be visualized around 20 weeks gestation by gray-scale imaging but a precise diagnosis of a particular cord abnormality may be difficult and time consuming. At the end of the second trimester or during the third trimester of pregnancy the umbilical cord anatomy can be examined in detail without difficulty (Figure 12.16). However, various factors such as a oligohydramnios or multiple loops in the cord can make accurate visualization of the cord vessels impossible, even near term. High resolution color Doppler imaging has an important role in early and accurate diagnosis of cord abnormalities and is also of clinical value in viewing invasive procedures such as amniocentesis or cordocentesis (Figures 12.18 and 12.19).

Abnormal vessel numbers

The absence of one umbilical artery is amongst the most common congenital fetal malformations with an incidence of approximately 1% of all deliveries[13]. Fetal major anatomic defects are largely responsible for the high fetal and neonatal loss from this pathology[13]. Fetal malformations are present in about 50% of the cases of single umbilical artery and can affect any organ system. The incidence of intrauterine growth retardation is significantly elevated among fetuses with a single umbilical artery and may be present without other congenital anomalies in 15–20% of the cases[13]. Table 12.3 summarizes the retrospective results of the comparison of sonographic and postnatal findings in 80 cases of single umbilical artery syndrome. In this context, minor malformations of the musculoskeletal system or of the genitourinary tract are often misdiagnosed by ultrasonography, in particular, when they are isolated. Color Doppler imaging (Figure 12.20) has an important role in early and accurate diagnosis of single umbilical artery[14].

During the second month of fetal development, the right umbilical vein regresses and the left umbilical vein and the two umbilical arteries become the vessels found in the normal cord. The persistence of a right umbilical vein is an uncommon finding which can be associated with numerous and occasionally lethal fetal malformations[15]. This cord abnormality is easily recognized during the second trimester and is an indicator for more depth scanning.

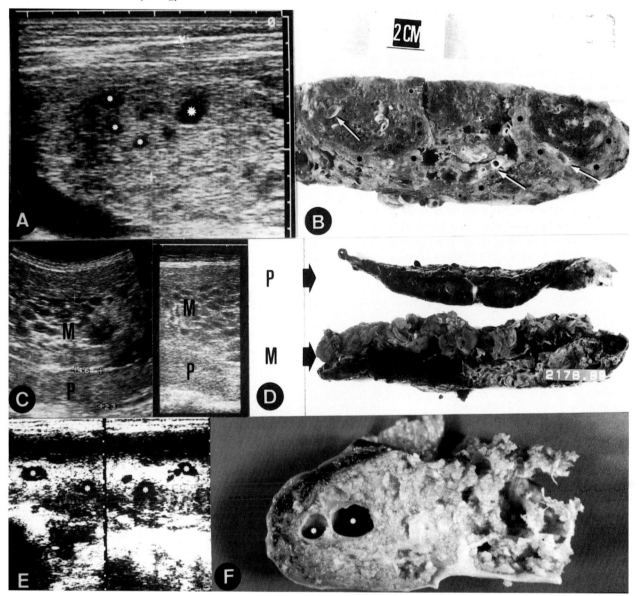

Figure 12.14 (**A**) Longitudinal sonogram at 22 weeks of gestation showing enlarged placenta containing multiple sonolucent spaces (*). The fetus was anatomically normal. (**B**) Pathologic examination demonstrated diffuse mesenchymal hyperplasia with myxoid degeneration of the stem villi and dilatation of the main fetal vessels (arrows). (**C**) Sonogram at 25 weeks of a molar mass (M) and a normal placenta (P) in a twin pregnancy combining a classical mole and a normal placenta and fetus. (**D**) Pathologic examination confirmed the presence of a normal placenta (P) and a complete mole (M). (**E**) Transverse sonograms of an enlarged placenta containing multiple sonolucent spaces of various sizes and shapes (*). The pregnancy was complicated by severe asymmetrical fetal growth retardation, oligohydramnios and early pregnancy-induced hypertension. (**F**) Pathologic investigation revealed a triploid syndrome with focal swelling of the villous tissue (*). (Reproduced from ref. 2 with permission)

Abnormalities of the cord position and insertion

Prolapse of the umbilical cord is an obstetrical emergency characterized by protrusion of the umbilical cord through the cervix into the vagina[16]. Cord prolapses are more likely to occur in premature pregnancies, or in pregnancies with a long umbilical cord, with the presenting part unengaged or in those complicated by polyhydramnios. Looping of the cord may occur around the fetal neck, body or shoulder and is an uncommon cause of fetal death, however, in monoamniotic twins a significant proportion of the high mortality can be attributed to umbilical cord problems[16]. Color Doppler imaging can easily

demonstrate the cord location early in pregnancy (Figures 12.21 and 12.22).

Velamentous insertion of the cord or placenta velamentosa is a well defined pathologic entity with a frequency around 1% of pregnancies[8]. The relation between this abnormal cord insertion and associated developmental defects is a matter of some debate[8]. From a clinical point of view, attachment of the cord to the extraplacental membranes is important because of the risk of severe fetal hemorrhage during labor. Antenatal diagnosis of attachment of the cord to the membranes rather than the placental mass can be also easily performed before labor by means of color Doppler imaging[17,18].

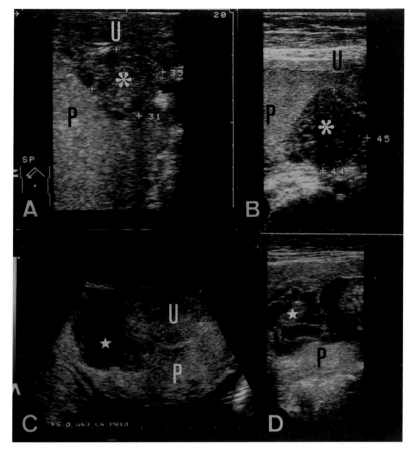

Figure 12.15 Composite compound scan of the uterus (U) and the placenta (P) showing a heterogeneous and hypoechoic placental lesion (*), at 17 (**A**) and 22 (**B**) weeks gestation corresponding to a thrombosis. For comparison, (**C**) a retroplacental hematoma (star) at 32 weeks, 2 weeks after an invasive procedure and (**D**) a recent marginal hematoma (star) at 18 weeks. (Reproduced from ref. 10 with permission)

Cord tumors and other abnormalities

Umbilical cord tumors are infrequent postnatal findings. From a pathologic point of view, primary cord tumors can be divided into angiomyxomas or hemangiomas derived from embryonic vessels, teratomas derived from germ cells, and vestigial cysts derived from remnants of the allantois or of the omphalomesenteric duct[8]. Raised maternal serum α-fetoprotein can be the earliest prenatal clue to the development of a cord tumor[4,19].

A cord angiomyxoma appears sonographically as a heterogeneous mass made up of a strong echogenic area (Figure 12.23), embedding the umbilical vessels (Figures 12.24 and 12.25) and surrounded by large echo-poor areas[4,16,19]. The prenatal diagnosis of a cord teratoma has never been reported but this type of tumor should be mainly composed of dense tissue[8]. Conversely, vestigial cysts appear sonographically as a single fluid-filled mass (Figure 12.26). Vestigial cysts and pseudocysts can sometimes be associated with small abdominal wall defects and a precise early prenatal diagnosis can be more difficult to establish[20,21].

Several conditions causing simple or complex multicystic masses of the cord can mimic a cord tumor on gray-scale imaging. These conditions include cord hematomas, ectasia of the umbilical vein, pseudocysts (Figure 12.27) and true knots[16,21]. Vestigial cysts and pseudocysts having similar sonographic features it is not possible to differentiate them *in utero*.

Cord hematomas are rare antenatal findings and are usually located near the fetal umbilicus[8]. Mechanical trauma of the cord such as prolapse, torsion, strangulation, dissecting aneurysm or accidental laceration of umbilical cord vessels during an invasive procedure are all potential causes of cord hematoma. These hematomas have a similar sonographic evolution as placental hematomas (hyperechoic in early stage with subsequent decrease of echogenicity). Thrombosis of an umbilical vessel may also be secondary to localized increased resistance in the umbilical circulation in cases of torsion, compression, or knotting of the hematoma[8]. Intense echogenic material within the lumen of the umbilical vessels is the main sonographic finding[16].

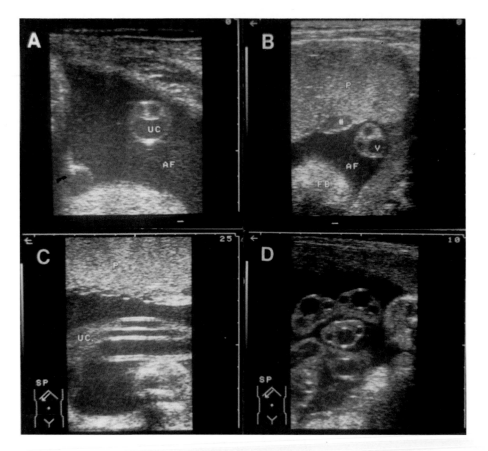

Figure 12.16 Transverse and longitudinal scans at 28–32 weeks of gestation showing the normal anatomy of the umbilical cord (UC) with two arteries and one vein (V); P, placenta; AF, amniotic fluid; FB, fetal body

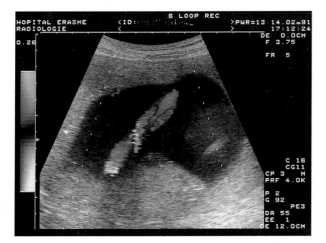

Figure 12.17 Color flow mapping of the umbilical cord at 20 weeks of gestation

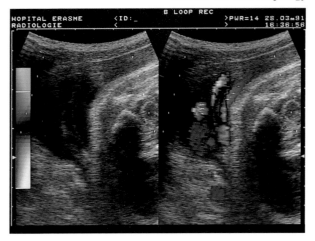

Figure 12.18 Free umbilical cord loops at 22 weeks of gestation clearly visualized by means of color Doppler imaging

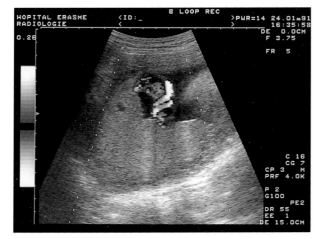

Figure 12.19 Color flow mapping of the placental insertion of the umbilical cord

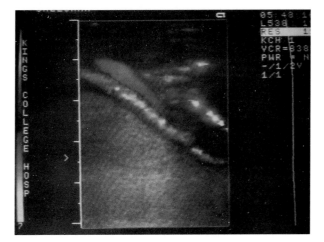

Figure 12.20 Color flow image of single umbilical artery cord (placental insertion) at 18 weeks, associated with multiple fetal malformations and oligohydramnios. (Reproduced from ref. 14 with permission)

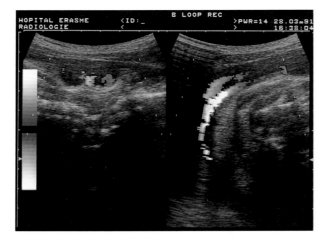

Figure 12.21 Longitudinal and transverse sonograms at 30 weeks showing cord loops around the fetal neck

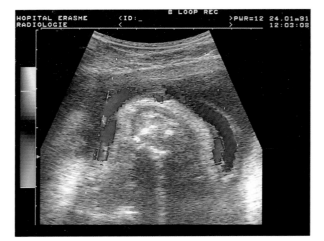

Figure 12.22 Color flow mapping at 36 weeks showing cord loops surrounding the fetal neck

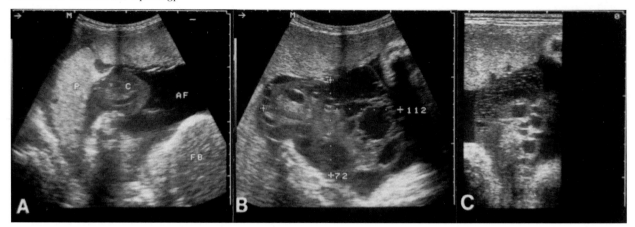

Figure 12.23 Heterogeneous multicystic mass of the cord involving the entire length of the cord at 36 weeks of gestation. The lesion is made of hyperechoic zones (**A**) surrounded by hypoechoic areas (**B**) and (**C**) and corresponds to an angiomyxoma of the cord

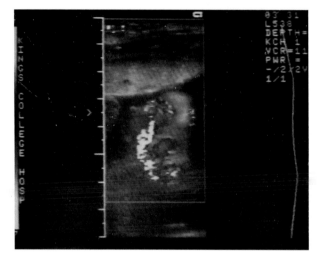

Figure 12.24 Color flow image of the cord tumor described in Figure 12.23, showing an abnormal vascular pattern at the placental insertion. (Reproduced from ref. 14 with permission)

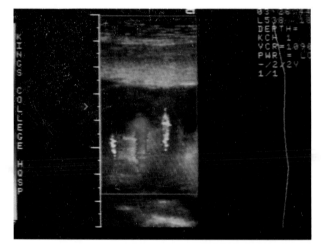

Figure 12.25 Color flow image of the same lesion showing the three vessels separated by a hyperechoic structure corresponding to the tumoral tissue

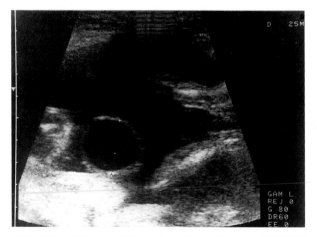

Figure 12.26 Sonogram of the cord near the fetal insertion at 32 weeks showing a hypoechoic round mass corresponding to an allantoid duct cyst. Blood flow within the mass was excluded by color flow imaging

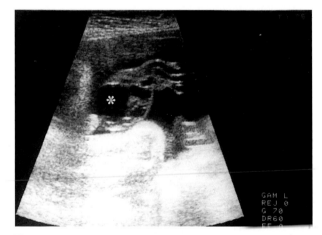

Figure 12.27 Transverse scan of the umbilical cord showing a large hypoechoic (*) mass corresponding to focal edema of the Wharton's jelly (pseudocyst)

REFERENCES

1. Grannum, P.A.T., Berkowitz, R.L. and Hobbins, J.C. (1979). The ultrasonic changes in the maturing placenta and their relation to fetal pulmonic maturity. *Am. J. Obstet. Gynecol.*, **133**, 915–22

2. Jauniaux, E. and Campbell, S. (1990). Sonographic assessment of placental abnormalities. *Am. J. Obstet. Gynecol.*, **163**, 1650–8

3. Proud, J. and Grant, A.M. (1987). Third trimester placental grading by ultrasonography as a test of fetal wellbeing. *Br. Med. J.*, **294**, 1641–4

4. Jauniaux, E., Moscoso, G., Campbell, S., Gibb, D., Driver, M. and Nicolaides, K.H. (1990). Correlation of ultrasound and pathologic findings of placental anomalies in pregnancies with elevated maternal serum alpha-fetoprotein. *Eur. J. Obstet. Gynecol. Biol. Reprod.*, **37**, 219–30

5. Jauniaux, E., Jurkovic, D., Kurjak, A. and Hustin, J. (1990). Assessment of placental development and function. In Kurjak, A. (ed.) *Transvaginal Color Doppler*, pp.53–65. (Carnforth: Parthenon Publishing)

6. Jauniaux, E., Jurkovic, D., Campbell, S., Kurjak, A. and Hustin, J. (1991). Investigation of placental circulations by color Doppler ultrasound. *Am. J. Obstet. Gynecol.*, **164**, 466–8

7. Jurkovic, D., Jauniaux, E., Kurjak, A., Hustin, J., Campbell, S. and Nicolaides, K.H. (1991). Transvaginal color Doppler assessment of the uteroplacental circulation in early pregnancy. *Obstet. Gynecol.*, **77**, 365–9

8. Fox, H. (1978). *Pathology of Placenta*. (Philadelphia: WB Saunders)

9. Thompson, R.S. and Trudinger, B.J. (1990). Doppler waveforms pulsatility index and resistance pressure and flow in the umbilical placental circulation: an investigation using a mathematical model. *Ultrasound Med. Biol.*, **16**, 449–58

10. Jauniaux, E., Gibb, D., Moscoso, G. and Campbell, S. (1990). Sonographic diagnosis of a large intervillous thrombosis associated with elevated maternal serum alpha-fetoprotein. *Am. J. Obstet. Gynecol.*, **163**,1558–60

11. Jauniaux, E., de Lannoy, E., Moscoso, G. and Campbell, S. (1990). Diagnostic prénatal des pathologies molaires associées à un foetus: revue de la littérature récente à propos d'un cas. *J. Gynecol. Obstet. Biol. Reprod.*, **19**, 941–6

12. Jauniaux, E. and Campbell, S. (1990). Fetal growth retardation with abnormal blood flows and placental sonographic lesions. *J. Clin. Ultrasound*, **17**, 210–14

13. Jauniaux, E, De Munter, C., Pardou, A., Elkhazen, N., Rodesch, F. and Wilkin, P. (1989). Evaluation echographique du syndrome de l'artere ombilicale unique: une serie de 80 cas. *J. Gynecol. Obstet. Biol. Reprod.*, **18**, 341–8

14. Jauniaux, E., Campbell, S. and Vyas, S. (1989). The use of color Doppler imaging for prenatal diagnosis of umbilical cord anomalies: report of three cases. *Am. J. Obstet. Gynecol.*, **161**, 1195–7

15. Jeanty, P. (1990). Pesistent right umbilical vein: an ominous prenatal finding. *Radiology*, **177**, 735–8

16. Romero, R., Pilu, G., Jeanty, P., Ghidini, A. and Hobbins, J.C. (1989). *Prenatal Diagnosis of Congenital Anomalies*, pp.385–402. (Norwalk, Connecticut: Appleton & Lange)

17. Nelson, L.H., Melone, P.J. and King, M. (1990). Diagnosis of vasa previa with transvaginal and color flow Doppler ultrasound. *Obstet. Gynecol.*, **76**, 506–9

18. Harding, J.A., Lewis, D.F., Major, C.A., Crade, M., Patel, J. and Nageotte, M.P. (1990). Color flow Doppler: a useful instrument in the diagnosis of vasa previa. *Am. J. Obstet. Gynecol.*, **163**, 1566–8

19. Jauniaux, E., Moscoso, G., Chitty, L., Gibb, D., Driver, M. and Campbell, S. (1990). An angiomyxoma involving the whole length of the umbilical cord: prenatal diagnosis by ultrasonography. *J. Ultrasound Med.*, **9**, 419–22

20. Jauniaux, E., Donner, C., Thomas, C., Francotte, J., Rodesch, F. and Avni, E. (1988). Umbilical cord pseudocyst in trisomy 18. *Prenat. Diagn.*, **8**, 557–63

21. Jauniaux, E., Jurkovic, D. and Campbell, S. (1991). Sonographic features of an umbilical cord abnormality combining a cord pseudocyst and a small omphalocele. *Eur. J. Obstet. Gynecol. Biol. Reprod.*, **40**, 245–8

13 Color Doppler in Obstetrics: First Trimester

A. Kurjak and R. Matijevic

More than any method available so far, ultrasound has enabled us to obtain direct information on embryo differentiation and growth. The application of high-frequency transvaginal sonography offers new opportunities in scanning during the first trimester of pregnancy. Remarkable progress in evaluation of that period of pregnancy has been obtained by means of transvaginal color Doppler. Color Doppler is a recently developed diagnostic tool which gives reliable information on early embryonic development and embryonal and fetal vessels. Embryonic, placental and maternal blood flow in the first and early second trimester of pregnancy are visualized much better by the transvaginal ultrasound approach than by any other diagnostic method. This approach, combined with high-resolution ultrasound, makes it possible to distinguish the fine structures and the developmental events occurring in embryonic life.

The value of transvaginal sonography for morphologic studies of early pregnancy has been well documented. The introduction of color Doppler flow imaging has allowed direct visualization of blood flow, which is superimposed on a conventional B-mode image. The transvaginal color Doppler technique and pulsed Doppler technique open new possibilities in studying the flow velocity waveforms of the uterine artery, corpus luteum, peritrophoblastic area, fetal aorta, umbilical cord, heart and cerebral vessels during early pregnancy. Our experiences with color Doppler investigations of maternal–fetal hemodynamics and anatomy in the first trimester of normal and abnormal pregnancy have been summarized in this chapter.

By transvaginal sonography compared with transabdominal sonography, all of these structures can be visualized 1 week earlier (Table 13.1). Transvaginal high-resolution 5–6 MHz probes make possible a closer look at the early pregnancy through more detailed imaging of different embryonic structures. In the second trimester, especially in its late part, transabdominal sonography gives better

Table 13.1 Detection times for embryological structures

Structure	Gestational age
Gestational sac	4 to 5 weeks
Yolk sac	5 to 6 weeks
Fetal heart action	5 to 6 weeks
Fetal head	8 to 9 weeks
Choroid plexus	9 to 11 weeks

results. It is believed that science begins when the measurements start. So far no reliable method for non-invasive blood flow measurement in the embryonal period has been found. The transvaginal color Doppler technique has finally introduced a non-invasive measurement of blood flow of maternal vessels in early embryonic development as well as in blood flow studies in embryonal and fetal vessels in normal and abnormal early pregnancy.

The gestational sac can usually be detected at 4 weeks and 1–4 days from the last menstrual period (LMP). At that time it measures 4–5 mm in diameter and blood flow in the peritrophoblastic area can be observed by transvaginal color Doppler (Figures 13.1–13.3). Clear and accurate display of the gestational ring, and presence of peritrophoblastic flow on its periphery, are suggestive of a normal intrauterine pregnancy. There is no significant difference in ultrasound findings comparing the 5th and 6th gestational weeks. At 5 weeks from the LMP color accurately indicates the position of embryonal heart, while blood flow in the peritrophoblastic area can be visualized in each case. Multiple pregnancy can easily be diagnosed (Figures 13.4 and 13.5) and the color flow signal of heart action (Figures 13.6–13.8) and/or umbilical cord flow gives the important information of whether there is a living embryo. At this time embryo passes 5 mm and the crown–rump length can be measured reliably. The main characteristic of the 7th gestational week is detection of the umbilical cord (Figure 13.9), and using the color Doppler technique, the flow in the umbilical cord can be seen and studied by means of

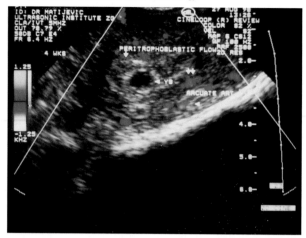

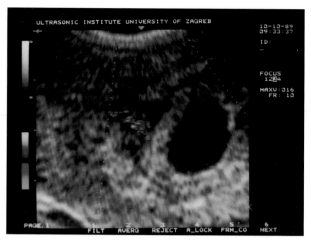

Figure 13.1 Early pregnancy, 4 weeks of amenorrhea, central anechogenic zone is gestational sac, and on the upper part is color-coded peritrophoblastic flow. On the right side is color signal of flow in arcuate arteries

Figure 13.2 Anechogenic structure on the right side of gestational sac, color-coded area (red and blue) represents peritrophoblastic flow; 4 weeks of pregnancy

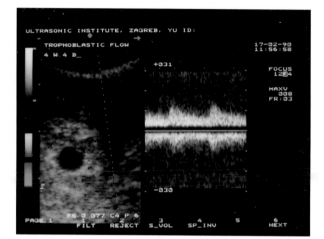

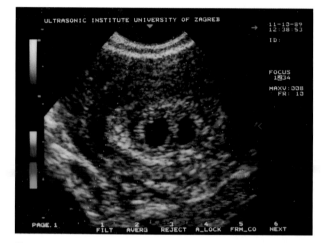

Figure 13.3 Four weeks and 4 days from the last menstrual period, duplex color and pulsed-wave Doppler scan of gestational sac (anechogenic structure in uterus on the B-mode), and pulsed-wave Doppler signal on the right side, give information of a high-velocity, low-resistance flow

Figure 13.4 Two gestational sacs with color-coded peritrophoblastic flow (up), 5 weeks from the last menstrual period

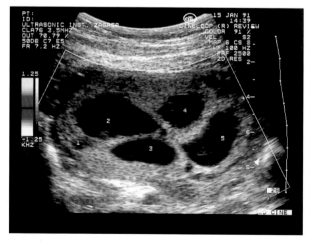

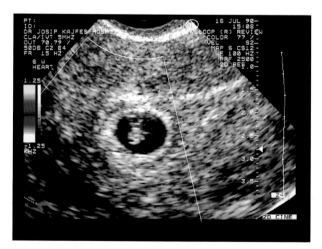

Figure 13.5 Multiple pregnancy: five gestational sacs are visible

Figure 13.6 Early pregnancy, 6 weeks from the last menstrual period. Gestational sac in the middle with color-coded (red) heart action

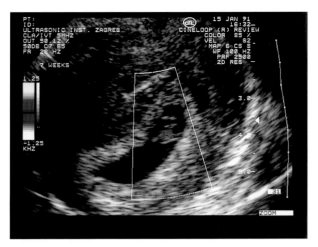

Figure 13.7 Transvaginal scan of gestational sac from Figure 13.10 with clearly visible heart action coded by color Doppler

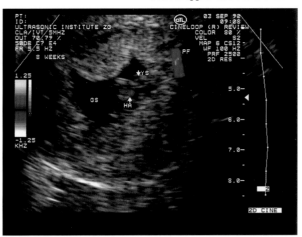

Figure 13.8 Eight weeks from the last menstrual period, clearly visible gestational sac (GS), yolk sac (YS) and color-coded heart action (HA)

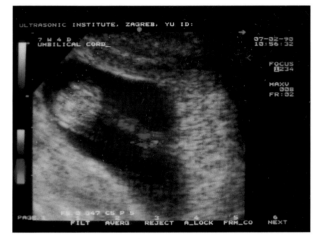

Figure 13.9 Pregnancy 7 weeks and 4 days from the last menstrual period, gestational sac with embryonic echo, black and white umbilical cord, and superimposed color-coded flow in the same

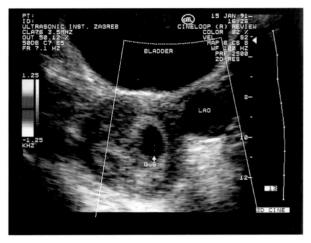

Figure 13.10 Early pregnancy 7 weeks from the last menstrual period and corpus luteum cyst on left ovary (LAO). Urinary bladder is on the top, and gestational sac (GS) in the uterus; color-coded (red) corpus luteum cyst flow, (transabdominal probe)

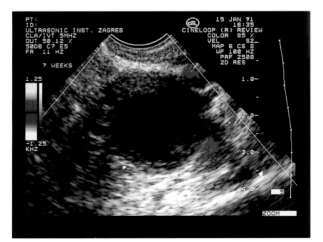

Figure 13.11 Transvaginal scan of the corpus luteum cyst from Figure 13.10 on the left ovary, and color-coded flow on the same

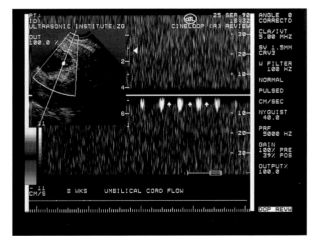

Figure 13.12 Duplex scan of early pregnancy, on the small part in left upper corner is B-mode superimposed by color Doppler picture of gestational sac and umbilical cord. Right side pulsed-wave Doppler analysis of flow signal in umbilical cord, clearly visible absence of diastolic flow. Resistance index is equal to 1

pulsed-wave Doppler. At this time luteal cysts can be clearly detected, as well as luteal blood flow (Figures 13.10 and 13.11). Umbilical cord flow is characterized by the absence of diastolic flow in the low volume umbilical cord (Figures 13.12 and 13.13). Both insertions of the umbilical cord can easily be seen (Figures 13.14 and 13.15) and embryonal anatomy can be clearly visualized after the 9th gestational week (Figures 13.16 and 13.17). The fetal aorta has been the second structure in which blood flow can be recognized during the early embryonic period (Figure 13.18). Using pulsed-wave Doppler analysis the absence of end diastolic flow is also noticed, and the resistance index (RI) is equal to 1 (Figure 13.19). The presence of carotid arteries (Figures 13.20 and 13.21) and cerebral arteries can be shown after 9 weeks of gestation, and the pulsed-Doppler waveform analysis can be done. Analysis of intracranial vessels shows absence of end diastolic flow – a normal finding for early pregnancy.

ECTOPIC PREGNANCY

The ectopic pregnancy has been one of the major problems in gynecology. The advantage of transvaginal sonography is best shown in its ability to visualize a live extrauterine pregnancy before its rupture or before abortion occurs. Embryonic structures such as fetal pole and heart beats; or extraembryonic structures such as the yolk sac and tiny placenta may be recognized by the attentive sonographer. In suspicious cases, (i.e. absence of menstrual bleeding for a few weeks, positive finding β–human chorionic gonadotropin and suspicious adnexal mass without typical ultrasound morphology) color can be of help in making a final diagnosis (Figures 13.22–13.24). The color can help to characterize the nature of the adnexal mass, thus permitting preoperative diagnosis when the ectopic embryo and its characteristic heart beats can not be visualized. Transvaginal color Doppler is expected to have direct implications for diagnosis and therapy of ectopic pregnancy.

PATHOLOGY OF THE EARLY INTRAUTERINE PREGNANCY

Missed abortion

After the 6th gestational week it is relatively easy to make this diagnosis using color Doppler techniques.

The absence of fetal movements and absence of a color flow signal from the fetal heart at its expected position can help in the recognition of this pathologic condition (Figures 13.25–13.27). There is no statistically significant difference in pulsed-wave Doppler analysis of peritrophoblastic flow comparing this pathologic condition to normal early pregnancy.

Blighted ovum

The diagnosis of blighted ovum can be done as early as the end of the 5th gestational week by means of the color Doppler technique (Figure 13.28). The criteria are well known, and easily detectable by conventional ultrasound (i.e. absence of the embryo; irregular shape of the gestational sac, size of the gestational sac in relation to the gestational age, discrepancy between uterine size and the gestational sac). Peritrophoblastic flow is present and does not show any statistically significant difference in measurement of resistance index of flow in the same area in comparison with normal pregnancy.

Hydatidiform mole

'Snowstorm-like' sonographic appearance is relatively easy to recognize and is a characteristic finding considered to be pathognomonic for this disorder. Transvaginal color Doppler sonography has made it possible to register the large volume of flow through small cystic structures inside the uterus (Figures 13.29–13.31). The pulsed-wave Doppler analysis of peritrophoblastic flow shows statistically significant differences in RI in comparison with normal pregnancy and all other pathologies of early pregnancy.

Further investigation will affirm transvaginal color Doppler imaging as a diagnostic tool for the evaluation of normal and abnormal early pregnancy (Figures 13.32–13.36). In the future, transvaginal color flow will most certainly become a part of routine work in the examination of early pregnancy, and that future starts today.

READING LIST

1. Kurjak, A., Zalud, I. and Crvenkovic, G. (1990). Transvaginal color Doppler in normal and abnormal early pregnancy. Presented at the 7th congress of European federation of societies for ultrasound in medicine and biology. Jerusalem, May 5–10,

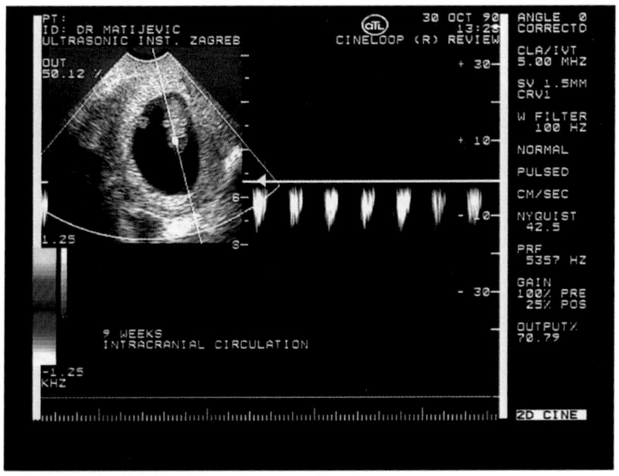

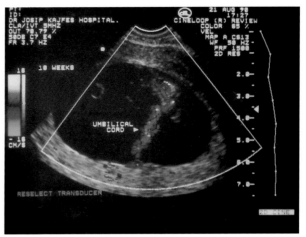

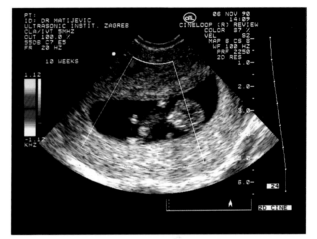

Figure 13.13 Duplex scan, early pregnancy 9 weeks of gestation. On the small part in left upper corner is B-mode image of embryo and sample volume is on the color-coded area from fetal head. On the right side is pulsed-wave analysis and clearly visible diastolic flow absence. Resistance index is equal to 1

Figure 13.14 Full length of umbilical cord coded by color Doppler and both insertions, fetal and placental at 10 weeks of gestation

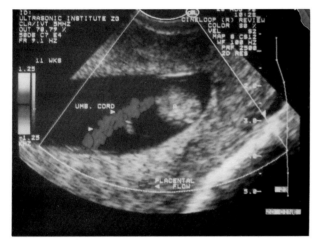

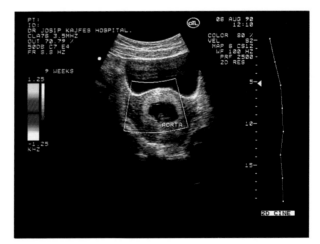

Figure 13.15 Full length of umbilical cord, both insertions fetal and placental are seen

Figure 13.16 Fetal anatomy with head, body, and all four extremities; color-coded umbilical cord

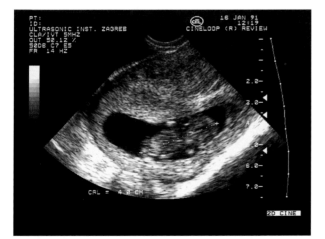

Figure 13.17 Black and white scan of fetal anatomy, 11 weeks from the last menstrual period. Clearly visible complete fetal anatomy and crown–rump length is shown

Figure 13.18 Transabdominal scan of early pregnancy, 9 weeks from the last menstrual period. Longitudinal scan of aorta coded by red color

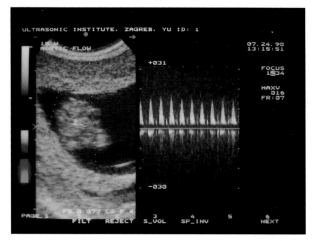

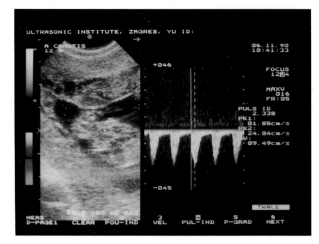

Figure 13.19 Duplex scan, early pregnancy 9 weeks from the last menstrual period. On the left side B-mode scan superimposed with color Doppler. Clearly visible embryonic echo and color-coded fetal aorta. On the right side pulsed-wave Doppler analysis with absence of diastolic flow; resistance index equal to 1

Figure 13.20 Duplex scan, early pregnancy 12 weeks of gestation, color-coded carotid artery and pulsed-wave Doppler signal show diastolic flow

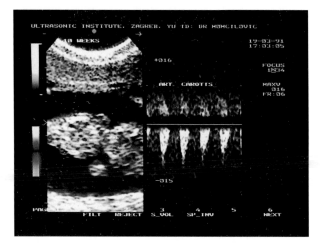

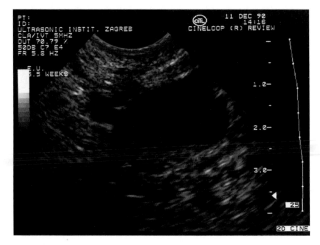

Figure 13.21 Duplex scan, early pregnancy 10 weeks of gestation, color-coded carotid artery and pulsed-wave Doppler signal show absence of diastolic flow

Figure 13.22 Suspected mass in right adnexa, 5 weeks and 5 days from the last menstrual period

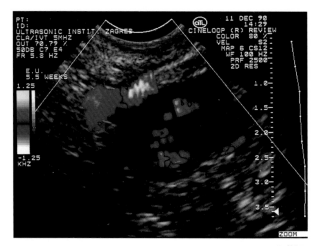

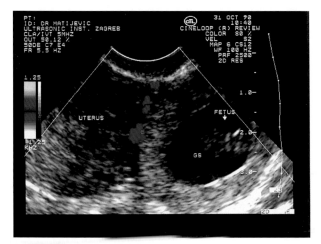

Figure 13.23 Color Doppler coded 'hot' area in suspected mass from Figure 13.22: diagnosis ectopic pregnancy

Figure 13.24 Transvaginal scan, empty uterus on the left side and extrauterine pregnancy in right Fallopian tube with normal developed fetus in gestational sac (GS). Color-coded area represents flow which is very helpful for detection of extrauterine pregnancy when anatomy is not clearly visible

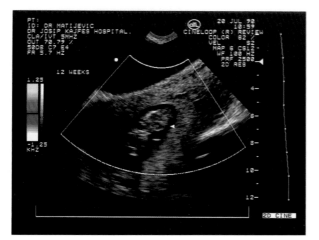

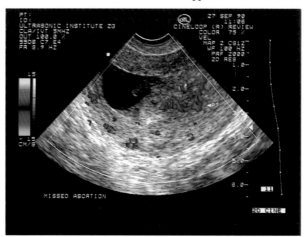

Figure 13.25 Transvaginal scan of pregnancy 12 weeks from the last menstrual period. By transabdominal ultrasound a diagnosis of missed abortion was made, but with transvaginal scan superimposed with color Doppler fetal heart action signal was present

Figure 13.26 Case of missed abortion, gestational sac in uterus, echogenic structure represents embryo, but without any heart action. Very intensive flow in intervillous space

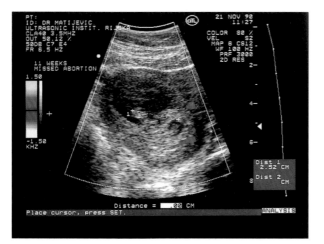

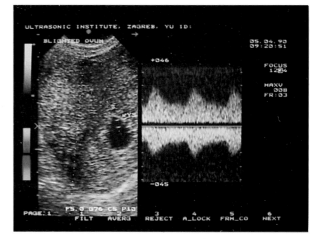

Figure 13.27 Missed abortion in resorption. Color-coded peritrophoblastic flow

Figure 13.28 Duplex scan, on the left side B-mode scan superimposed with color Doppler, empty gestational sac and color-coded peritrophoblastic flow. On the right side pulsed-wave Doppler analysis

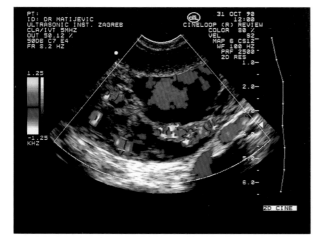

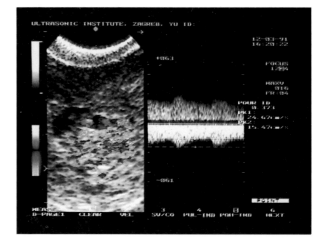

Figure 13.29 Whole uterine cavity is full with color coded 'hot' areas which represents hydatidiform mole. Pulsed-wave Doppler analysis showed low-resistance high-velocity waveform analysis; resistance index = 0.31

Figure 13.30 'Hot' areas inside uterine cavity represent hydatidiform mole. Pulsed-wave Doppler analysis of this area showed resistance index = 0.37

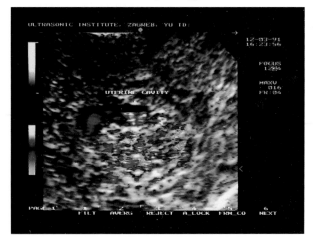

Figure 13.31 Close up of uterine cavity from Figure 13.30 showing 'hot' areas

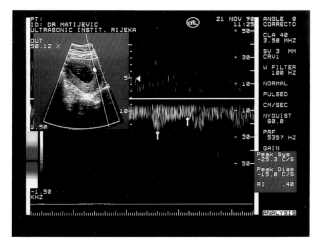

Figure 13.32 Duplex scan of abnormal early pregnancy, empty gestational sac on the B-mode scan superimposed with color Doppler on the left upper corner and peritrophoblastic flow. Right side of the picture shows pulsed-wave signal of peritrophoblastic flow, lower resistance than in normal pregnancy

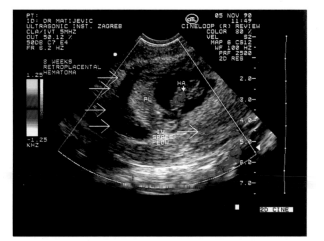

Figure 13.33 Transvaginal scan of early pregnancy, 8 weeks from the last menstrual period, clearly visible gestational sac with embryo and heart action (HA) coded by color Doppler. On the right side color-coded area is peritrophoblastic flow, and anechogenic structure on the left represents retroplacental hematoma

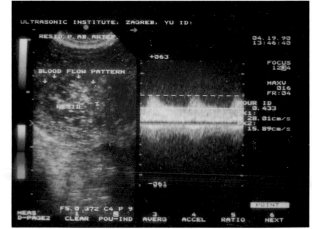

Figure 13.34 Duplex scan, left part B-mode scan superimposed with color Doppler. Flow pattern on the picture represents residual blood vessels in tissue after artificial abortion. Right part shows pulsed-wave Doppler analysis, high-velocity low-resistance flow, resistance index = 0.43

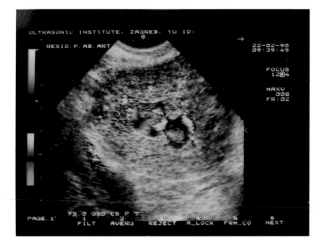

Figure 13.35 Color Doppler scan, residual tissue in uterine cavity after artificial abortion

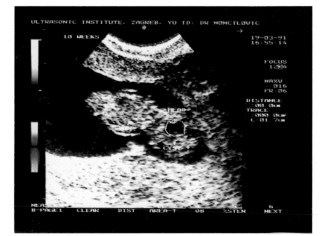

Figure 13.36 Ten weeks of gestation, cystic structure inside fetal head, heart action color-coded red

Abstr. p.71.

2. Kurjak, A., Crvenkovic, G. and Takeuchi, H. (1991). Assessment of early pregnancy. In Kurjak, A. (ed.) *Transvaginal Color Doppler*, pp.41–51. (Carnforth: Parthenon Publishing Group)

3. Timor-Tritsch, I.E., Rottem, S. and Thaler, I. (1988). Review of transvaginal ultrasonography. A description and clinical application. *Ultrasound Q.*, **6**, 1

4. Schulman, H., Fleischer, E., Farmakaides, G., Bracero, I., Rochelsen, B. and Grunteld, L. (1986). Development of uterine artery compliance in pregnancy as detected by Doppler ultrasound. *Am. J. Obstet. Gynecol.*, **155**, 1031

5. Jurkovic, D., Jauniaux, E., Kurjak, A., Hustin, J., Campbell, S. and Nicolaides, K.H. (1991). Transvaginal color Doppler assessment of the uteroplacental circulation in early pregnancy. *Obstet. Gynecol.*, **77**, 30

6. Kurjak, A., Zalud, I., Salihagic, A., Crvenkovic, G. and Matijevic, R. (1991). Transvaginal color Doppler in the assessment of abnormal early pregnancy. *J. Perinat. Med.*, in press

7. Hansmann, M., Hackeloer, B.J. and Staudach, A. (1985). *Ultrasound Diagnosis in Obstetrics and Gynecology: Pregnancy (First Trimester)*, p.35. (Berlin, Heidelberg, New York, Tokyo: Springer Verlag)

14 Color Doppler in Obstetrics: Second and Third Trimesters

A. Kurjak and R. Matijevic

Ultrasound is already an essential component of obstetric evaluation. The new technique of color Doppler has been introduced in obstetrics to make a clear sonographic appearance of almost the whole fetal, maternal and placental circulation. The blood flow through all fetal and maternal structures in pregnancy has been the main point of interest for clinicians, since a lot of pathological cases could be discovered by studying this. Color Doppler imaging has introduced direct visualization of blood flow, displayed simultaneously with the conventional B-mode image. Detection of blood flow and blood vessels by color Doppler compared to those obtained by B-mode and duplex systems alone is easier, faster and more accurate. The use of transabdominal probes for the second and third trimester of pregnancy seems to be more convenient.

The first application of pulsed Doppler technique, providing quantification of blood flow in fetal vessels, was reported in 1977 by FitzGerald and Drumm. They demonstrated Doppler frequency shift waveforms from the umbilical artery. This technique has been used in the last few years for investigation of some fetal circulation components, e.g. umbilical cord, fetal aorta, fetal heart, great vessels and cerebral circulation. The only disadvantage of this method was the dimension limit of the vessel of interest. Color Doppler superimposed on B-mode provides visualization of small blood vessels, makes examination time shorter, and pulsed Doppler examination more precise. Color Doppler has also provided detection of blood flow in small branches, undetectable by B-mode real-time imaging or conventional pulsed Doppler technique.

NORMAL ANATOMY

Prenatal diagnosis of fetal malformations has been one of the main fields of application of ultrasound in obstetrics. The routine evaluation of fetal anatomy was made possible by means of high-resolution, real-time scanners. Color Doppler superimposed on a conventional B-mode image has provided more accurate and precise analysis of the fetal anatomy. Blood flow through all fetal vessels can be detected, and functional analysis can be done. Location of some fetal blood vessels, especially those small in diameter, might be very difficult even using high-resolution, real-time equipment. In these cases color Doppler is extremely helpful for location of the blood vessels and functional analysis of their flow can be done. Pulsed-wave Doppler analysis of flow in umbilical cord and fetal aorta has been a good guide for evaluation of biometrically suspected cases of intrauterine growth retardation (IUGR). In cases of IUGR it has been noticed that there is an increase of resistance in fetal circulation (increase of A/B ratio (where A is top systolic velocity and B is end diastolic velocity), resistance index (RI) and pulsatility index (PI)). The same results could be noticed in intracerebral circulation and uteroplacental circulation. As well as in these vessels, detection of the blood flow by means of color Doppler could be done in nearly all parts of the fetal circulation. The examination of the fetal cranium may begin from the 11th or 12th weeks of gestation. The cerebral vascular system is easily detectable and a lot of blood flow analysis can be done. Our preliminary results obtained from fetal intracerebral arteries between 10 and 13 weeks of gestation, showed that the PI is significantly higher compared to the results of the same flow in the second and third trimesters of pregnancy.

Aorta and main arteries

Using fetal heart pulsation as a landmark, the fetal chest can be easily recognized. In the second and third trimesters of pregnancy this pulsatility could be recognized by real-time equipment as well, but much more easily by color Doppler instrumentation. The fetal aorta in the second and third trimesters can be easily recognized in longitudinal scans (Figures 14.1–14.7). Recent years have witnessed a surge of interest in the application of Doppler ultrasound velocimetry as a fetal diagnostic tool. Fetal aortal flow waveform analysis is of remarkable help in distinction between normal and abnormal conditions in pregnancy, especially in suspected cases of IUGR. The first step in this analysis is location of the descending part of the aorta. The color flow signal is extremely helpful for the location of the aorta, especially in early pregnancy. Both the aortic root, with brachycephalic vessels, and the descending aorta, can be identified easily, as well as visualization of abdominal blood vessels.

Umbilical cord

The umbilical cord is one of the basic fields of interest for all scientists, because a lot of pathologies of pregnancy can be discovered by its functional study. It is well known that waveform analysis of blood flow in the umbilical artery in normal pregnancy shows relatively high systolic peak and low diastolic end velocities. Being very mobile the umbilical cord can be easily displayed with real-time devices, especially if there is more amniotic fluid. Color Doppler has provided visualization of the umbilical cord, as well as identification of both insertions, placental and fetal (Figures 14.8–14.16). Towards the end of the pregnancy, when the fetus fills the uterine cavity almost completely, it might be difficult to find the cord. In these cases the umbilical cord color flow signal is remarkably helpful. Pulsed-wave Doppler analysis of umbilical artery flow showed end diastolic flow, but in cases of IUGR the absence of this flow is noticed. Introducing this technique we found new non-invasive diagnostic methods for evaluation of some pathological conditions during pregnancy. Some malformations of the umbilical cord (i.e. single umbilical artery, tumors etc.) could also be diagnosed by means of the color Doppler technique.

Placenta

The placenta is the organ responsible for fetal nutrition and homeostasis, and is essential for fetal growth and development. The placenta is not completely formed in the first two trimesters of pregnancy. Pulsed-wave Doppler has often been used for functional analysis of the placental blood vessels. Yet, in many cases it has been quite difficult to visualize placental vessels. Color Doppler allows their identification in normal cases as well as in cases of their pathology (Figures 14.17–14.20). The visualization of blood vessels overlapping the internal cervical os in cases of placenta previa (Figure 14.21) can also be done by color Doppler instrumentation.

Urinary system

The fetal kidneys can be ultrasonically visualized as early as the 12th to 14th weeks of gestation, and a routine visualization is possible after the 16th week from the last menstrual period. Applying color Doppler techniques in the third trimester of pregnancy, the renal vascular system can easily be identified (Figures 14.22–14.24). The urinary bladder is easily recognized as a small ovoid cystic structure in the fetal pelvis. The urinary bladder circulation, vessels circuiting the fetal urinary bladder, can also be detected using color Doppler technology (Figures 14.25 and 14.26).

PATHOLOGY

As well as its uses in the evaluation of normal blood flow, color Doppler gives a clear sonographic picture of abnormal and pathologic conditions, describing anatomical details that would be necessary for diagnosis. It can be used for elucidation of anomalous fetal circulation in cardiac malformations as well as in extracardiac malformations. In cases of cystic hygroma (Figures 14.27–14.31), fetal ascites, meningomyelocele (Figure 14.32), omphalocele (Figure 14.33), ileojejunal atresia (Figure 14.34), sacrococcygeal teratoma and different urogenital abnormalities (Figures 14.35–14.39), color superimposed on conventional B-mode image gives information for diagnosis of specific pathologic conditions, providing visualization of some special anatomical details.

In cases of urogenital malformations, the multicystic kidney is the most common of all neonatal abdominal masses. The diagnosis of multicystic kidney is suggested by the presence of multiple cysts. The cysts are usually only a few centimeters in diameter, but they can be up to 6 cm.

The renal artery and vein can be visualized and because of their anatomical position can help to distinguish this pathologic condition from sonographically similar abnormalities. In cases of

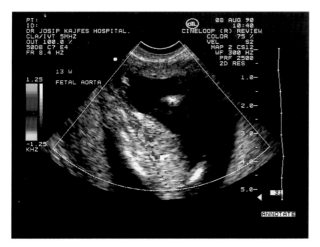

Figure 14.1 Longitudinal scan through 13-week-old fetus, with fetal heart and fetal aorta coded by color Doppler. Color-coded red signal from flow in the placental vessels on the left; transabdominal probe (TA)

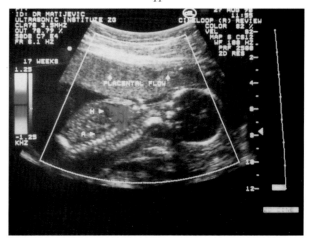

Figure 14.2 Pregnancy at 17 weeks, placental flow on the top, fetus *in utero*, head on the right side and thorax on the left side, with color-coded fetal heart action (H) and fetal aortal flow (A) (TA)

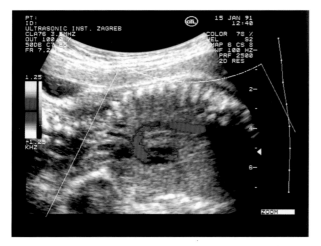

Figure 14.3 Aortic arch, 29 weeks of pregnancy: ascendent and transverse parts coded red, and descendent part coded blue. Two areas; first on the ascendent part and second on the descendent part without any color signal because of insonation of ultrasound beam at angle of 90° (TA)

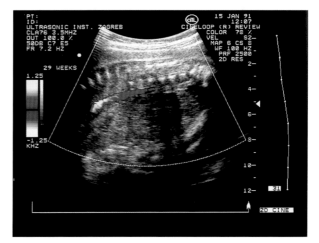

Figure 14.4 Longitudinal scan of fetal aorta, thoracic part with color-coded flow at 29 weeks of pregnancy (TA)

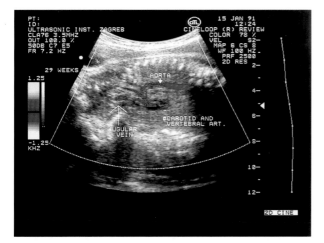

Figure 14.5 Pregnancy at 29 weeks: longitudinal scan through fetal thorax, aortic arch and origin of carotid and vertebral artery (#), color-coded (blue) jugular vein (TA)

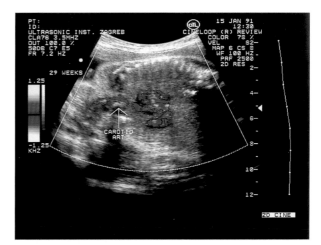

Figure 14.6 Pregnancy 29 weeks, color-coded fetal heart in the middle, and carotid artery (red). Blue coded signal on the right is from descendent part of fetal aorta (TA)

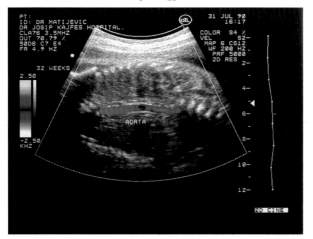

Figure 14.7 Full length of fetal aorta, 32 weeks of pregnancy: example of color Doppler principles; color-coded flow towards the probe (red) and from the probe (blue). Small part of the aorta in the middle without color is the point of insonation of the ultrasound beam at an angle of 90°, and there has been no Doppler effect (TA)

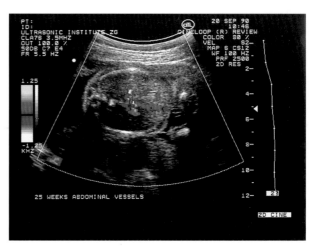

Figure 14.8 Transverse scan through fetal abdomen at level of umbilical vein: color-coded abdominal blood vessels at 25 weeks (TA)

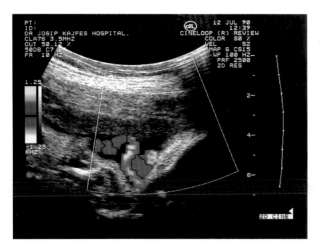

Figure 14.9 Transabdominal scan 28 weeks from the last menstrual period, umbilical cord color-coded flow in two arteries (red), and one vein (blue) (TA)

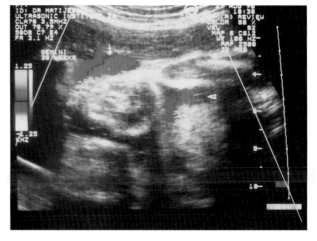

Figure 14.10 Color-coded two umbilical cords in twin pregnancy: on both sides two arteries (red) and one vein (blue) are clearly visible (TA)

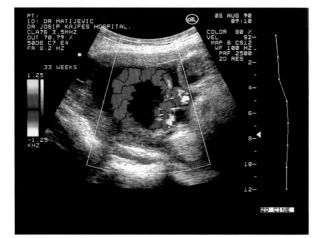

Figure 14.11 Umbilical cord at 33 weeks of pregnancy: color-coded two arteries (red) and one vein (blue). On the right side aliasing was present (TA)

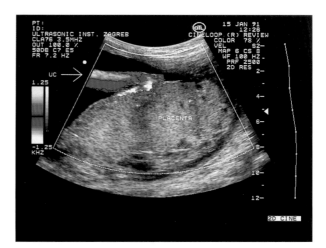

Figure 14.12 Third trimester of pregnancy, placental insertion of umbilical cord, coded by color Doppler (TA)

150

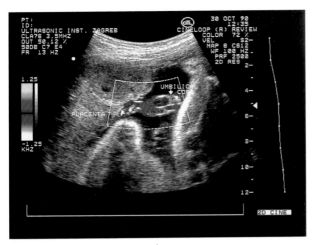

Figure 14.13 Placental insertion of umbilical cord at 27 weeks of pregnancy: color can be a good guide for cordocentesis (TA)

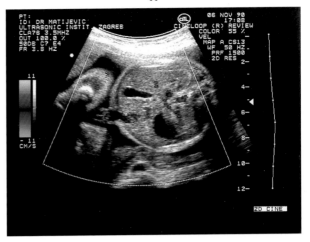

Figure 14.14 Transverse scan through fetal abdomen at 28 weeks of gestation at level insertion of umbilical cord: color-coded aorta near the spine, stomach (down), and hepatic vessels (TA)

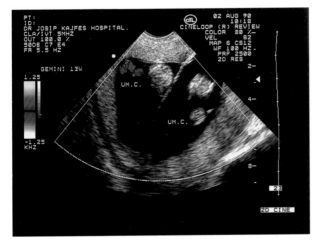

Figure 14.15 Multiple pregnancy, 13 weeks from the last menstrual period: two gestational sacs and two fetuses *in utero* are clearly visible. Color-coded flow in both umbilical cords (um. c.) (red and blue) (TA)

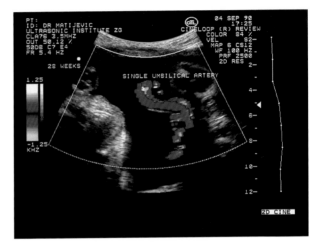

Figure 14.16 Single umbilical artery, 28 weeks of pregnancy: color-coded flow in one artery (red) and one vein (blue) (TA)

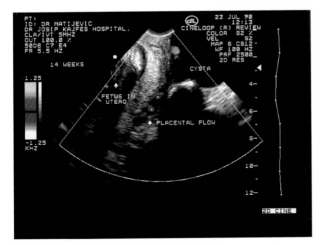

Figure 14.17 Pregnancy at 14 weeks, including fetus *in utero* with heart action (blue and red), placental flow and cystic structure in right adnexa (CYSTA), represents corpus luteum cyst (TA)

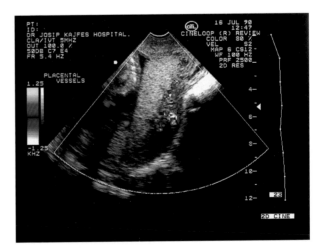

Figure 14.18 Color-coded placental vessels: fetus is in uterine cavity on the left, and color-coded umbilical cord appears red (TA)

151

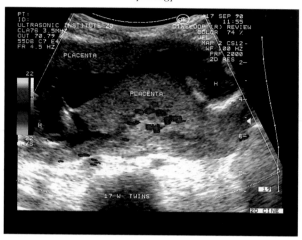

Figure 14.19 Twin pregnancy at 17 weeks: two different placentas with their own vascularization coded red and blue (TA)

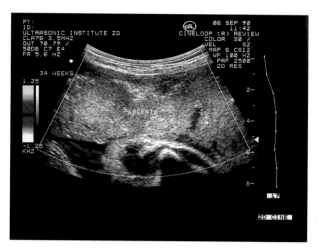

Figure 14.20 Placental flow at 34 weeks of pregnancy: color-coded placental blood vessels (TA)

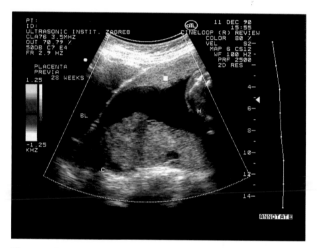

Figure 14.21 Placenta previa at 28 weeks of pregnancy: urinary bladder on the left (BL), and fetal head on the right (H); C = uterine cervix (TA)

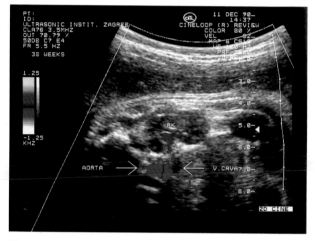

Figure 14.22 Pregnancy at 38 weeks, transverse scan through fetal abdomen: right kidney in the middle (RK), color-coded abdominal aorta and vena cava: renal artery (red) and flow in right kidney (TA)

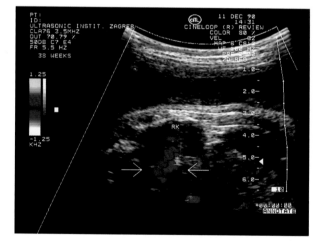

Figure 14.23 Pregnancy at 38 weeks, transverse scan through fetal abdomen, right kidney (RK) in the middle, color coded renal artery (red) and renal vein (blue) as well as flow in right kidney

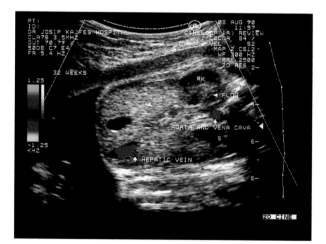

Figure 14.24 Transverse scan through fetal abdomen at 32 weeks of pregnancy: right kidney (RK) with renal artery and vein (FLOW), and hepatic vein coded blue, stomach (S) and aorta with vena cava on the right side (TA)

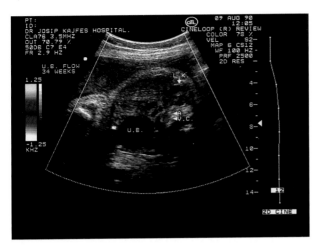

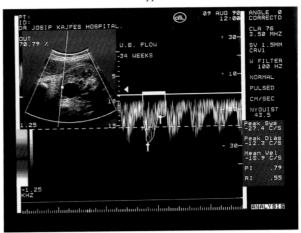

Figure 14.25 Transverse scan through fetal abdomen on level of urinary bladder (U.B., the anechogenic ovoid structure on the left), with color-coded urinary bladder artery (blue) and vein (red); LK = left kidney, A = aorta, V.C. = vena cava (TA)

Figure 14.26 Pulsed-wave Doppler signal of urinary bladder vessels (artery), resistance index = 0.55 and pulsatility index = 0.79 (TA)

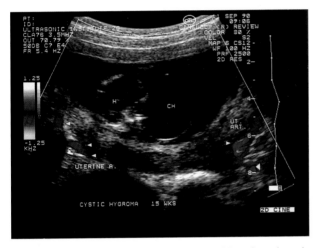

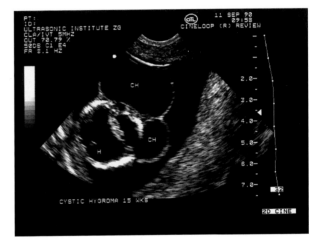

Figure 14.27 Pregnancy at 15 weeks: fetal head (H), and anechogenic cystic structure, cystic hygroma (CH). Below, on both sides color-coded uterine arteries appear (TA)

Figure 14.28 Same cystic hygroma as Figure 14.27 in black and white transvaginal scan, head (H) and two cystic structures (CH) top and right. Transvaginal (TV) sonography can display more details than the transabdominal sonography in the first part of the second trimester

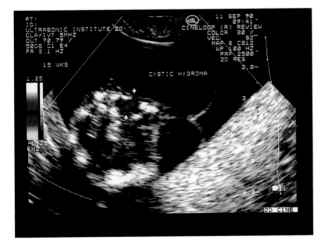

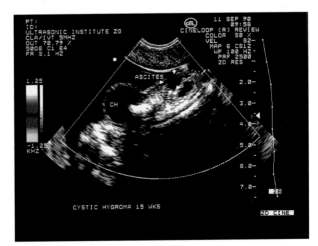

Figure 14.29 Same case of cystic hygroma as in Figure 14.27, transvaginal color Doppler scan, two cystic structures top and right and color-coded vertebral artery flow (TV)

Figure 14.30 Transvaginal scan of 15-week-old fetus, longitudinal scan through complete fetus, fetal spine, cystic hygroma (CH) and fetal ascites (TV)

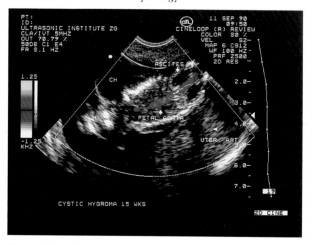

Figure 14.31 Pregnancy at 15 weeks, fetus *in utero* with huge anechogenic structure on its neck (CH), a cystic hygroma, complete longitudinal scan through fetal aorta coded red, and two anechogenic structures below diaphragm, ascites (TA)

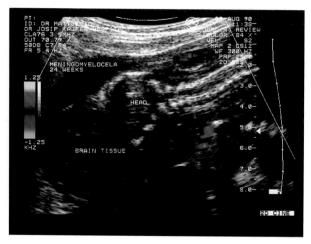

Figure 14.32 Pregnancy at 24 weeks, on the left side fetal head and spine with protruded brain tissue are visible – meningomyelocele – fetal heart action color-coded (red and blue) (TA)

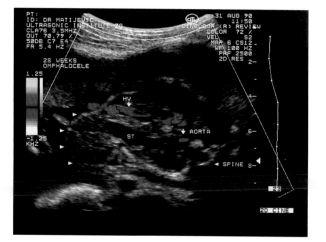

Figure 14.33 Transverse scan through fetal abdomen 28 weeks of pregnancy, includes rounded structure on the left – omphalocele – with protruded stomach (ST): color-coded umbilical vein (HV) and aorta (TA)

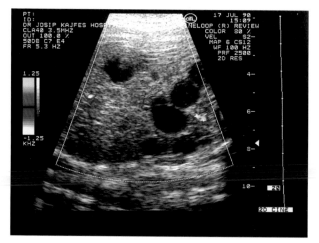

Figure 14.34 Transverse scan through fetal abdomen at 37 weeks of pregnancy, few anechogenic structures show ileojejunal atresia with color-coded mesenteric blood vessels (TA)

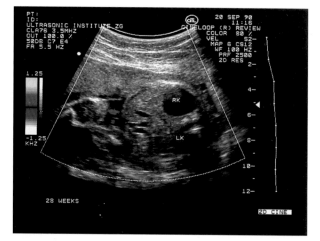

Figure 14.35 Anechogenic structure on the right kidney (RK) completely destroying normal kidney tissue at 28 weeks of pregnancy; LK – left kidney (TA)

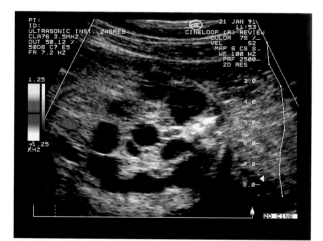

Figure 14.36 Pregnancy at 38 weeks, transverse scan through fetal abdomen at the level of the kidneys. Multiple anechogenic cystic structures represent multicystic kidney (TA)

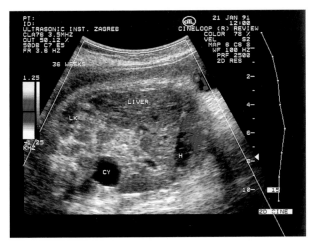

Figure 14.37 Pregnancy at 36 weeks, transverse scan through fetal abdomen, liver on the top and left kidney (LK) on the top left. On the bottom left anechogenic cystic structure represents ovarian cyst (CY); H = heart (TA)

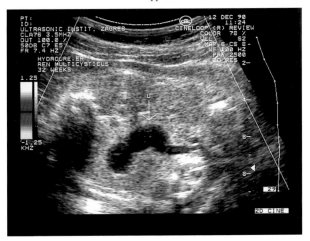

Figure 14.38 Pregnancy at 34 weeks, scan through fetal abdomen at level of the kidneys, hydroureter-like anechogenic structure in the center (TA)

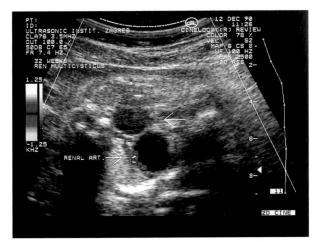

Figure 14.39 Multicystic kidney at 32 weeks of pregnancy: two anechogenic cystic structures in the center and color-coded (red) renal artery (TA)

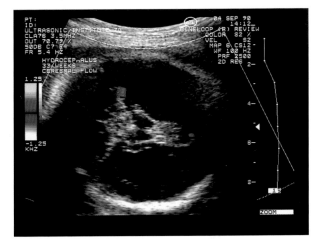

Figure 14.40 Fetal head, transverse scan at 27 weeks of pregnancy showing dilated brain ventricles. Color-coded (red) middle cerebral artery, and anterior communicant artery (blue) (TA)

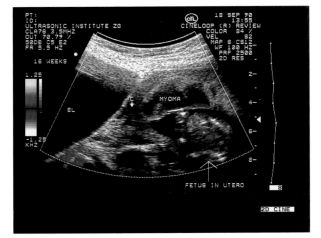

Figure 14.41 Pregnancy at 16 weeks, urinary bladder on the left (BL), fetus *in utero* and myoma on anterior wall of uterus near to cervix (C). Fetal heart action is coded red and blue. (TA)

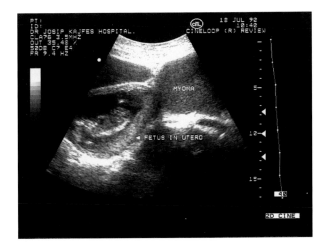

Figure 14.42 Pregnancy at 11 weeks, fetus *in utero* on the left, and myoma on the right (TA)

hydrocephaly (Figure 14.40), a pathological condition characterized by an abnormal increase in cerebrospinal fluid causing subsequent ventricular dilatation and enlargement of the cranial vault, color Doppler techniques visualize cerebral blood vessels, and these vessels could be further functionally analyzed by pulsed Doppler. The identification of these vessels is simple, and that is the new view for functional analysis. Detection of myoma in pregnancy and functional analysis of blood flow in the same can help in the prognosis of its growth and also in the prognosis of the pregnancy (Figures 14.41 and 14.42).

Color Doppler techniques open a new approach to second and third trimesters pregnancy studies. Blood flow waveform analysis of the fetal vascular system can easily be done because the location of blood vessels is easier and more accurate. The application of color Doppler is still in its infancy, but time will show the value of the information it can provide. The benefits of this method are more than obvious, many revolutionary changes have taken place and it is quite impossible to imagine the great potential this technique can provide.

READING LIST

1. Kurjak, A., Jurkovic, D., Alfirevic, Z. and Zalud, I. (1990). Transvaginal color Doppler imaging. *J. Clin. Ultrasound*, **18**, 277

2. FitzGerald, D.E. and Drumm, J.E. (1977). Noninvasive measurement of fetal circulation using Doppler ultrasound: a new method. *Br. Med. J.*, **2**, 1450

3. Joupplila, P. and Kirkinen, P. (1984). Increased vascular resistance in the descending aorta of the human fetus in hypoxia. *Br. J. Obstet. Gynaecol.*, **91**, 863

4. Reed, K.L., Meijboom, E.J., Sahn, D.J., Scagnelli, S.A., Valdes-Cruz, L.M. and Shenker, L. (1986). Cardiac Doppler flow velocities in human fetuses. *Circulation*, **73**, 41

5. Allan, L.D., Chita, S.K., Al-Ghazali, W., Crawford, D. and Tynan, M. (1987). Doppler echocardiographic evaluation of the normal human fetal heart. *Br. Heart J.*, **57**, 528

6. Machado, M.V.L., Chita, S.C. and Allan, L.D. (1987). Acceleration time in the aorta and pulmonary artery measured by Doppler echocardiography in the midtrimester fetus. *Br. Heart J.*, **58**, 15

7. Reed, K.L., Anderson, C.F. and Shenker, L. (1987). Fetal pulmonary artery and aorta: two dimensional Doppler echocardiography. *Obstet. Gynecol.*, **69**, 175

8. Wladimiroff, J.W., Tonge, H.M. and Stewart, P.A. (1986). Doppler ultrasound assessment of cerebral blood flow in the human fetus. *Br. J. Obstet. Gynecol.*, **93**, 471

9. Veile, J.C. and Cohen, I. (1990). Middle cerebral artery blood flow in normal and growth-retarded fetuses. *Am. J. Obstet. Gynecol.*, **62**, 391

10. Van den Wijngaard, J.A.G.W., Groenenberg, I.A.L., Wladimiroff, J.W. and Hop, W.C.J. (1989). Cerebral Doppler ultrasound of the human fetus. *Br. J. Obstet. Gynaecol.*, **96**, 845

11. Kurjak, A., Zalud, I., Jurkovic, D., Alfirevic, Z. and Miljan, M. (1989). Transvaginal color Doppler in the assessment of pelvic circulation. *Acta Obstet. Gynecol. Scand.*, **68**, 131

Section II

Ultrasound in Gynecology

15 Normal and Abnormal Anatomy of Female Pelvis

I. Zalud and A. Kurjak

SONOGRAPHY OF THE UTERUS

The ability of sonography to depict subtle changes in the myometrium and endometrium makes it the diagnostic modality of choice for the evaluation of many uterine disorders. With sonography, the uterus can be imaged in several scanning planes. With real time, the sonographer can alter the scanning plane and gain settings for optimal depiction of the endometrium and myometrium (Figures 15.1–15.17).

Sonographic evaluation of the uterus should be performed when the patient has a fully distended bladder. A fully distended bladder displaces gas-filled bowel loops from the pelvis and places the uterus in a more horizontal plane. This orientation of the uterus relative to the transducer is advantageous since the uterus can then be imaged utilizing the better characteristics of axial, rather than lateral resolution.

Sonography can accurately depict the position, size, shape and texture of the uterus. The uterus is centrally located and the most accessible organ for ultrasound evaluation. The uterine cervix is the middle structure while the body is usually situated slightly to the left or right. The fundus is usually anteriorly flexed when compared to the cervix (anteflexed). Although a retroflexed uterus is sometimes a normal variant, this uterine configuration should arouse suspicion of posterior compartment pathology. Because of the posterior position and curved surface of the fundus, it may be difficult to obtain detailed images of the fundal portion of a retroflexed uterus and the endometrial layer may not be seen. The size and shape of the uterus varies according to the patient's pubertal status, age and parity. Before puberty occurs, the uterus measures 1.0–3.3 cm in length and 0.5–1.0 cm in width. The cervix and isthmus comprise a greater proportion of the uterus (up to two-thirds of the total length) and are thicker than the fundus. In contrast, the normal postpubertal uterus measures 7 cm in length, 4 cm in width and height and has a relatively thicker fundus and shortened cervix. The multiparous woman typically has a uterus that measures an average of 1.2 cm greater in all directions as compared to the nulligravid individual. A postmenopausal woman has a uterus that is smaller then the normal postpubertal woman. The average dimension of the postmenopausal uterus ranges from 3.5 to 6.5 cm long and 1.2 to 1.8 cm thick.

The texture of the normal myometrium is consistent throughout all age groups and is of a homogeneous, low to medium echogenicity. The innermost layers of the endometrium appear as a central linear echogenicity, most prominent during menses. The endometrium thickens from 2–3 mm in the proliferative phase to 3–6 mm in the secretory phase. The hypoechoic texture of the endometrium, that is most frequently seen in the proliferative phase, is related to the particular arrangement of the enlarging glands and stromal edema. A small amount of intraluminal fluid can be observed during the periovulatory and secretory phases of the cycle. The endometrium appears thickened and echogenic during the secretory phase.

The normal uterus has well-defined contours and a pear-shaped configuration. The uterine shape, contour and internal texture should be carefully evaluated in every patient because minor pathological changes can change some of the characteristics of the normal uterus before their clear visualization and distinction. The vagina can also be easily identified as a midline structure. The mucosal attachment of the vagina produces a strong, thin linear echo which can be easily seen in longitudinal section.

Congenital uterine anomalies can cause numerous clinical symptoms such as dysmenorrhea, metrorrhagia, repeated spontaneous abortions and infertility. Sonographically it is possible to detect accurately all kinds of uterine anomalies, even minor abnormalities such as uterus arcuatus. The diagnosis of uterine abnormalities is based on clear visualization of the uterine cavity echo in transverse section. In cases involving a suspected uterine anomaly the examination should be performed in the secretory

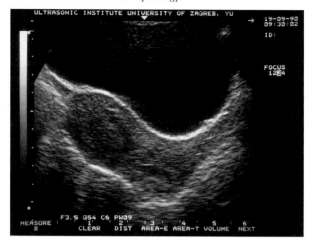

Figure 15.1 The scan of a normal uterus and vagina. The uterus is anteverted and the fundus is more anterior than the cervix. The uterine fundus is larger than the cervix

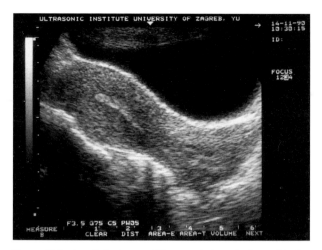

Figure 15.2 Longitudinal scan of the normal uterus in the proliferative part of the menstrual cycle

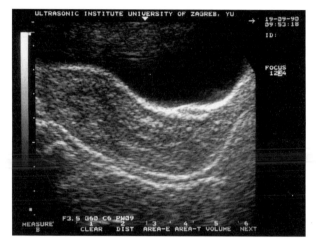

Figure 15.3 Longitudinal scan of the uterus in the luteal part of the menstrual cycle

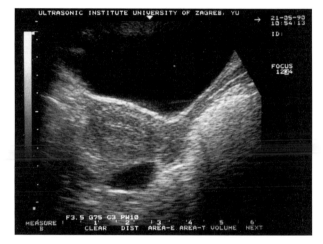

Figure 15.4 Typical finding in the case of retroverted uterus. Corpus and fundus are more posterior in comparison with cervix and vagina

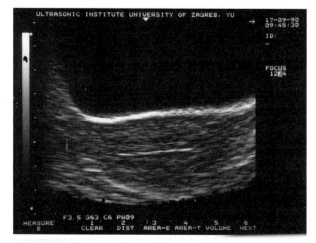

Figure 15.5 Transverse sonogram of a normal uterus. The contour is clearly outlined and the texture displays homogeneous and moderate echogenicity. The central cavity echo is clearly visible

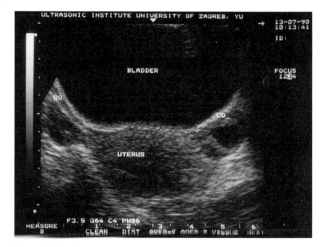

Figure 15.6 Another example of the normal uterus. Both ovaries (LO and RO) are seen in close proximity to the uterus

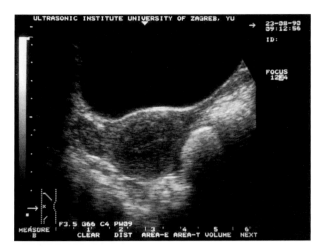

Figure 15.7 Transverse scan of the normal uterus in the early proliferative part of menstrual cycle

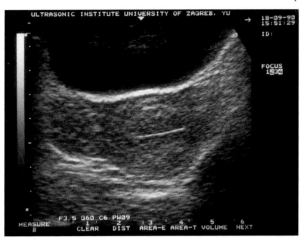

Figure 15.8 The uterus in the late proliferative part of menstrual cycle; central endometrial echo is clearly visible

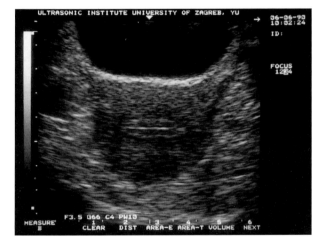

Figure 15.9 Preovulatory ring is a typical sign of forthcoming ovulation

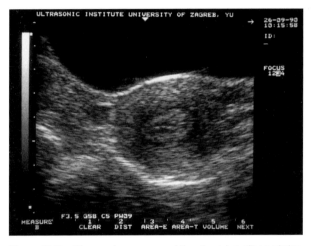

Figure 15.10 Ultrasound appearance of the uterus just after ovulation; endometrium is thin and echogenic

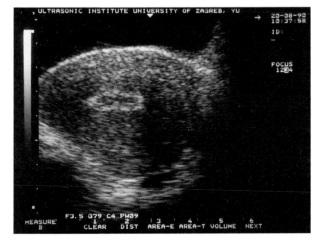

Figure 15.11 The uterus in the early secretory part of menstrual cycle; endometrium is easily visualized

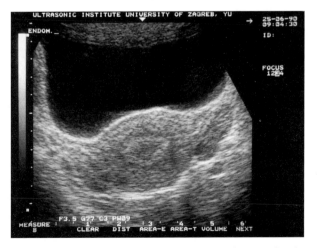

Figure 15.12 The uterus in the late secretory part of menstrual cycle; endometrium is still thin but not so echogenic

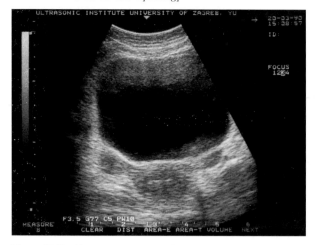

Figure 15.13 Transverse sonogram of a normal prepubertal uterus: the uterus is considerably smaller than in the generative age. Both ovaries are also visualized

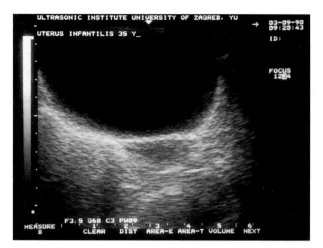

Figure 15.14 Infantile uterus in 35-year-old infertile patient

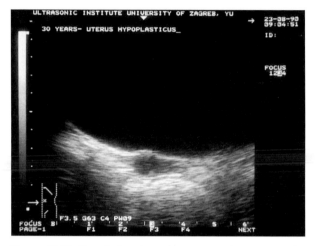

Figure 15.15 Hypoplastic uterus in a case of severe ovarian insufficiency. The endometrium is hardly recognizable

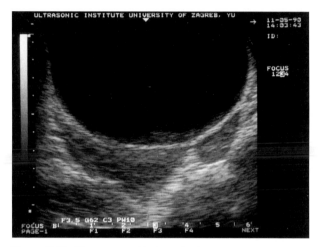

Figure 15.16 The uterus and both ovaries in menopausal patient. The uterus is significantly smaller than in generative period

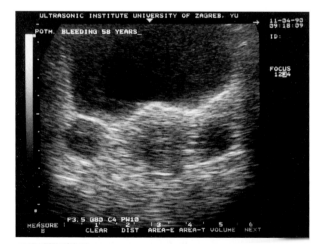

Figure 15.17 Postmenopausal uterus and ovaries

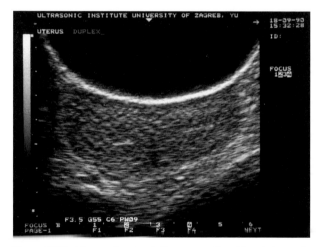

Figure 15.18 Uterus subseptus: in the upper portion of the uterine cavity the separation of the unique endometrial echo is visible. The displayed uterine septum is of similar echogenicity as compared to the myometrium

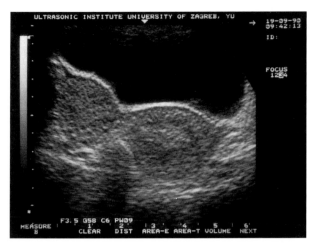

Figure 15.19 Uterus bicornis unicollis: the transverse section displays two distinct cavities and two separate uterine horns

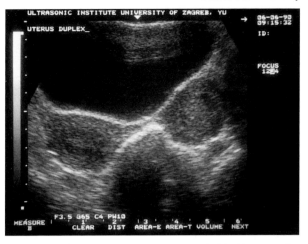

Figure 15.20 Transverse sonogram of the uterus didelphis: two uterine bodies and two separate uterine cavities are demonstrated

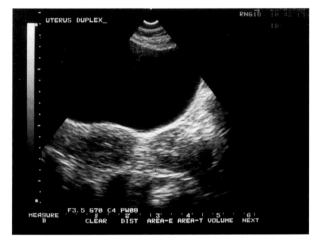

Figure 15.21 Sonogram of uterus bicornis with an atretic left horn

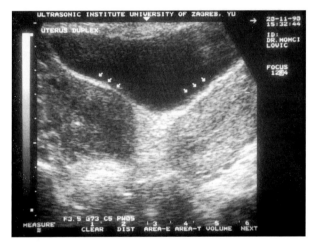

Figure 15.22 Uterus duplex: two complete, separate uteri are visualized

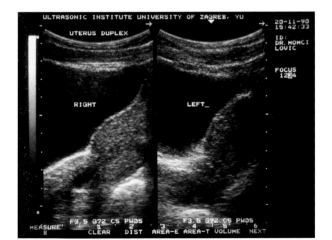

Figure 15.23 The same patient: left and right uterus visualized on a longitudinal scan

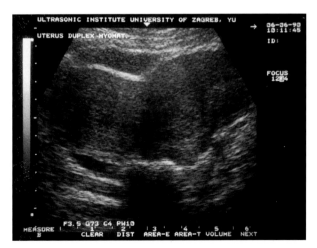

Figure 15.24 Typical appearance of myomatosus uterus duplex: both uteri are of inhomogeneous texture

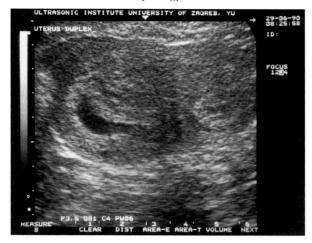

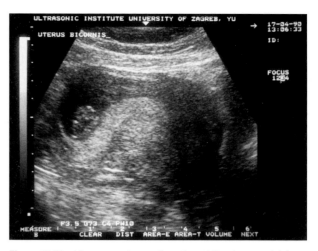

Figure 15.25 Transverse sonogram of a 5-week gestation showing the gestational sac in the right horn of a bicornuate uterus. The left horn is empty with pseudogestational endometrial reaction

Figure 15.26 Uterus arcuatus: an 8-week gestational sac containing a normally developed embryo is observed in the right horn. The left horn is empty

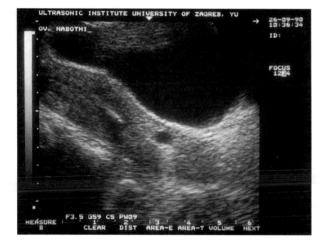

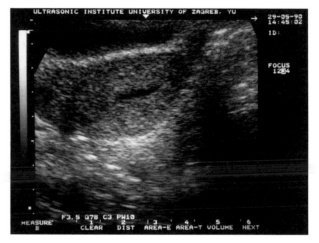

Figure 15.27 Small anechogenic structure detected in the cervical part of the uterus representing Nabothian cyst

Figure 15.28 Transverse scan of the uterus: typical appearance of intrauterine bleeding

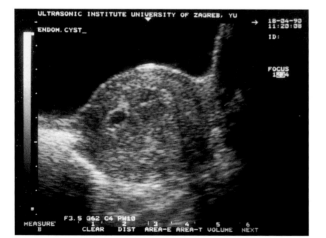

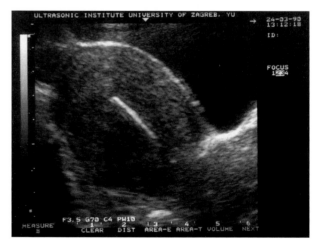

Figure 15.29 Endometrial cyst: it should not be mistaken for an early intrauterine gestation

Figure 15.30 Transverse sonogram of the uterus showing a correctly placed intrauterine device (IUD)

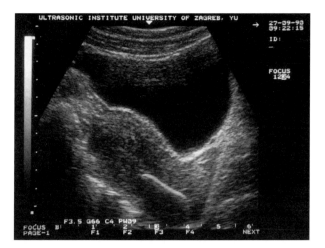

Figure 15.31   Partially expelled IUD

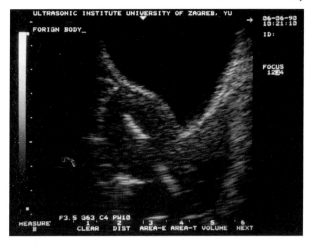

Figure 15.32   Foreign intrauterine body detected on longitudinal scan of the uterus

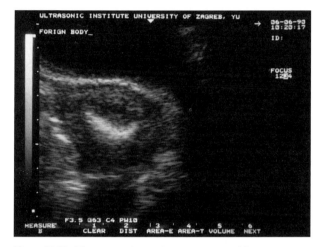

Figure 15.33   The same patient and transverse scan of the uterus

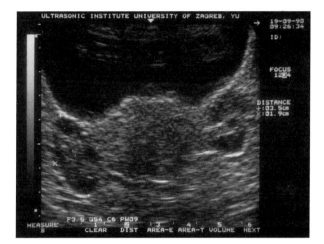

Figure 15.34   Transverse scan showing a normal uterus and both ovaries. The ovaries are of ovoid or fusiform shape, and display a lower echogenicity as compared to the uterus. Small cyst affecting ovarian texture homogenicity can be seen almost regularly

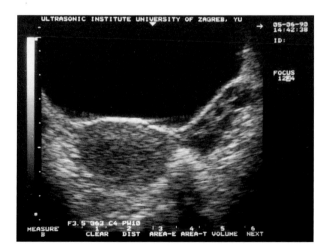

Figure 15.35   The oblique scan through the left ovary exhibits a normal shape and texture. Developing follicles are also demonstrated

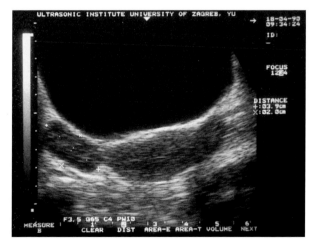

Figure 15.36   Normal-sized right ovary

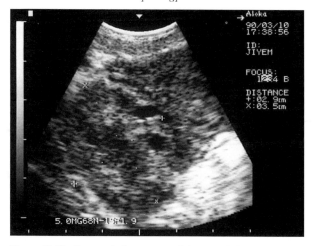

Figure 15.37 Transvaginal sonogram of the normal-sized right ovary: better resolution is one of the major advantages of the transvaginal approach

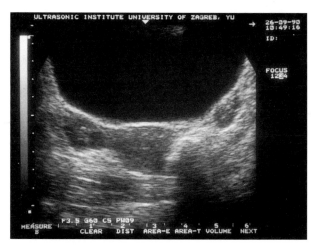

Figure 15.38 Transverse scan of the normal prepubertal uterus and both ovaries which are smaller than in the generative period

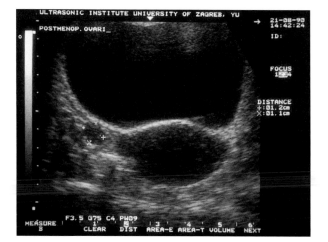

Figure 15.39 Normal postmenopausal ovary is smaller than in the generative period

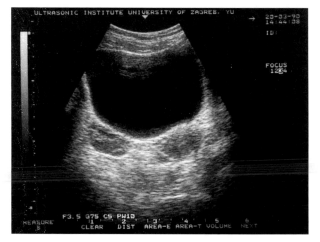

Figure 15.40 Both ovaries are visualized in a patient after hysterectomy

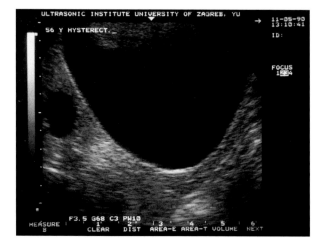

Figure 15.41 Small cyst was detected in the right ovary after hysterectomy and left adnexectomy

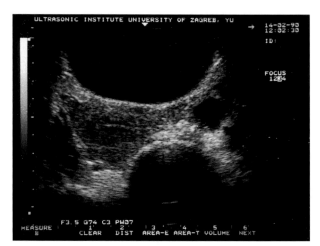

Figure 15.42 Transverse sonogram of the uterus and the left ovary showing a developing follicle. The follicle appears as a small, round cystic structure with well-defined walls and clear fluid within

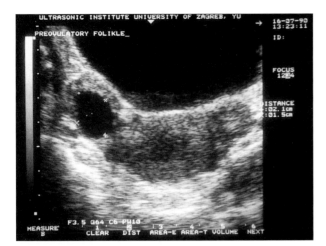

Figure 15.43 Typical finding of the preovulatory follicle

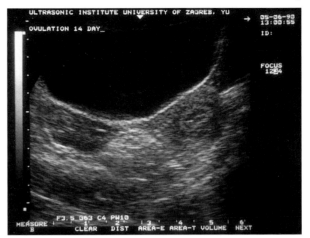

Figure 15.44 Disappearance of the follicle just after ovulation

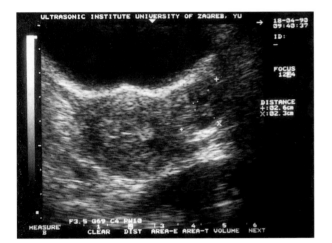

Figure 15.45 Corpus luteum on the left ovary

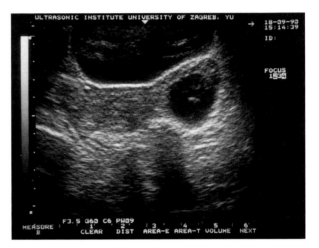

Figure 15.46 Corpus luteum cyst on the left ovary

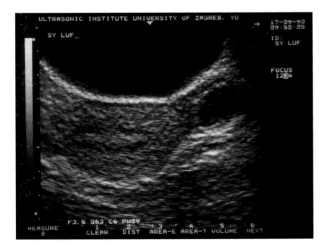

Figure 15.47 A case of luteinized unruptured follicle syndrome: ultrasound monitoring of follicular growth revealed complete luteinization of the preovulatory follicles and acyclic follicular persistence

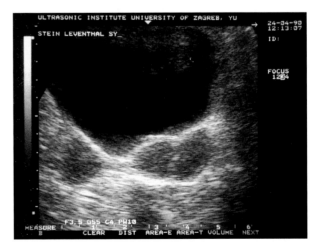

Figure 15.48 Stein–Leventhal syndrome: transverse sonogram of a patient with amenorrhea and hirsutism. Both ovaries are enlarged and polycystic. The uterus is small and the transverse uterine diameter is smaller than the longitudinal ovarian diameter

phase of the cycle when the endometrium is highly echogenic and clearly visualized. The uterine anomaly is then recognized as the presence of two separate uterine cavities (uterus bicornis, uterus duplex) or as the splitting of the single endometrial echo in the upper portions of the uterus in transverse section (uterus arcuatus) (Figures 15.18–15.33).

Other uterine abnormalities include endometrial polyps and hyperplasia which are demonstrated as a highly echogenic and thick endometrium. The diagnosis of Nabothian cysts which appear as small anechoic cysts close to the endocervical canal is useful in cases of high cyst which cannot be detected on vaginal examination.

Foreign bodies and intrauterine contraceptive devices are easily demonstrated by ultrasound. The characteristic finding is the presence of high-level echoes and posterior shadowing.

SONOGRAPHY OF THE ADNEXAL REGION

The pelvic soft tissue structures are examined by direct contact scanning through the abdominal wall or by transvaginal sonography (Figures 15.34–15.41). For detailed visualization of pelvic structures the urinary bladder should be fully distended. Adequate filling is usually achieved by a water load given orally to the patient 1–2 h prior to the examination, although occasionally diuretics or retrograde filling of the bladder through catheterization may be necessary. Assessment of pelvic pathology should not be made sonographically without definite identification of the bladder. Transvaginal sonography does not require full bladder techniques.

The adnexa consists of the broad ligament, Fallopian tubes and ovaries. The broad ligament and Fallopian tubes cannot be clearly distinguished by ultrasound under physiological conditions. The ovaries are seen in 95–99% of cases by serial transverse scans. The location of the ovaries is extremely variable in normal patients because of their flexible attachment to the uterus and lateral pelvic wall. This is the reason why it is quite unusual to demonstrate both ovaries in one transverse section. If the uterus is inclined to the right or left one ovary is seen close to or even behind the uterus, while the contralateral one is positioned relatively far and laterally at a variable distance. In cases of retroflected uterus the ovaries are typically located anteriorly and superiorly to the uterine fundus.

Ovarian size can be measured from the

ultrasonogram with reasonable accuracy. Ovaries are considered to measure less than one-half the size of the normal uterus and if greater than 30 mm in two axes they are considered enlarged. Ovarian enlargement is seen with cysts, cystic tumors, solid tumors, ovarian hematoma and, rarely, massive edema of the ovary.

The ovaries are generally hypoechoic as compared to the uterus because of multiple small follicles present in the cortical area. The medulla and capsule exhibit a higher echogenicity as compared to the cortex. The growing follicle is easily demonstrated as a hypoechoic, cystic structure within the ovarian tissue, with a well-defined wall and a characteristic daily growth rate.

Detection of ovulation

This is essential for the treatment of infertility. In the past ovulation could only be detected by a hormone profile. Now, however, ultrasound is an accepted diagnostic method in this field. Serial ultrasound assessment of ovarian follicular growth is an accurate, rapid, non-invasive technique for use in intensive investigation of patients complaining of infertility. The ultrasonic changes seen are:

(1) Demonstration of growing follicles with measurement of their number and size.

(2) Demonstration of intrafollicular structures – cumulus oophorus, corpus luteum.

(3) Demonstration of the uterine endometrial reaction to follicular growth.

(4) Quantitative flow measurement in ovarian and uterine vessels.

The commonest finding after ovulation is the disappearance of the follicle or its modification into an irregular and more solid structure representing the corpus luteum. (Figures 15.42–15.48).

READING LIST

1. Bernaschek, G. and Deutinger, J. (1989). Endosonography in obstetrics and gynecology: the importance of standardized image display. *Obstet. Gynecol.*, **74**, 917

2. Dodson, M.G. and Deter, R.L. (1990). Definition of anatomical planes for use in transvaginal sonography. *J. Clin. Ultrasound*, **18**, 239

3. Fleischer, A.C., Gordon, A.N., Entman, S.S. and

Kepple, D.M. (1990). Transvaginal scanning of the endometrium. *J. Clin. Ultrasound*, **18**, 337

4. Kurjak, A. (1986). *Atlas of Ultrasonography in Obstetrics and Gynecology*. (Zagreb: Mladost)

5. Kurjak, A. and Zalud, I. (1991). Female pelvis. In Kurjak, A., Fuckar, Z. and Gharbi, H. (eds.) *Atlas of Abdominal and Small Parts Ultrasonography*, pp.217–34. (Zagreb: Naprijed)

6. Lewit, N., Thaler, I. and Rottem, S. (1990). The uterus: a new look with transvaginal sonography. *J. Clin. Ultrasound*, **18**, 331

7. Mendelson, E.B., Bohm-Velez, M., Joseph, N. and Neiman, H.L. (1988). Gynecologic imaging: comparison of transabdominal and transvaginal sonography. *Radiology*, **166**, 321

8. Sanders, R.C. (ed.) (1985). *The Principles and Practice of Ultrasonography in Obstetrics and Gynecology*. (Norwalk: Appleton Century Crofts)

9. Timor-Tritsch, I.E. and Rottem, S. (1991). *Transvaginal Sonography*, 2nd edn. (New York, Amsterdam, London: Elsevier)

10. Timor-Tritsch, I.E. and Rottem, S. (1988). Review of transvaginal ultrasonography: a description with clinical application. *Ultrasound Q.*, **6**, 1

16 Adnexal Tumors

A. Kurjak and I. Zalud

Sonography has an important role in the evaluation of a patient with a suspected or palpable pelvic mass. The list below summarizes features of a pelvic mass that are clinically relevant and that can be determined by sonography:

(1)   Origin, size and location of pelvic mass;

(2)   Internal consistency;

(3)   Definition of walls; and

(4)   The presence or absence of ascites or other metastatic lesions.

Prediction of whether or not a mass is benign or malignant according to its sonographic appearance is only moderately reliable.

The commonest anomaly of the ovaries recognized by ultrasound is the polycystic ovary (Figures 16.1–16.4). The ovaries are regularly enlarged and filled with numerous small cysts measuring 3–8 mm in diameter. If polycystic ovaries are associated with amenorrhea, hirsutism and uterine hypoplasia, the ultrasonic finding is highly indicative of Stein–Leventhal syndrome.

In clinical practice, adnexal tumors are most commonly divided into four categories based on the complexity of tumor appearance. Every category has a relative specificity and should always be viewed within the framework of other clinical findings.

A completely cystic adnexal mass represents the first category and is defined according to the following criteria: anechoic cyst content, well-defined walls of varying thickness and posterior acoustic enhancement. The commonest type of adnexal mass which meets these criteria is the functional ovarian cyst (Figures 16.5 and 16.6). These cysts originate from the unruptured follicle or from the corpus luteum and are unilateral with a smooth, thin wall. Their size rarely exceeds 10 cm and normal ovarian tissue can be seen along part of the cyst wall. Paraovarian cysts which develop from Gartner's duct have the same appearance as functional cysts and are only occasionally distinguishable from them. Paraovarian cysts can measure only 2–3 cm, but more often grow to be quite large. Hydrosalpinx (Figures 16.7–16.12) and tubo-ovarian abscesses (Figures 16.13–16.25) often appear as a cystic mass. A smaller hydrosalpinx usually assumes a fusiform shape (Figure 16.8), but if large it is of a rather round shape (Figure 16.9). A tubo-ovarian abscess can ˙ be differentiated from hydrosalpinx by the demonstration of ovarian tissue incorporated within the abscess wall.

The second morphological group of adnexal masses comprises predominantly cystic structures containing internal echoes such as septa, solid tissue, or any other echogenic material. The commonest adnexal mass in this group is ovarian cystadenoma (Figures 16.26–16.37). Serous and mucinous cystadenomas are the commonest ovarian epithelial tumors, having a very specific ultrasonic appearance. They are usually large with echogenic, linear, internal septa which are more pronounced in the mucinous type. Dermoid cysts appear extremely variable, but a cystic mass containing a cone of solid tissue with a highly echogenic focus and posterior shadowing is a pathognomonic finding. Tubo-ovarian abscesses can contain echoes or fluid levels representing the layering of purulent debris, whereas endometriomas (Figures 16.38–16.41) contain echogenic blood clots.

Complex tumors with a dominant solid component include most of the masses listed in the previous category such as dermoid cysts (Figures 16.42 and 16.43), ectopic pregnancy, endometriosis (Figures 16.44 and 16.45) and cystadenomas. Other ovarian neoplasms, e.g. endometrioid carcinoma, clear cell carcinoma, dysgerminoma, granulosa cell and Sertoli–Leydig cell tumors, exhibit a solid, partly cystic ultrasonic appearance.

Solid ovarian tumors are included in the fourth category (Figures 16.46–16.76). The commonest tumor types being solid are malignant teratoma and adenocarcinoma. Non-genital metastatic tumors can also be demonstrated as solid adnexal masses.

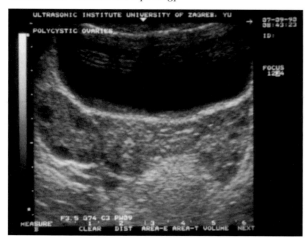

Figure 16.1 Typical appearance of polycystic ovaries

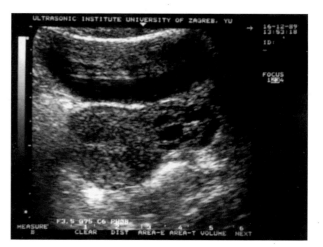

Figure 16.2 Enlarged and polycystic left ovary

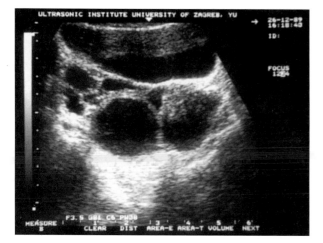

Figure 16.3 Large polycystic ovary

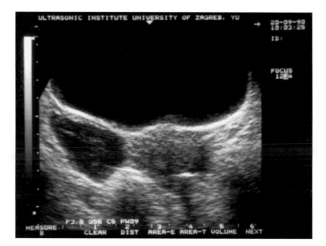

Figure 16.4 Enlarged microcystic right ovary

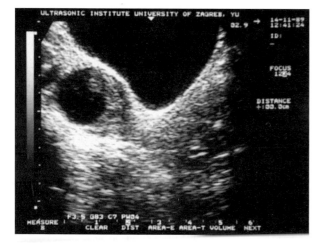

Figure 16.5 Simple follicular cyst in the right ovary: the patient was referred for ultrasound detection of ovulation, but the follicle did not rupture and developed into a cyst

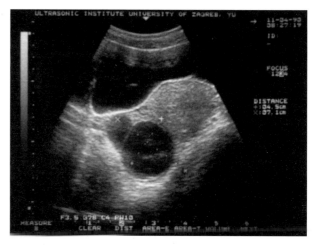

Figure 16.6 Large cyst in the right ovary: the cyst is simple, bilocular with thin and well-defined borders and no internal echoes. A case of physiological ovarian cyst

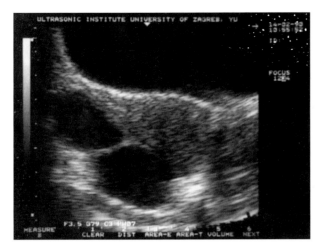

Figure 16.7 Hydrosalpinx: the sonogram displays a cystic, bilocular structure (right) with no internal echoes and a fusiform shape typical of hydrosalpinx

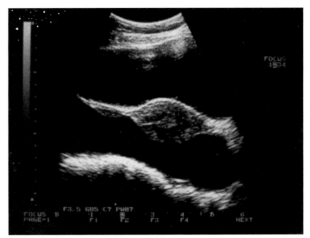

Figure 16.8 Hydrosalpinx presenting a fusiform shape

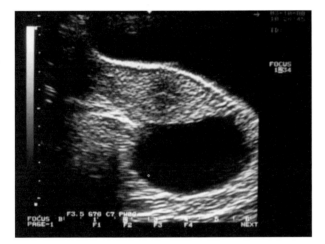

Figure 16.9 Hydrosalpinx (left) presenting a rounded shape

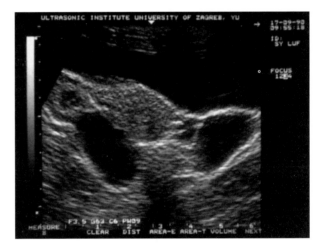

Figure 16.10 Bilateral hydrosalpinx

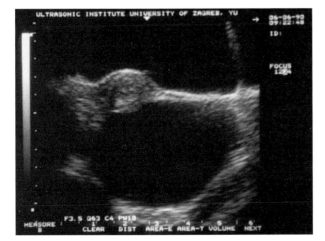

Figure 16.11 Extremely dilated left Fallopian tube

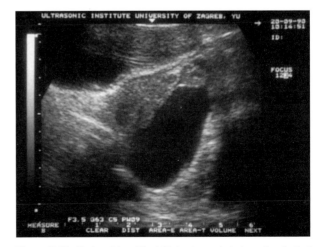

Figure 16.12 Hydrosalpinx of the left tube demonstrated on a longitudinal scan

173

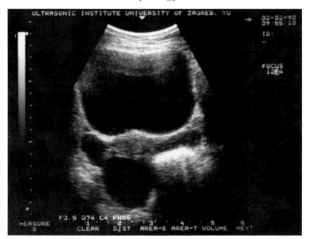

Figure 16.13 Sonogram demonstrating a purulent accumulation in the pouch of Douglas after abdominal surgery

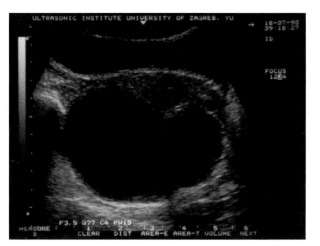

Figure 16.14 Transverse sonogram showing a large tubo-ovarian abscess occupying the pouch of Douglas

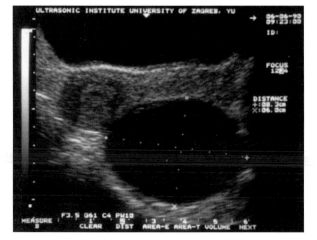

Figure 16.15 Large abscess displacing the uterus in the cul-de-sac

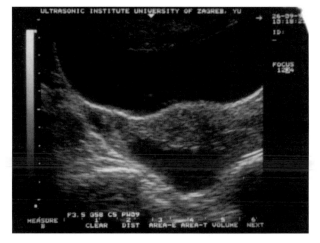

Figure 16.16 Pyosalpinx appearing as a fusiform structure on the right. Note the irregularities of the cyst wall and internal echoes

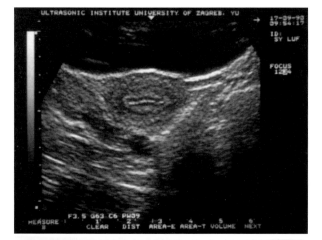

Figure 16.17 Chronic tubal inflammation

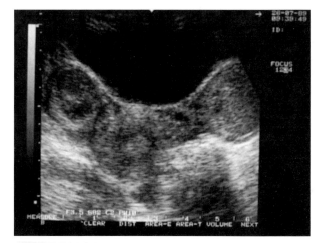

Figure 16.18 Subacute adnexitis: the uterus can be distinguished from the structures in the left and right adnexal regions. The formation of a tubo-ovarian abscess has started

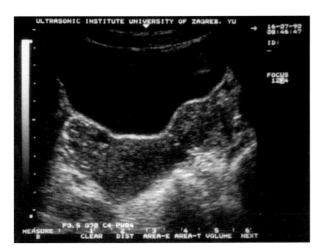

Figure 16.19 Acute pelvic inflammation: the transverse sonogram demonstrates a large complex solid, cystic mass in both adnexal regions. The uterine contour can hardly be distinguished from the structure

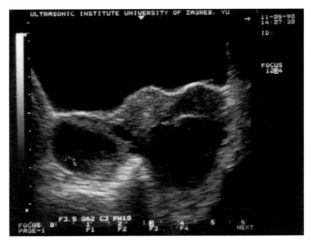

Figure 16.20 Bilateral acute adnexitis: note the formation of complex masses on both sides of the uterus which can hardly be outlined. The ovaries can not be visualized

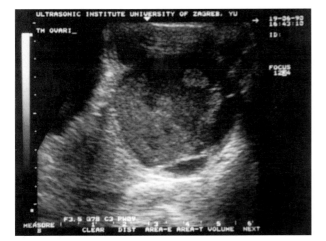

Figure 16.21 Oblique sonogram showing a large tubo-ovarian abscess left and above the uterus

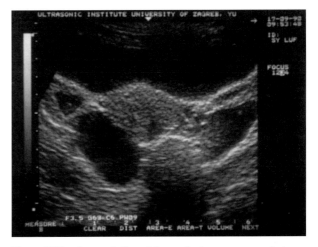

Figure 16.22 Abscess in the cul-de-sac: the transverse scan displays a cystic structure with low-level internal echoes

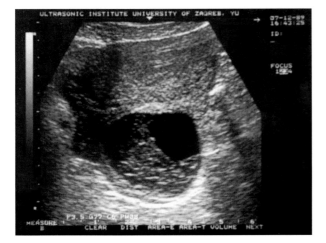

Figure 16.23 Longitudinal sonogram exhibiting the complex internal structure of the tubo-ovarian abscess

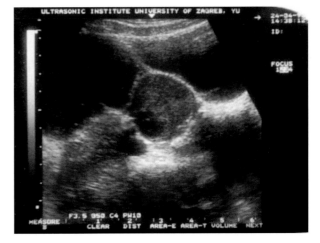

Figure 16.24 The large echogenic tumor on the left represents a large tubo-ovarian abscess occupying the pouch of Douglas and fixed bowel loops in a patient suffering from chronic pelvic infection

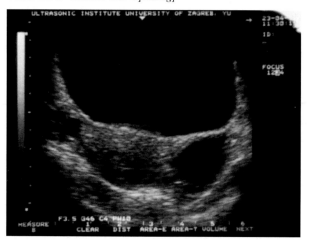

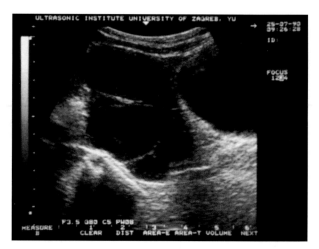

Figure 16.25 Tubo-ovarian abscess (left): unilocular cystic structure appearing as a follicular cyst at first sight; however, wall irregularities and thickness are pathognomonic of abscess and cannot be observed in case involving simple cyst

Figure 16.26 Mucinous cystadenoma exhibiting the characteristics of a complex, predominantly cystic ovarian mass

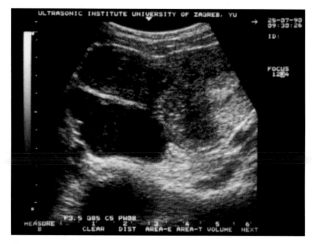

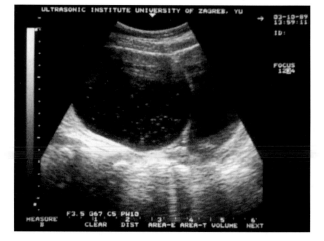

Figure 16.27 Mucinous cystadenoma (right) resembling a cyst with a well-defined septum

Figure 16.28 Middle-sized mucinous cystadenoma with well-defined septum on a longitudinal scan

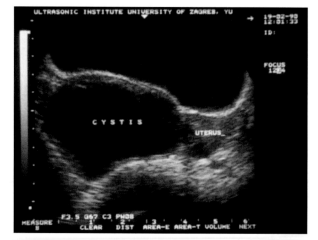

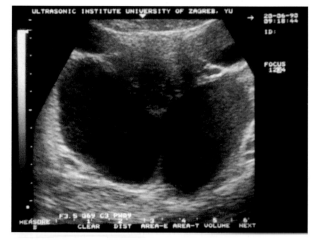

Figure 16.29 Mucinous adenoma (right) of fusiform shape

Figure 16.30 Bilocular cystadenoma

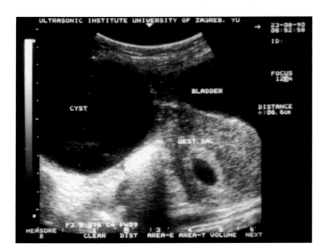

Figure 16.31 Large cystadenoma (right) in the 5th week of gestation: gestation sac is seen below bladder

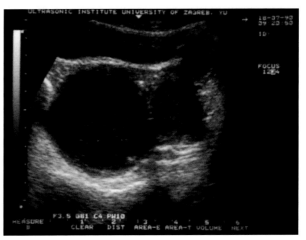

Figure 16.32 Papillary serous cystadenoma: the sonogram shows a large complex predominantly cystic mass

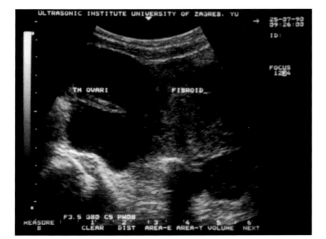

Figure 16.33 Uterine fibroma and serous cystadenoma with septum on the right ovary

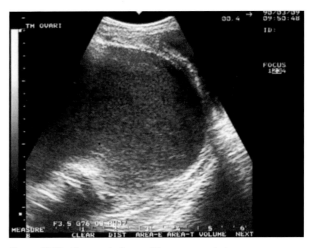

Figure 16.34 Transvaginal scan of the serous cystadenoma

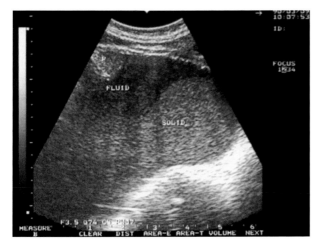

Figure 16.35 Transvaginal scan of complex adnexal mass with solid part, fluid and papillary proliferation

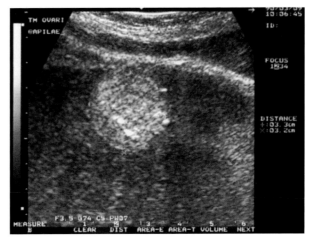

Figure 16.36 The same patient showing papillary proliferation

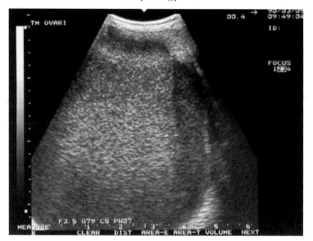

Figure 16.37 Mucinous cystadenoma detected by transvaginal ultrasound

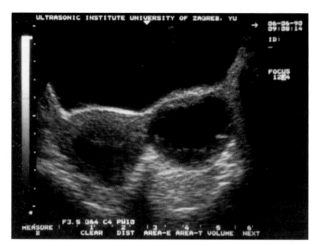

Figure 16.38 Large endometrioma (left) with pronounced internal echoes: such a finding cannot be distinguished from a tubo-ovarian abscess and the diagnosis was made on laparotomy

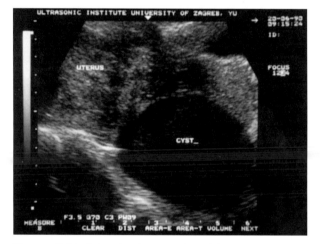

Figure 16.39 Extremely large endometriotic cyst which is indistinguishable from a large hydrosalpinx because of its round shape, absence of internal echoes and wall thickness

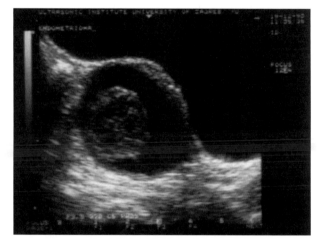

Figure 16.40 Another example of an endometriotic cyst with clearly visible intracystic echoes

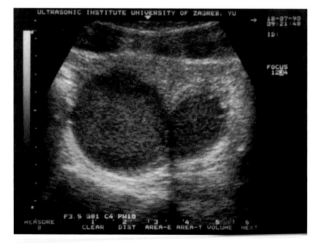

Figure 16.41 Two endometriotic cysts with high-level internal echoes

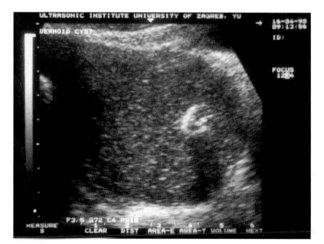

Figure 16.42 A dermoid tumor of completely solid appearance on the transverse sonogram: the strong echo represents the teeth and is a common finding typical of this tumor type

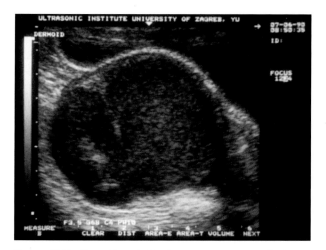

Figure 16.43 Dermoid cyst: the transverse sonogram displays a complex, predominantly solid tumor on the left. Note the echogenicity of the solid tumor parts

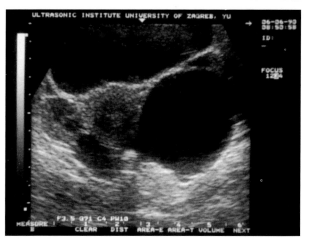

Figure 16.44 Endometriosis: transverse sonogram showing a large cyst in the left and a smaller one in the right ovary. Note the presence of an additional small cyst in the retrouterine space

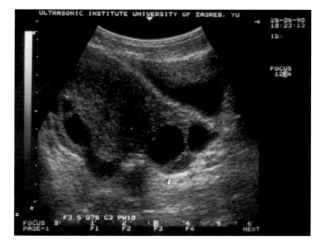

Figure 16.45 A case of endometriosis with an irregular cyst in the retrouterine region and two small cysts in the left ovary: small intraovarian endometriotic cysts sometimes cannot be distinguished from developing follicles and a proper diagnosis can be made only by monitoring follicular growth and ovulation

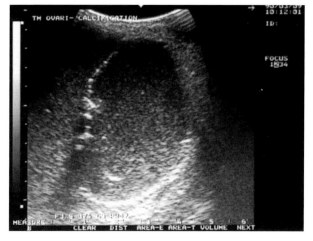

Figure 16.46 Calcification of the septum

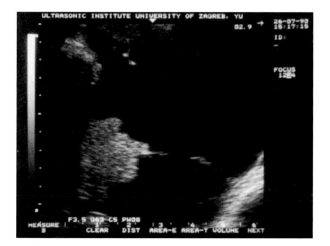

Figure 16.47 Bizarre appearance of adnexal mass: however, benign nature was confirmed on histopathology

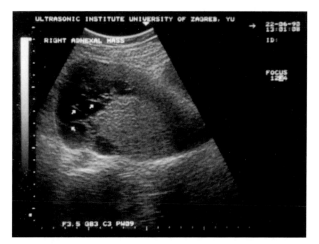

Figure 16.48 Complex adnexal mass of the right ovary: septa indicated by arrows

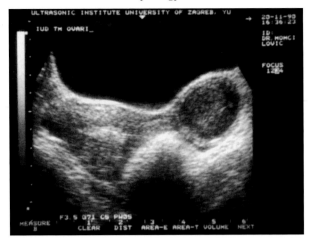

Figure 16.49 Predominantly solid ovarian tumor and an intrauterine device

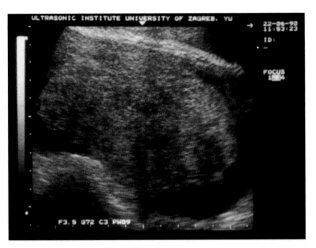

Figure 16.50 Large solid adnexal mass with hypoechoic area on the periphery representing hemorrhage

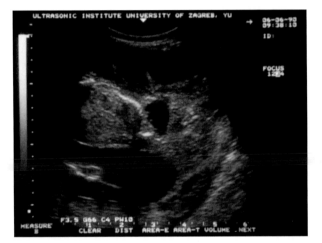

Figure 16.51 Large complex adnexal mass with necrosis, hemorrhage and calcifications

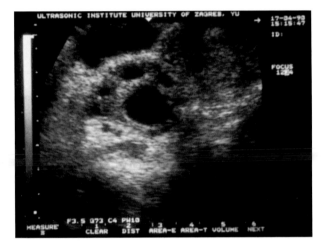

Figure 16.52 Minimally enlarged cystic right ovary

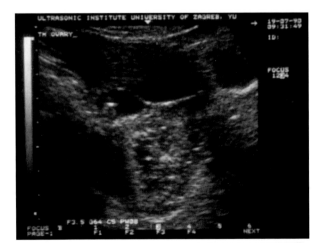

Figure 16.53 Benign ovarian tumor with secondary changes

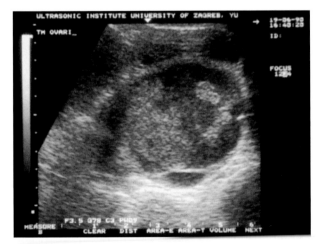

Figure 16.54 Benign ovarian tumor with papillary proliferations

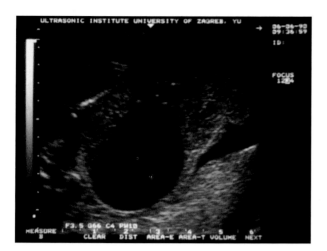

Figure 16.55 Unilocular ovarian mass and free fluid in cavum Douglasi

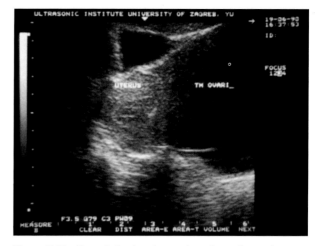

Figure 16.56 Hypoechoic adnexal mass situated very close to the uterus

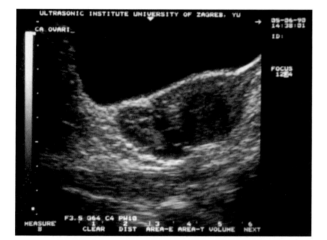

Figure 16.57 Minimally enlarged right ovary in clinically healthy postmenopausal woman; cystadenocarcinoma grade Ia was diagnosed on histopathology

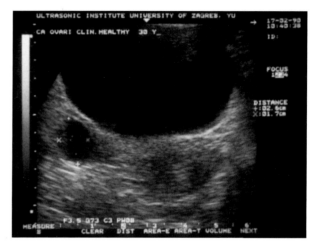

Figure 16.58 Another example of the initial stage of ovarian carcinoma in an otherwise clinically healthy 30-year-old woman: only a small cyst was detected in the right ovary. Such a finding is indistinguishable from benign ovarian lesions

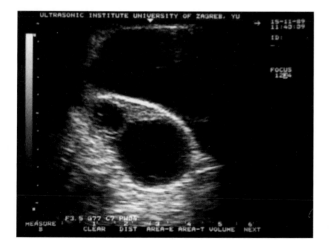

Figure 16.59 An oblique scan of slightly enlarged left ovary with bilocular cyst with smooth and regular walls. There was no typical finding for ovarian malignancy

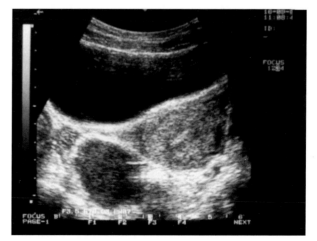

Figure 16.60 Minimally enlarged and solid right ovary: ovarian cancer was diagnosed on histopathology

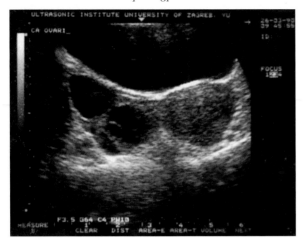

Figure 16.61 Ovarian cancer presented as multilocular cystic right ovary

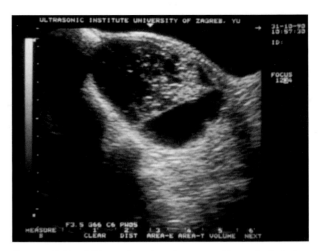

Figure 16.62 Solid cystic adnexal mass with marked texture irregularities: the diagnosis of ovarian malignancy was confirmed after surgery

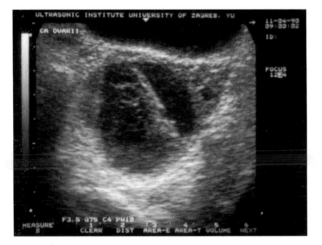

Figure 16.63 Malignant teratoma of the left ovary: note the pronounced echogenicity of the predominantly solid tumor detected in a young patient

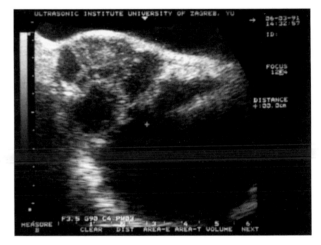

Figure 16.64 A case of ovarian cancer associated with ascites

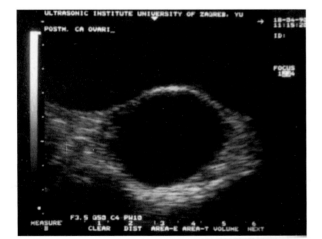

Figure 16.65 Cystic ovarian tumor in postmenopausal woman proved to be a cancer

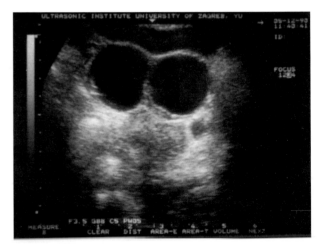

Figure 16.66 Bilocular ovarian cyst: ovarian cancer was diagnosed on histopathology

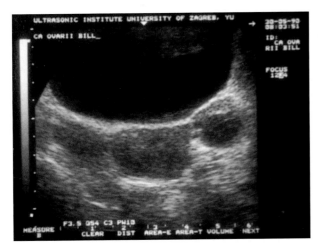

Figure 16.67 Bilateral ovarian cancer diagnosed at an early stage

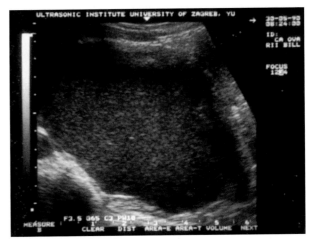

Figure 16.68 Cystadenocarcinoma: the large cystic tumor in the left adnexal region could not be differentiated from mucinous cystadenoma

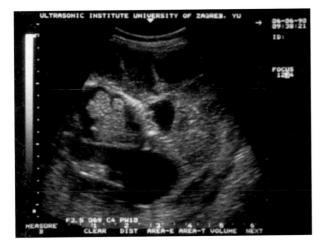

Figure 16.69 Bizarre appearance of an adnexal mass in a case of ovarian carcinoma

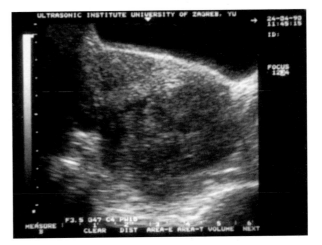

Figure 16.70 Adenocarcinoma of the left ovary appearing as a completely solid tumor

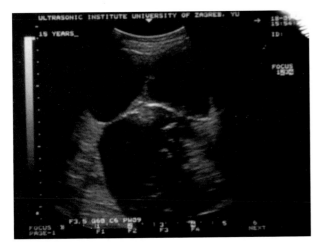

Figure 16.71 Irregularly shaped multilocular cystic structure with internal echoes representing a malignant teratoma

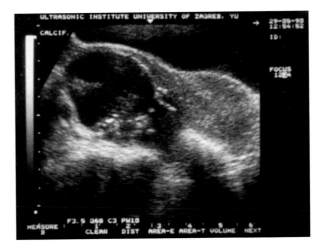

Figure 16.72 Metastatic ovarian mass: note the area of necrosis and calcification

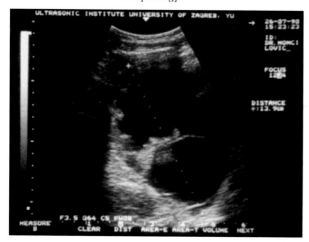

Figure 16.73 Bizarre appearance of adnexal mass: note papillary proliferations. The primary cancer was in the thyroid gland

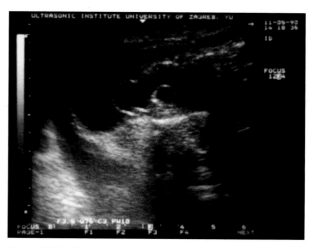

Figure 16.74 Metastatic rectal cancer detected in left adnexal region

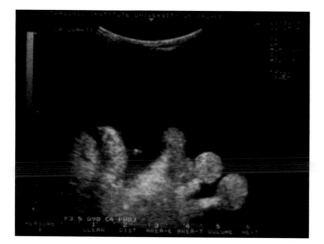

Figure 16.75 Metastatic ovarian cancer with pronounced papillary proliferations

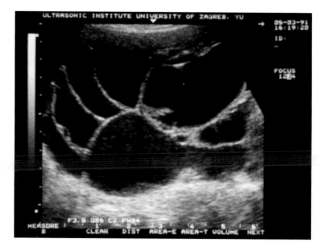

Figure 16.76 Different ultrasound appearance of the same ovarian cancer in the advanced stage

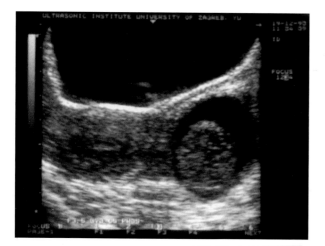

Figure 16.77 Chronic pelvic inflammation: the transverse scan shows an incapsulated abscess and bowel loops fixed by adhesions

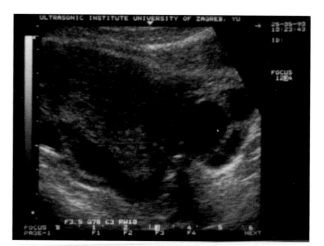

Figure 16.78 Longitudinal sonogram demonstrating complex solid cystic structures in both adnexal regions and occupying the pouch of Douglas in a patient with chronic pelvic inflammation. The adhesion led to bowel loop fixation in the lesser pelvis

Pelvic inflammatory disease (Figures 16.77 and 16.78) affects the normal appearance of pelvic anatomy considerably, particularly that of the adnexal region, and it should also be briefly outlined here even though the diagnosis of pelvic infection is primarily a clinical one. Pelvic adhesions can be recognized as slight thickenings of the adnexa and are rarely seen. The presence of pelvic adhesions is easily confirmed by the visualization of bowel loops within the lesser pelvis which can imitate the ovarian neoplasms and cannot be displaced even by an overdistended bladder.

The number of false-positive and false-negative sonograms in pelvic-mass assessment has been estimated to be less than 5%. The majority of errors in the sonographic evaluation of pelvic masses can be attributed to poor scanning technique (improper transducer angulation or gain settings), lesions that are below the scanning resolution of the equipment, or misinterpretation of bowel or pelvic masses. The information obtained by ultrasound is complementary to other radiographic studies for the complete evaluation of a patient prior to surgical intervention. When 'conservative' management is deemed appropriate, serial sonographic examinations can be performed to assess the enlargement or regression of a mass. It should be remembered that the major source of a wrong diagnosis in gynecology lies in the non-critical overinterpretation of ultrasonic findings.

READING LIST

1. Barber, H.R.K. (1984). Ovarian cancer: diagnosis and management. *Am. J. Obstet. Gynecol.*, **150**, 910

2. Bhan, V., Amso, N., Whitehead, M.I. *et al.* (1989). Characteristics of persistent ovarian masses in asymptomatic women. *Br. J. Obstet. Gynaecol.*, **96**, 1384

3. Campbell, S., Goessens, L., Goswamy, R. and Whitehead, M.I. (1982). Real-time ultrasonography for the determination of ovarian morphology and volume. A possible early screening test for ovarian cancer. *Lancet*, **1**, 425

4. Fleischer, A.C. (1988). Transvaginal sonography helps find ovarian cancer. *Diagn. Imaging*, **10**, 124

5. Jacobs, I.J., Stabile, I., Bridges, J. *et al.* (1988). Multimodal approach to screening for ovarian cancer. *Lancet*, **1**, 268

6. Moyle, J.W., Rochester, D., Sider, L. *et al.* (1983). Sonography of ovarian tumors: predictability of tumor type. *Am. J. Roentgenol.*, **141**, 985

7. Rottem, S., Levit, N., Thaler, I., Yoffe, N., Bronstein, M., Manor, D. and Brandes, J.M. (1990). Classification of ovarian lesions by high-frequency transvaginal sonography. *J. Clin. Ultrasound*, **18**, 359

8. Sharp, F., Mason, W.P. and Leake, R.E. (1990). *Ovarian Cancer*. (London: Chapman and Hall Medical)

17 Uterine Tumors

I. Zalud and A. Kurjak

Conventional B-mode ultrasound has improved the accuracy of clinical non-invasive diagnosis of uterine tumors. Uterine fibroids or leiomyoma are the commonest acquired uterine disorders (Figures 17.1–17.17). Fibroids can be found in more than 30% of women over the age of 35. These benign tumors are responsible for the wide spectrum of clinical complaints, e.g. menorrhagia, menstrual pain, acute pain if infarction occurs, pressure sensation, urinary retention or obstipation. Leiomyomas are usually multiple and they all originate out of the myometrium of the uterine body and fundus. Very rarely myomas are located in the cervix. Tumor growth can cause its displacement, and myomas are therefore classified as intramural, subserous, or submucous. Intramural tumors are the most common and submucosal the least common.

The diagnosis of uterine fibroma is based on texture changes, distortion of the uterine contour and uterine enlargement. The typical sonographic appearance of leiomyomas consists of mildly to moderately echogenic intrauterine masses that cause nodular distortion of the uterine outline. Small intramural or submucous leiomyomas may be recognized by their distortion of the normally linear central endometrial echoes. The solid nature of a fibroid often may cause an indentation on the bladder or rectum.

The echogenicity of a fibroid depends upon the relative ratio of fibrous tissue to smooth muscle. With a more fibrous component, there is increased echogenicity of the nodule. The sonographic texture of fibroids also depends on the type and presence of degeneration and upon the vascular supply. Uterine enlargement is a constant but not pathognomonic sign of uterine fibroma. Secondary tumor changes are very common (necrosis, hemorrhage, calcification or degeneration) and cause a wide spectrum of ultrasonic images.

The most common cause of calcification within the uterus is calcific degeneration within a fibroid. Twenty-five per cent of one series of 75 cases of fibroids had calcifications. The pattern of calcification varied from a few small foci to a large rim of globular calcification. Other types of degeneration within leiomyomas that produce sonographically recognizable changes in uterine texture include cystic, myxomatous and hyaline degeneration. Among these, hyaline degeneration is the most common and appears as anechoic areas within a fibroid.

Leiomyomas that are pendunculated can be confused with other adnexal masses if their pedicle is not visualized. The most common location of pedunculated leiomyomas is superior to the uterine fundus. Submucous leiomyomas may be difficult to differentiate from intramural leiomyomas. Fibroids may be particularly difficult to detect in the retroverted uterus. Because the uterine fundus curves posteriorly in the retroverted uterus, this area may appear to be relatively sonolucent.

Serial sonographic evaluation of leiomyomas can be of significant value to the clinician. Follow-up scans of the fibroid uterus of a pregnant woman may help assess the growth and accelerated degeneration of this mass. Since fibroids should regress after menopause, serial sonograms can objectively document enlargement or regression of leiomyomas in the older woman.

Adenomyosis or internal endometriosis is characterized by ingrowths of the endometrium into the myometrium (Figures 17.18–17.26). Adenomyosis is more often than not a diffuse process, but occasionally large adenomyomas can be seen. This condition can be diagnosed sonographically because of a thickened and 'Swiss cheese' appearance of the myometrium due to areas of hemorrhage and clotting within the muscle. The uterus is slightly enlarged, with small cystic structures which affect uterine texture homogenicity. The uterus can be generally hypoechoic, and sometimes large cysts are seen. The diagnosis of adenomyosis is more reliable when the uterine finding is associated with cysts of various sizes in the adnexal region or retrouterine space.

In ultrasonic terms uterine malignancies can hardly be distinguished from fibromas. Typical findings include uterine enlargement and non-homogeneous

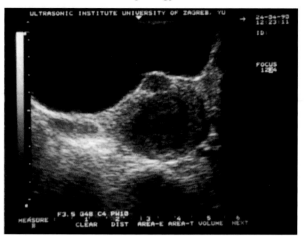

Figure 17.1 Small subserous myoma detected on anterior uterine border

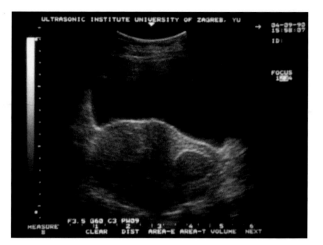

Figure 17.2 Multiple leiomyomas of the uterus affecting the normal shape and texture of the uterus: the uterus is of round shape and displays hypoechogenicity as compared to the normal myometrium. The uterine cavity is not recognizable

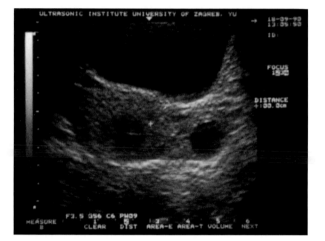

Figure 17.3 Necrotic myoma in the posterior uterine wall appearing as a cyst of similar characteristics to a cyst in the left ovary

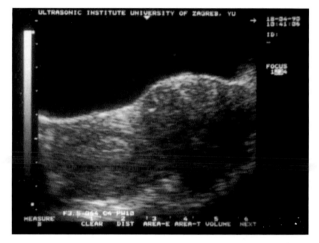

Figure 17.4 Uterine sonogram demonstrating the uterine body on the right and a subserous myoma (on the left) appearing as a solid adnexal tumor

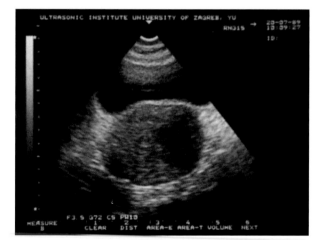

Figure 17.5 Moderately enlarged uterus with intramural myoma on the left side

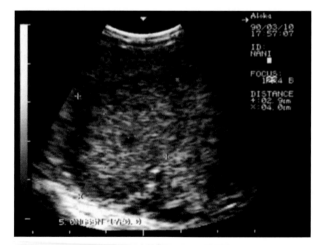

Figure 17.6 Large intramural myoma detected by transvaginal sonography

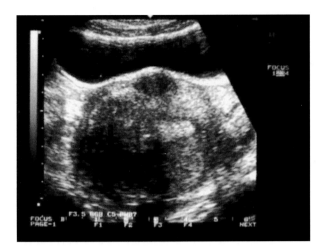

Figure 17.7 Small subserous (anterior) and very large intramural (on the right side) myomas

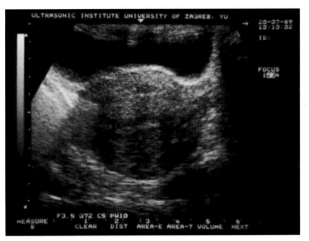

Figure 17.8 Enlarged uterus with numerous small myomas which affected normal uterine tissue

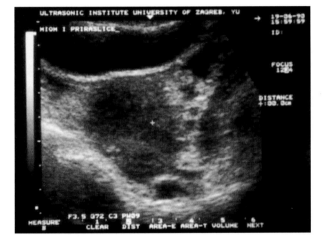

Figure 17.9 Myomatous uterus and chronic pelvic inflammatory disease presented by calcified synechias

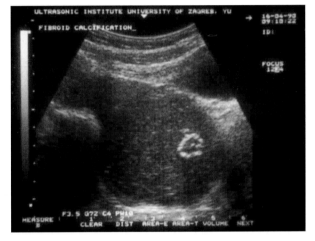

Figure 17.10 Intramural uterine myoma with marked calcifications on the surface of the tumor. Note the shadowing behind the calcifications

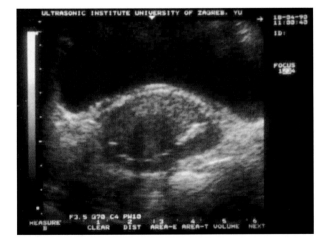

Figure 17.11 Numerous calcifications situated on the posterior uterine wall

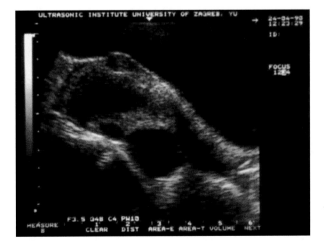

Figure 17.12 Necrotic myoma in the posterior uterine wall appearing as a cyst

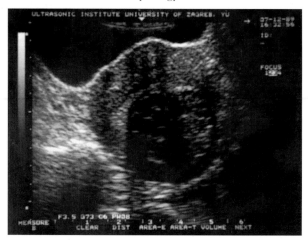

Figure 17.13 Intramural myoma appearing as a cyst because of calcifications on the anterior surface of the tumor which can be accidentally misinterpreted as adenomyoma

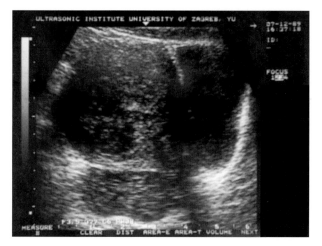

Figure 17.14 Large uterine myoma with secondary changes: degeneration, calcification and necrosis. The texture of the tumor is inhomogeneous and exhibits strong echoes with shadowing (calcifications) and irregular cystic areas (degeneration and necrosis)

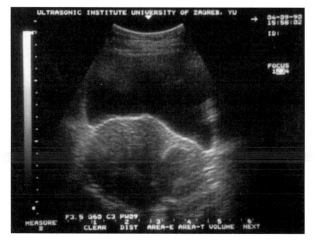

Figure 17.15 Subserous calcified myoma on the left uterine side

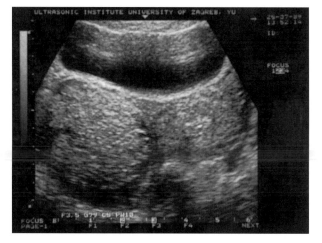

Figure 17.16 Lateral scan of a large pedunculated myoma shows secondary changes in the tumor

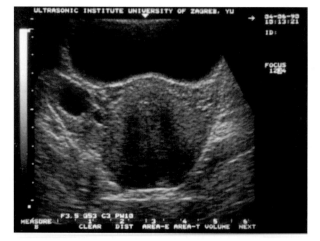

Figure 17.17 Multiple small necrotic intrauterine myomas

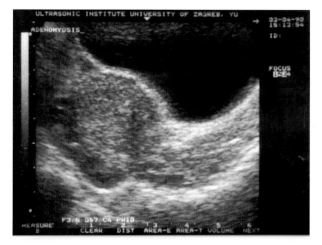

Figure 17.18 Adenomyosis: the uterus is hypoechoic and the homogenicity of uterine texture is affected by small cystic areas which contain blood

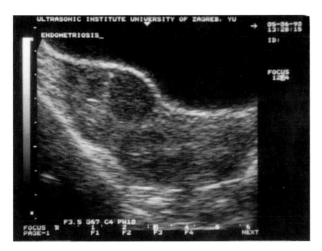

Figure 17.19 Adenomyosis uteri: a large adenomyoma can be observed in the anterior and posterior uterine walls

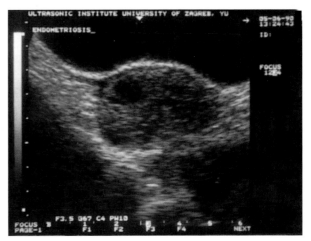

Figure 17.20 The same uterus on transverse scan

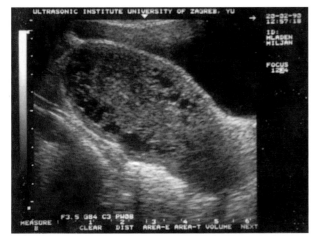

Figure 17.21 Another typical finding in the case of adenomyosis

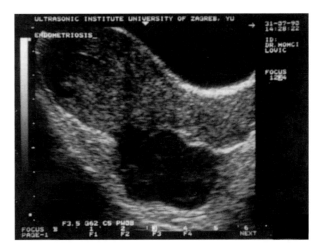

Figure 17.22 Typical finding of adenomyosis with endometriosis: the uterus is markedly hypoechoic and several large cysts are visible in the retrouterine space

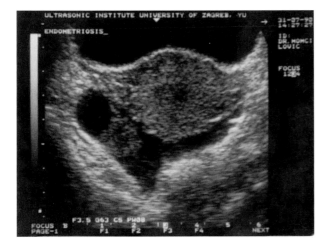

Figure 17.23 The same uterus on transverse scan

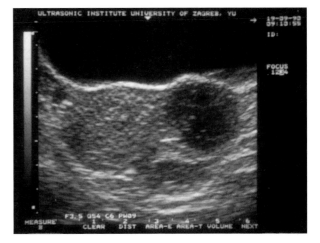

Figure 17.24 Endometriotic cyst in the left ovary associated with adenomyosis

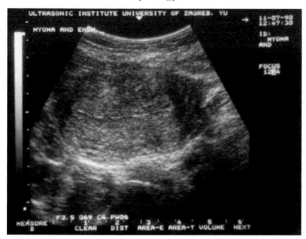

Figure 17.25   A case of uterine myoma associated with endometriosis

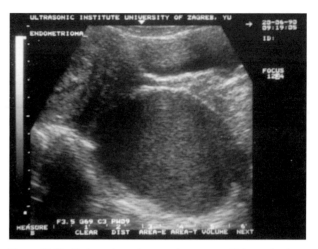

Figure 17.26   Endometrioma: large cystic structure with internal echoes visualized on the left side very close to the uterus

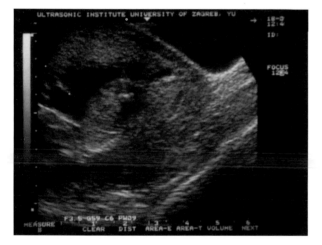

Figure 17.27 Extremely large uterine tumor with pronounced degeneration, necrosis and hemorrhage: the diagnosis of uterine sarcoma was confirmed on histopathology

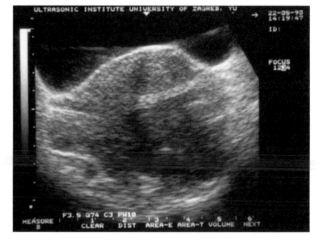

Figure 17.28   Uterine sarcoma: the texture of the tumor is irregular and almost half of the tumor tissue shows signs of necrosis and degeneration

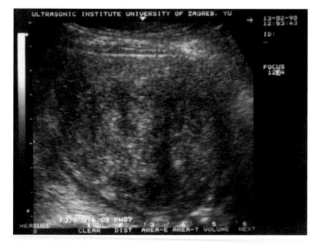

Figure 17.29 Sarcoma botryoides diagnosed in a 16-year-old girl: enlarged uterus with large areas of degeneration

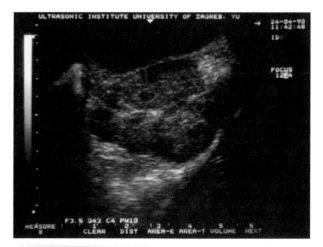

Figure 17.30   Malignant tumor has destroyed normal uterine tissue

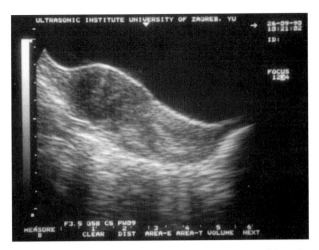

Figure 17.31 Example of malignant uterine tumor originated from the fundal part of the uterus

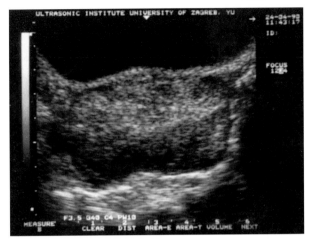

Figure 17.32 Example of advanced stage of cervical carcinoma

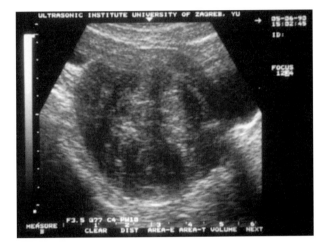

Figure 17.33 Endometrial carcinoma: large inhomo-geneous uterus, myometrium and endometrium could not be distinguished

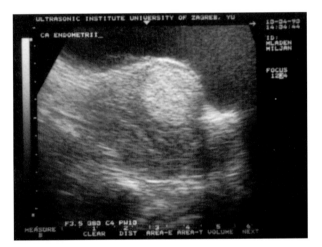

Figure 17.34 Hyperechogenic uterine mass representing endometrial cancer

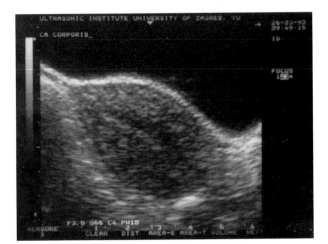

Figure 17.35 An example of initial stage of corporeal carcinoma: uterine texture is minimally affected

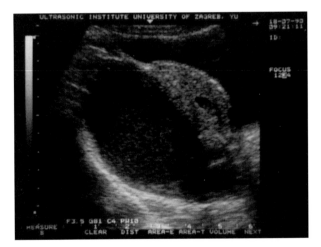

Figure 17.36 Advanced stage of corporeal carcinoma has destroyed normal uterine texture

tumor texture due to necrosis and other secondary changes (Figures 17.27–17.36). The commonest uterine malignancy is endometrial carcinoma which accounts for 90% of malignant uterine body growth. Postmenopausal bleeding associated with an ultrasound finding of uterine enlargement, thick endometrium and hypoechoic and non-homogeneous texture is highly suggestive of this malignancy. Uterine sarcomas are responsible for 3% of uterine malignancies. These tumors usually originate from leiomyomas and exhibit a similar echo pattern. Ultrasound is of limited value in diagnosing cervical carcinoma.

READING LIST

1. Andolf, E. and Jorgensen, C. (1990). A prospective comparison of transabdominal and transvaginal ultrasound with surgical findings in gynecologic disease. *J. Ultrasound Med.*, **9**, 71

2. Bowie, J. (1977). Ultrasound of gynecologic pelvic masses: the indefinite uterus sizes and other patterns associated with diagnostic error. *J. Clin. Ultrasound*, **5**, 323

3. Fleischer, A.C., Dudley, B.S., Entman, S.S., Baxter, J.W., Kalemeris, G.C. and James, A.E. (1987). Myometrial invasion by endometrial carcinoma: sonographic assessment. *Radiology*, **162**, 303

4. Johnson, M., Graham, M. and Cooperburg, P. (1982). Abnormal endometrial echoes: sonographic spectrum of endometrial pathology. *J. Clin. Ultrasound*, **1**, 181

5. Kurjak, A. (ed.) (1990). *Handbook of Ultrasonography in Obstetrics and Gynecology*. (Boca Raton: CRC Press)

6. Steel, W.B. and Cochrane, W.J. (eds.) (1984). *Gynecologic Ultrasound*. (New York, Edinburgh, London, Melbourne: Churchill Livingstone)

18 Ultrasound in Ectopic Pregnancy

I. Zalud, A. Kurjak and V. Dukic

Ectopic pregnancy is a serious clinical condition responsible for almost 30% of maternal deaths. In spite of the absence of specific clinical symptoms and tests, every suspected ectopic pregnancy case should be evaluated with extreme care. Clinical diagnosis has been based on the classic triad of pelvic pain, adnexal mass and vaginal bleeding. However, these symptoms are present in less than 50% of cases. Culdocentesis has also been performed in initial patient evaluation. The aspiration of blood from the pouch of Douglas which fails to clot within 15 min is a relatively reliable sign and it is positive in 75% of patients with ectopic pregnancy. Specific radioimmunoassay pregnancy tests which detect the β-human chorionic gonadotropin subunit in very low concentrations are also a helpful diagnostic tool. The positive pregnancy test is a reliable sign of pregnancy, but alone it is not sufficient to discriminate between ectopic and pathologic intrauterine pregnancies. Furthermore, early diagnosis of any ectopic pregnancy still remains a challenge. Although diagnostic ultrasound has played an increasing role recently in the assessment of patients suspected of having ectopic pregnancy, its major place has been excluding an intrauterine gestation in patients confirmed to be pregnant.

The sonographic findings that may be encountered in patients with ectopic pregnancy are divided into those that are considered 'diagnostic' and those thought to be 'suggestive'. The 'diagnostic' signs are: absence of intrauterine gestational sac bordered by two layers of decidua; extrauterine and extraovarian adnexal mass; fetal heart beats and motions. The 'suggestive' features of ectopic pregnancy are: 'enlarged' uterus with thick, echogenic endometrium in the case of unruptured pregnancy; and blood or organized clot in cul-de-sac, or pericolic recesses in the case of ruptured pregnancy. The sonographic diagnosis of an ectopic pregnancy can be made with greater confidence if more than one sonographic sign is present (Figures 18.1–18.14).

Because the size of the ectopic pregnancy can be small (less than 1 cm in size), its sonographic detection as an adnexal mass is variable. In most patients with an unruptured ectopic pregnancy, an adnexal mass separate from the ovary that has a small anechoic center can be identified. Rarely, fetal heart motion can be detected within the ectopic gestational sac which arises from a live fetus. In addition, the uterus in a patient with an ectopic pregnancy typically has an echoic endometrium, a sign of a decidual thickening associated with ectopic pregnancy. Such a finding is described as a 'pseudogestational sac' (Figure 18.12). In contrast to the two concentric rings of decidua that can be identified in an early intrauterine pregnancy, the decidual cast of an ectopic pregnancy has only one layer of decidua. A double decidual sac can occasionally be mimicked by separation of the decidua from the myometrium prior to expulsion of a decidual cast associated with an ectopic pregnancy. A double decidual sac can also be encountered in patients with an incomplete abortion. Furthermore, approximately 6% of the patients with a single decidual layer had a viable intrauterine pregnancy. Obviously, 'pseudogestational sac' may be the source of many diagnostic failures, both positive and negative. The sonographic detection of the double decidua is highly dependent upon the resolution of the scanner used and the scanning ability and experience of the individuals who perform the examination.

Besides meticulous sonographic evaluation of the uterus and adnexa, one should carefully evaluate the cul-de-sac for the presence of intraperitoneal blood in patients suspected of having an ectopic pregnancy. The presence of fluid within the cul-de-sac most frequently indicates the presence of a ruptured ectopic pregnancy. The sonographic appearance of intraperitoneal blood varies from anechoic to hyperechoic, probably depending upon the amount of organization that has occurred within the clot. Unclotted blood is typically anechoic and becomes more echogenic as it organizes.

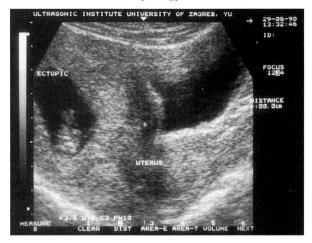

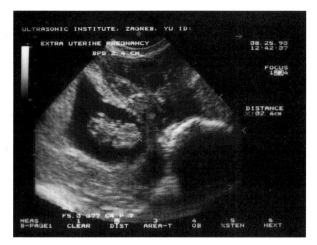

Figure 18.1 Transverse sonogram showing extrauterine pregnancy with an embryo at 9 weeks of gestation right of the empty uterus

Figure 18.2 Typical ultrasound finding in the case of extrauterine pregnancy: the ectopic gestational sac, embryonal echo and heart beats are clearly visualized

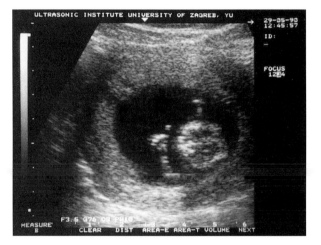

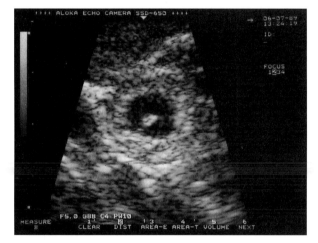

Figure 18.3 Normal live 12-week fetus found in the left upper part of the abdominal cavity

Figure 18.4 Ectopic gestation detected by transvaginal ultrasound at 5 weeks of amenorrhea

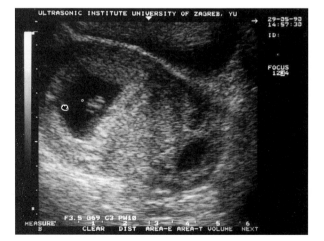

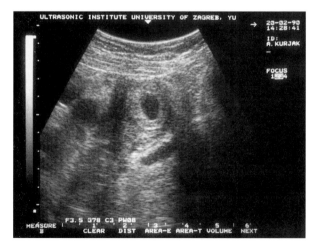

Figure 18.5 Heterotopic pregnancy: normal intrauterine pregnancy with a live embryo and empty ectopic gestational sac visualized in the left tube

Figure 18.6 Transvaginal sonogram displaying a small gestational sac without a visible embryonal pole between the uterus and the left ovary

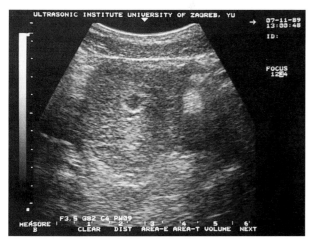

Figure 18.7 Empty uterus (left) and ectopic pregnancy as a solid ovarian tumor

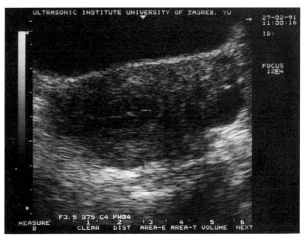

Figure 18.8 Empty uterus in a patient amenorrheic for 6 weeks: the thickened endometrium is easily recognized

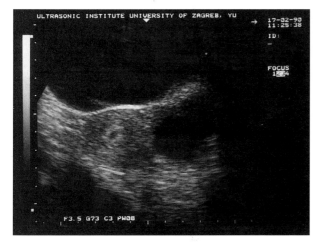

Figure 18.9 Transverse sonogram demonstrating an empty uterus with decidual reaction and cystic adnexal tumor representing an ectopic gestation

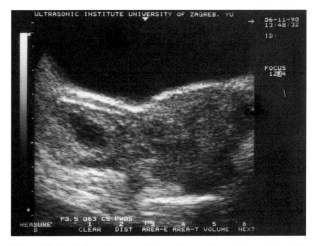

Figure 18.10 Enlarged uterus with a uterine cavity echo in a patient with severe pain in the lower abdomen: the ectopic gestational sac is visualized in the right tube. Note the presence of free fluid in the pouch of Douglas

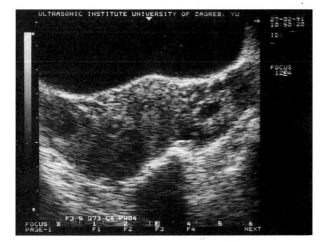

Figure 18.11 Ectopic gestational sac situated left of the uterus: the embryo is not visible

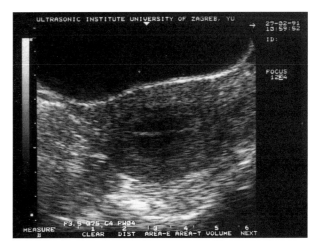

Figure 18.12 The same patient: empty and slightly enlarged uterus with typical 'pseudogestational' reaction

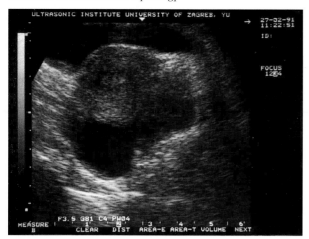

Figure 18.13 The same patient: free fluid was visualized in the pouch of Douglas

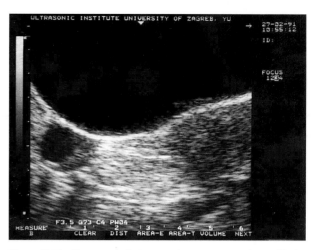

Figure 18.14 The same patient: corpus luteum cyst was detected in the contralateral ovary

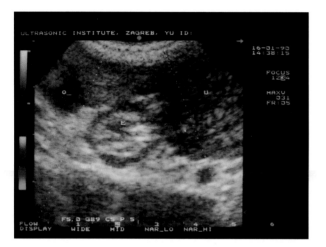

Figure 18.15 A transvaginal scan of an empty uterus, the right ovary and a solid adnexal mass suspected to be an ectopic gestation: this is a non-specific ultrasound finding; O = right ovary, E = ectopic pregnancy, U = empty uterus

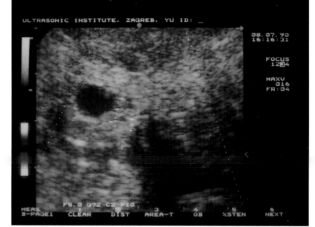

Figure 18.16 A highly vascularized adnexal mass suspected to be an ectopic pregnancy: transvaginal color Doppler helps to diagnose the ectopic pregnancy in the presence of non-specific ultrasound findings

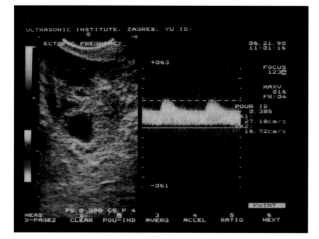

Figure 18.17 Transvaginal color Doppler shows ectopic blood flow. Pulsed Doppler (right) shows high velocity and very low resistance of flow (RI = 0.385). These are typical Doppler findings of ectopic pregnancy. The diagnosis was confirmed by surgery

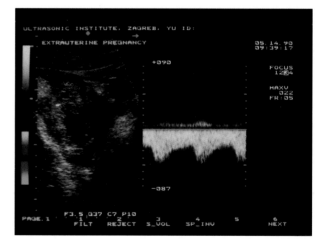

Figure 18.18 Another example of an ectopic pregnancy diagnosed by transvaginal color and pulsed Doppler

The detection of an intrauterine gestational sac can be achieved by the transvaginal approach earlier (usually as early as 16 days after conception) and easier than by the transabdominal route. When using a transabdominal probe, one may find it difficult to differentiate a 'pseudogestational sac' from a true gestational sac. Using transvaginal sonography these echoes are found to originate from local blood clots or from a central sonolucent area outlined by a thick endometrium. If an intrauterine gestation cannot be identified, one should proceed to scan the Fallopian tubes.

The first transabdominal Doppler study of ectopic pregnancy was recently reported. Transvaginal color Doppler can help to characterize the nature of the adnexal mass thus permitting preoperative diagnosis when the ectopic embryo and its characteristic heartbeat cannot be visualized (Figures 18.15–18.18). Ectopic pregnancy is defined as ectopic color flow, usually very prominent and randomly dispersed inside the solid part of the adnexal mass and clearly separated from ovarian tissue and corpus luteum. Pulsed Doppler waveform analysis shows a very low-impedance signal and calculated resistance index (RI) is below 0.40 due to increased end-diastolic flow. The brightness of color is usually high, indicating high velocity of ectopic flow.

Transabdominal ultrasound B-mode diagnosis for ectopic pregnancy is good enough only in typical cases. However, many ectopic pregnancies do not present a gestational sac and a live embryo. Transvaginal color Doppler is expected to have direct implications for the diagnosis and therapy of ectopic pregnancy, particularly when typical ultrasound morphology (gestational sac and embryonal heartbeat) is absent. Since Doppler appears to identify the viability and perhaps the invasiveness of the trophoblast more accurately than any other currently available diagnostic method, it may provide a foundation for a more selective management of ectopic pregnancy.

READING LIST

1. Cacciatore, B., Stenman, U.H. and Ylostalo, P. (1989). Comparison of abdominal and vaginal sonography in suspected ectopic pregnancy. *Obstet. Gynecol.*, **73**, 770
2. Fleischer, A.C., Cartwright, P.S., DiPetro, D.L. and James, A.E. (1985). Sonographic evaluation of ectopic pregnancy. In Sanders, R.C. (ed.) *The Principles and Practice of Ultrasonography in Obstetrics and Gynecology.* p.399. (Norwalk: Appleton Century Crofts)
3. Kadar, N. (1989). Transvaginal ultrasound for ectopics. *Fertil. Steril.*, **51**, 909
4. Kurjak, A., Zalud, I., Alfirevic, Z. and Jurkovic, D. (1990). The assessment of abnormal pelvic blood flow by transvaginal color Doppler. *Ultrasound Med. Biol.*, **16**, 437
5. Kurjak, A., Zalud, I. and Volpe, G. (1990). Conventional B-mode and transvaginal color Doppler in ultrasound assessment of ectopic pregnancy. *Acta Med. Iug.*, **44**, 91
6. Mahony, B.S., Filly, R.A., Nyberg, D.A. and Callen, P.W. (1985). Sonographic evaluation of ectopic pregnancy. *J. Ultrasound Med.*, **4**, 221
7. Nyberg, D.A., Mack, L.A., Jeffrey, R.B. and Laing, F.C. (1987). Endovaginal sonographic evaluation of ectopic pregnancy: a prospective study. *Am. J. Roentgen.*, **149**, 1181
8. Romero, R., Kadar, N., Jeanty, P., Copel, J.A., Chervenak, F.A., DeCherney, A. and Hobbins, J. (1985). Diagnosis of ectopic pregnancy: value of the discriminatory human chorionic gonadotrophin zone. *Obstet. Gynecol.*, **66**, 357
9. Rottem, S., Thaler, I., Levron, J., Peretz, B., Istkowitz, J. and Brandes, J. (1990). Criteria for transvaginal sonographic diagnosis of ectopic pregnancy. *J. Clin. Ultrasound*, **18**, 274
10. Taylor, K.J.W., Ramos, I.M., Feyock, A.L., Snower, D.P., Carter, D., Shapiro, B.S., Meyer, W.R. and DeCherney, A.H. (1989). Ectopic pregnancy: duplex Doppler evaluation. *Radiology*, **173**, 93
11. Kurjak, A., Zalud, I. and Schulman, H. (1991). Ectopic pregnancy: transvaginal color Doppler identifies trophoblastic flow in suspicious adnexa. *J. Ultrasound Med.*, **10**, 685

19 Color Doppler in Gynecology

A. Kurjak, I. Zalud and V. Dukic

More information can be obtained using Doppler ultrasound than can be gained from a morphological study alone. Furthermore, while color Doppler always indicates direction, velocity and type of blood flow, pulsed Doppler enables quantification of such flow. However, combination of high quality B-mode images, pulsed Doppler and color Doppler in the same vaginal probe produces a superb, simultaneous visualization of morphological and blood flow information from the female pelvic circulation.

NORMAL PELVIC BLOOD FLOW

Blood flow in the main pelvic vessels can be easily visualized and recognized (Figures 19.1–19.5). The artery and vein are distinguished according to the pulsation and brightness of color flow. The external iliac vessels are situated lateral to the ovary and present in prominent color due to high velocity blood flow. The internal iliac vessels can be visualized easily in the entire population. They can be observed in the side wall of the pelvis, often lying deep close to the ovary. Both the internal and external iliac arteries produce prominent and pulsating color flow, high velocity with typical reverse flow and very high impedance of flow. Common iliac vessels can only occasionally be seen because they are usually too far from the probe. If seen, they present a high velocity of blood flow with the most prominent reverse flow in diastole.

The color Doppler signal from the main uterine vessels may be seen in all patients lateral to the cervix. The small branches of the uterine artery can be followed by searching the corpus uteri, ascending along the lateral wall. Even small, terminal branches can be visualized in the direction of the ovary or of the myometrium. Waveform analysis showed high to moderate velocity. The resistance index depends on age, phase of menstrual cycle and any special conditions (e.g. pregnancy, tumor) and is usually very high.

It is difficult to visualize ovarian vessels, but an experienced operator using modern color Doppler equipment can detect them in most patients in the lateral upper pole of the ovary (Figures 19.6–19.9). Color flow is usually not prominent, velocity is low and resistance varies according to the menstrual cycle.

ABNORMAL PELVIC BLOOD FLOW (NEOVASCULARIZATION)

The importance of neovascularization was first recognized by Judah Folkman in 1971, when he proposed the hypothesis that increased cell population must be preceded by the production of new vessels. Folkman's hypothesis has been proved and is now universally accepted. Such abnormal tumor vascular morphology can be used as a valuable marker for tissue characterization. These vessels must be formed very early in the development of the tumor and therefore are early markers of the presence of a malignant tumor. New vessels are continually produced at the periphery of the tumor and therefore act as a marker of continued growth and proliferation. The amount and vascularity of the stroma vary greatly in different tumors. In general, rapidly growing tumors, particularly sarcomas, have a highly vascular stroma with little connective tissue. More slowly growing tumors are less well vascularized.

Intratumoral blood flow displayed on color Doppler images indicates that there is flow rapid enough to be detected. The presence of arteriovenous communications should be an important factor that produces sufficient velocity above the minimal threshold on color Doppler imaging. The technique may be useful in demonstrating pelvic tumors with rapid blood flow and in providing important hemodynamic information (Figures 19.10–19.36). Color Doppler can also depict the hemodynamic characteristics of the tumor, allowing echo sources of the hypoechoic zones to be separated

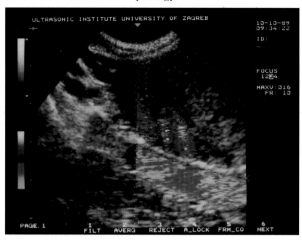

Figure 19.1   The color Doppler signal from both right uterine vessels seen laterally to the cervix

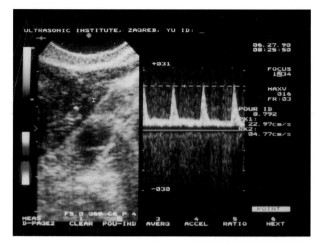

Figure 19.2   The uterine artery: pulsed Doppler (right) showing high to moderate velocity and a high resistance of blood flow. This is the normal finding for uterine blood flow

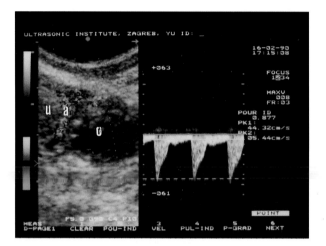

Figure 19.3   High-velocity and high-resistance (RI = 0.877) blood flow of the uterine artery: these are characteristic findings in the proliferative part of the menstrual cycle; U = uterus, A = left uterine artery, O = left ovary with follicle

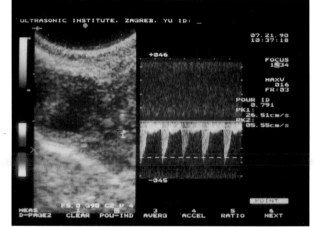

Figure 19.4   The uterine artery: an increased diastolic flow (RI = 0.791), indicating the luteal part of the cycle

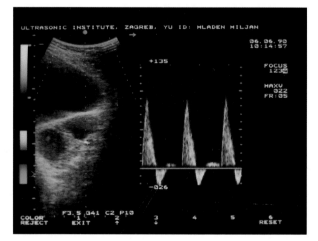

Figure 19.5   The internal iliac artery: pulsed Doppler waveform (right) shows high-velocity and high-resistance flow with characteristic normal finding of reverse flow

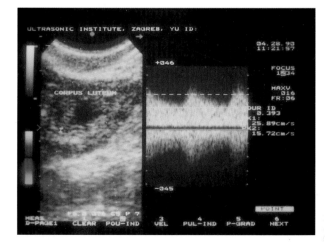

Figure 19.6   A color-coded blood flow of the corpus luteum: pulsed Doppler analysis (right) shows moderate velocity and increased diastolic flow. There is a typical very low-resistance (RI = 0.393) blood flow characteristic of the newly formed vessels of the corpus luteum

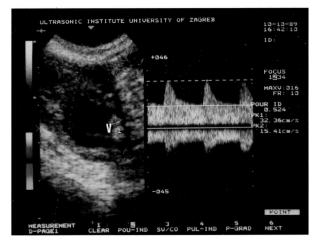

Figure 19.7 Small ovarian cyst: transvaginal color Doppler shows tumor blood flow. Pulsed Doppler (right) shows moderate-velocity and high-resistance flow (RI = 0.524). The benign nature of the adnexal tumor was proven by histopathology (V = vein)

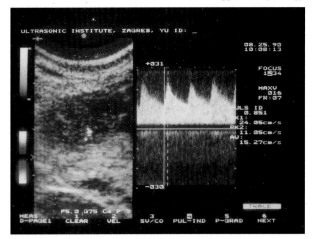

Figure 19.8 Normal size right ovary: superimposed color Doppler shows highly vascularized ovarian tissue in the luteal part of the menstrual cycle, even small newly formed vessels can be studied

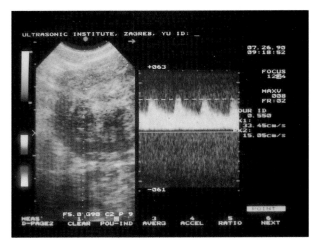

Figure 19.9 Enlarged ovary in a postmenopausal woman: color and pulsed Doppler analysis show moderate-velocity and moderate-resistance flow. The benign nature of the tumor was proven by histopathology

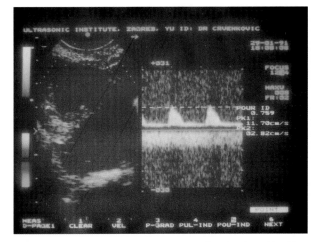

Figure 19.10 Suspected ovarian cancer: color Doppler shows blood flow on the tumor periphery. Pulsed Doppler (right) indicates a normal finding. The benign nature of the tumor (endometriosis) was confirmed by histopathology

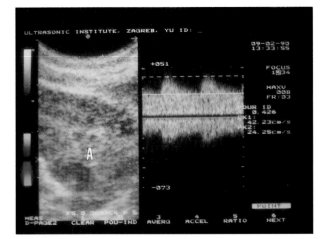

Figure 19.11 Color and pulsed Doppler show moderate-velocity and low-resistance blood flow; borderline case (A = artery)

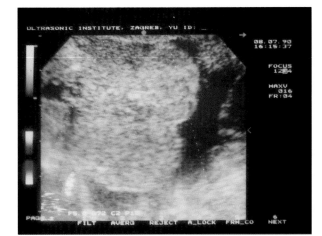

Figure 19.12 Tumor vasculature visualized by color Doppler

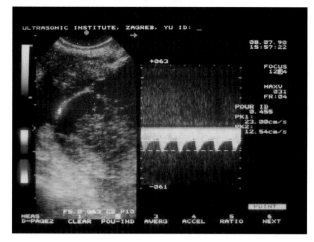

Figure 19.13 The same patient: pulsed Doppler extracted from the tumor septa shows moderate resistance of blood flow; borderline case

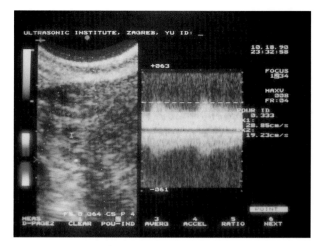

Figure 19.14 Transvaginal color Doppler shows tumor vessels: waveform (right) study shows a very low-velocity and very low-resistance blood flow. Ovarian cancer at stage Ia was confirmed on histopathology

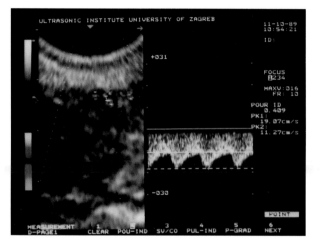

Figure 19.15 Color flow was visualized by transvaginal color Doppler. Pulsed Doppler (right) shows a very low resistance of blood flow. A malignant ovarian tumor was diagnosed

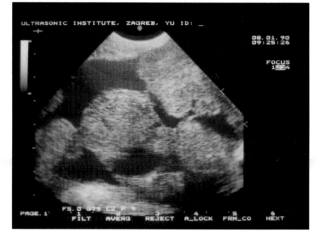

Figure 19.16 Huge complex adnexal mass diagnosed by B-mode ultrasound

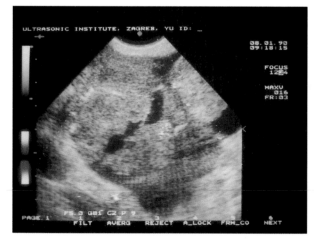

Figure 19.17 The same patient: color Doppler shows tumor vascularity

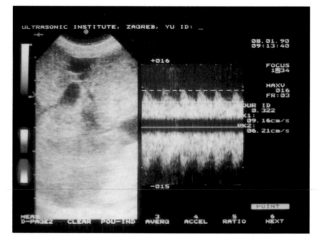

Figure 19.18 The same patient: pulsed Doppler (right) shows high-velocity but very low-resistance (RI = 0.322) blood flow. Cystadenocarcinoma stage III was diagnosed on histopathology

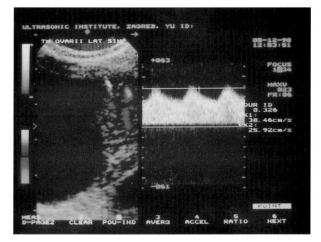

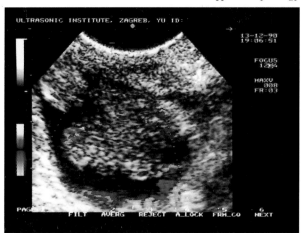

Figure 19.19 Bilocular cystic ovarian tumor: blood flow was detected in the tumor septa. Pulsed Doppler (right) was typical for a malignant adnexal mass

Figure 19.20 Metastatic adnexal mass: color Doppler shows tumor vascularity

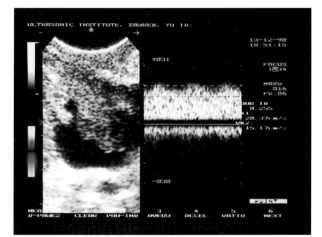

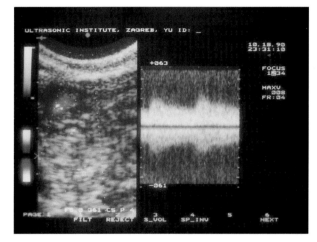

Figure 19.21 The same patient: pulsed Doppler shows very low-resistance blood flow (RI = 0.255)

Figure 19.22 Abundant color flow of newly formed tumor vessels

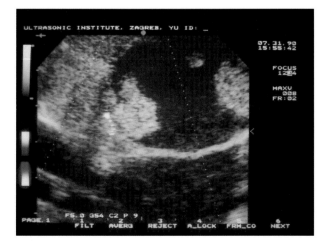

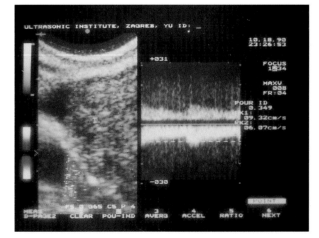

Figure 19.23 Transvaginal color Doppler presents tumor neovascularization of papillary proliferation

Figure 19.24 Small tumor vessels are detected by transvaginal color Doppler. Pulsed Doppler (right) analysis shows low velocity and very low resistance of blood flow. The Doppler findings strongly supported the diagnosis of ovarian malignancy. The final diagnosis was ovarian cystadenocarcinoma

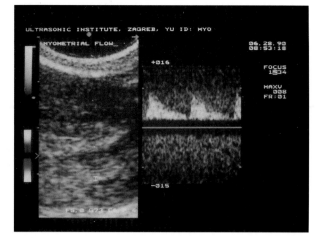

Figure 19.25 Normal myometrial blood flow detected by color and pulsed Doppler

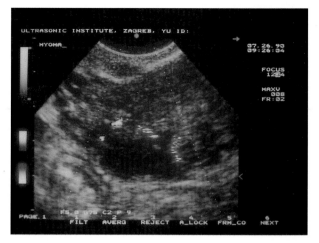

Figure 19.26 A uterine myoma: color Doppler detected increased uterine perfusion

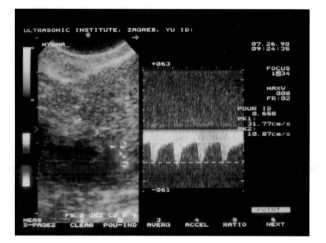

Figure 19.27 The same patient: pulsed Doppler (right) shows blood flow similar to the normal myometrial perfusion originating from the terminal branches of the uterine artery

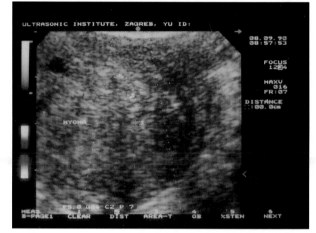

Figure 19.28 Color Doppler detected a good vascular supply to this uterine tumor

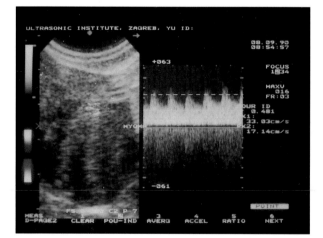

Figure 19.29 The same patient: the waveform analysis (right) indicates moderate-velocity and low-resistance blood flow. The diastolic component of cardiac cycle was increased. A borderline Doppler finding. The benign nature of the uterine mass was confirmed by histopathology

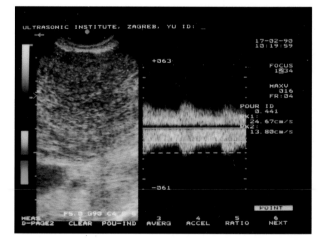

Figure 19.30 Adenomyosis uteri: small vessels were visualized by color Doppler. Pulsed Doppler (right) shows low-velocity and low-resistance blood flow

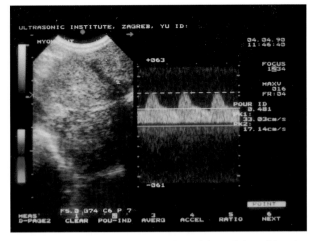

Figure 19.31 Color flow obtained on the periphery of the solid uterine mass suspected to be a myoma: pulsed Doppler (right) showed moderate-resistance (RI = 0.481) blood flow. A myoma was diagnosed by histopathology

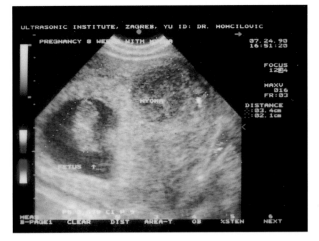

Figure 19.32 Myoma vascularization and early pregnancy at 8 weeks of gestation

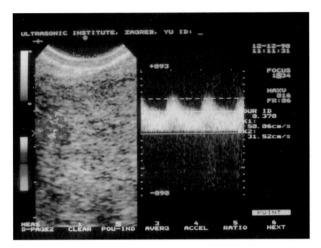

Figure 19.33 Uterine adenocarcinoma: the typical finding was the presence of irregular and thin vessels visualized by color Doppler. Pulsed Doppler (right) shows high-velocity and very low-resistance (RI = 0.370) blood flow

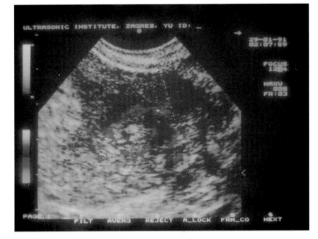

Figure 19.34 Randomly dispersed newly formed tumor vessels detected by color Doppler in a case of uterine malignancy

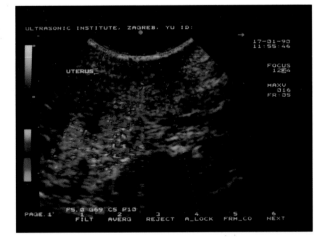

Figure 19.35 Abundant color flow in a patient with endometrial cancer

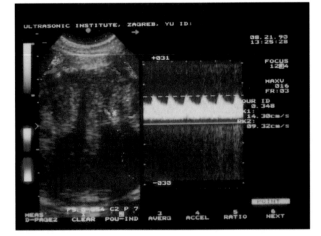

Figure 19.36 Enlarged and inhomogeneous uterus: color Doppler indicates tumor vascularity. Pulsed Doppler (right) shows very low-resistance (RI = 0.348) blood flow. Uterine sarcoma was diagnosed on histopathology

into compartment, vesicles and the blood pooling or hemorrhage surrounding them.

The differentiation of benign and malignant adnexal tumors *in vivo* still involves many clinical problems. However, there are known features that characterize this difference. Many of them, such as the mitotic index and pleomorphism, are of histologic nature and are not amenable to current imaging methods. One feature of malignancy is the bizarre vascular morphology which characterizes many malignant tumors. Transvaginal color Doppler sonography seems to produce a better characterization of pelvic tumor vascularity than any other currently available diagnostic method. The characteristic finding is the observation of small vascular channels within the solid part of the tumor. Being very thin and randomly dispersed within the tissue, such vessels are difficult to find unless transvaginal color Doppler is used.

The goal of transvaginal color Doppler sonography should be to identify ovarian tumors which are not significantly enlarged. Until now no one diagnostic method has been successful enough to detect ovarian cancer at an early stage. Consequently, there is no effective screening program for ovarian cancer and no simple diagnostic and therapeutic approach. Transvaginal color Doppler is a non-invasive method and its diagnostic sensitivity, specificity and accuracy seem to be clinically good enough for it to be a potential technique for use in a screening program. Color Doppler ultrasound is a pertinent diagnostic tool which can also be used to observe changes in the vascularity of gynecologic malignant tumors before and after treatment.

Transvaginal color Doppler can also be helpful in the diagnosis of uterine malignancy. When peripheral impedance was compared in cases of myoma uteri and carcinoma endometrii, a significantly lower resistance index was obtained in the latter.

READING LIST

1. Bourne, T., Campbell, S., Steer, C., Whitehead, M.I. and Collins, W.P. (1989). Transvaginal colour flow imaging: a possible new screening technique for ovarian cancer. *Br. Med. J.*, **299**, 1367
2. Folkman, J. (1985). Tumor angiogenesis. *Adv. Cancer Res.*, **43**, 175
3. Ginsburg, J. (1989). *The Circulation in the Female.* (Carnforth: Parthenon Publishing)
4. Goswamy, R.K. and Steptoe, P.C. (1988). Doppler ultrasound studies of the uterine artery in spontaneous ovarian cycles. *Hum. Reprod.*, **3**, 721–5
5. Hata, T., Hata, K., Senoh, D., Makihara, K., Aoki, S., Takamiya, O., Kitao, M. and Umaki, K. (1989). Transvaginal Doppler color flow mapping. *Gynecol. Obstet. Invest.*, **27**, 217
6. Kurjak, A. (1990). *Transvaginal Color Doppler.* (Carnforth: Parthenon Publishing)
7. Kurjak, A., Jurkovic, D., Alfirevic, Z. and Zalud, I. (1990). Transvaginal color Doppler imaging. *J. Clin. Ultrasound*, **18**, 227–34
8. Kurjak, A., Zalud, I., Alfirevic, Z. and Jurkovic, D. (1990). The assessment of abnormal pelvic blood flow by transvaginal color and pulsed Doppler. *Ultrasound Med. Biol.*, **16**, 437–42
9. Kurjak, A., Zalud, I., Jurkovic, D., Alfirevic, Z. and Miljan, M. (1989). Transvaginal color Doppler for the assessment of pelvic circulation. *Acta Obstet. Gynecol. Scand.*, **68**, 131–5
10. Taylor, K.J.W., Burns, P.N. and Wells, P.N.T. (1988). *Clinical Applications of Doppler Ultrasound.* (New York: Raven Press)
11. Taylor, K.J.W., Burns, P.N., Wells, P.N.I. and Conway, D.I. (1985). Ultrasound Doppler flow studies of the ovarian and uterine arteries. *Br. J. Obstet. Gynaecol.*, **92**, 240–6

20 Transvaginal Color Doppler in the Assessment of Infertility

A. Kurjak and S. Kupešić-Urek

Blood flow studies of the pelvic circulation represent the most recent development in the ultrasound assessment of infertile patients. Transvaginal color Doppler will become the technique of choice for scanning pelvic circulation in infertile patients because of the small distance between the probe and the vessels, its better resolution and patient's convenience, since a full bladder is not necessary for the examination.

The uterine artery blood flow can be easily seen just lateral to the cervix at the level of the cervicocorporeal junction. The use of blood flow studies in uterine arteries shows that there is a small amount of end diastolic flow in the uterine arteries in the proliferative phase. It is also recognized that in some infertile patients end diastolic flow is absent. A significant decline in resistance index (RI) begins prior to ovulation, and persistently lower RI persists until the onset of menstruation (Figures 20.1–20.7).

Transvaginal color Doppler facilitates the identification of small vascular branches. The accuracy of the measurement is increased because of the better resolution and unlimited examination time. By using transvaginal color Doppler it is possible to observe intraovarian (follicular and luteal) blood flow as well as to study the alterations of the endometrial blood flow under physiologic and pathophysiologic conditions. (Figures 20.8–20.24). The alterations of the endometrial blood flow may play an important role for predicting the optimum time for implantation. The potential use of color Doppler studies in the assessment of infertility is prediction of ovulation on the basis of detection of the changes in blood flow. It may help in the diagnosis of some ovulatory disorders, as well as in the detection of early complications in ovulation induction.

A study of the sequential changes of the uterine artery blood flow during the periovulatory period is shown in Figures 20.13–20.18. One 30-year-old woman, with secondary infertility but with apparently normal ovarian function, volunteered to participate in the study. Ovulation was detected on day 16 of the 32-day regular menstrual cycle and biphasic changes in basal body temperature were noted during the cycle. Figures 20.19–20.24 show the myometrial and endometrial flows in the same patient.

Transvaginal color Doppler might answer some interesting questions, for example, do blood flow changes play any role in infertility and whether inadequate vascularization is responsible for early pregnancy loss. This simplified examination technique, with its usefulness, promises exciting future developments.

READING LIST

1. Kurjak, A. (ed.) (1989). *Ultrasound and Infertility*. (Boca Raton: CRC Press)
2. Kurjak, A. and Kupešić-Urek, S. (1991). Infertility. In Kurjak, A. (ed.) *Transvaginal Color Doppler*, pp.33–40. (Carnforth: Parthenon Publishing)
3. Timor-Tritsch, I. and Rottem, S. (1991). *Transvaginal Sonography*, 2nd edn. (New York: Elsevier Science Publishers)
4. Kurjak, A., Zalud, I., Jurkovic, D., Alfirevic, Z. and Miljan, M. (1989). Color Doppler in the assessment of pelvic circulation. *Acta Obstet. Gynecol. Scand.*, **68**, 131
5. Goswamy, R.K., Williams, G. and Steptoe, P.C. (1988). Decreased uterine perfusion – a cause of infertility. *Hum. Reprod.*, **3**, 955

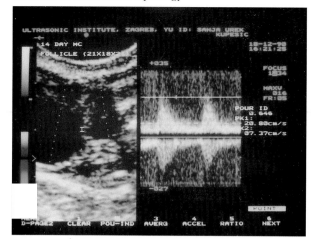

Figure 20.1 Illustration of ultrasonic diagnosis of ovulation after serial daily scanning, using transvaginal color Doppler. On day 14 of the 32-day regular menstrual cycle, there was an obvious increase in the follicular size and the mean diameter reached 21 mm (left). Flow velocity waveforms were obtained around the follicle (right)

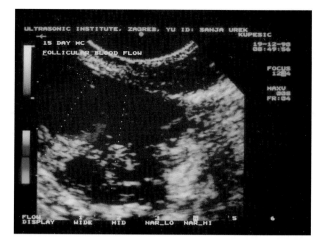

Figure 20.2 On the following day the size of the dominant follicle had increased and follicular blood flow could be easily detected

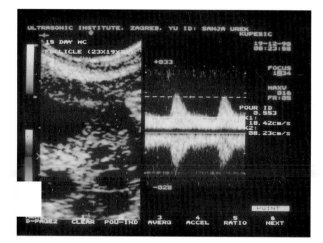

Figure 20.3 During the 15th day of the menstrual cycle the resistance index tended to decrease

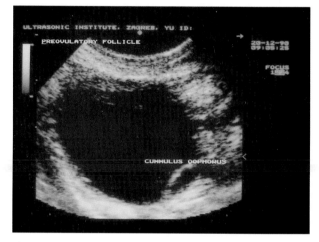

Figure 20.4 Transvaginal scan of the mature preovulatory follicle demonstrating the triangular echo of the cumulus oophorus

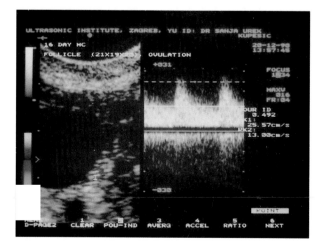

Figure 20.5 On day 16 of the 32 day regular menstrual cycle follicular size was gradually reduced. Blood velocity of the follicular flow tended to increase, while the resistance index decreased during the ovulation

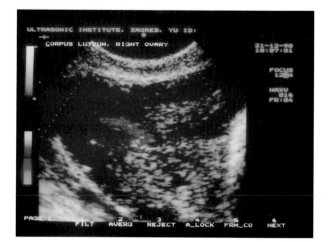

Figure 20.6 Follicle had completely disappeared when the examination was repeated on the following day

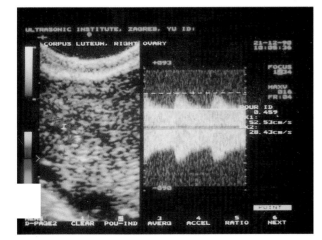

Figure 20.7 Demonstration of increased vascularity in the corpus luteum as seen by transvaginal color Doppler (left). Increased blood velocity and decreased resistance index represent the typical signs of ovulation and early corpus luteum blood flow (right)

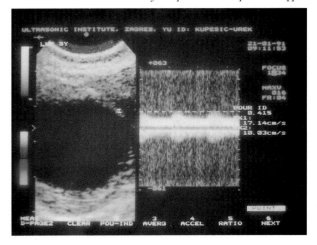

Figure 20.8 A mature ovarian follicle can be seen in the right ovary on day 14 of the cycle. The same finding persisted for a few days and diagnosis of luteinized unruptured follicle syndrome was made

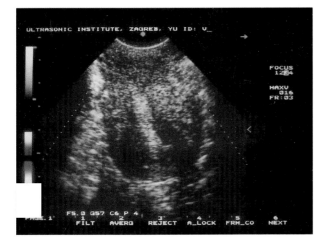

Figure 20.9 The same patient: the endometrium is echogenic and a small amount of fluid is present in the pouch of Douglas due to ovarian secretion

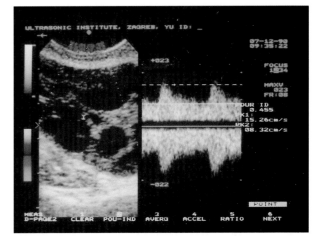

Figure 20.10 Transvaginal sonogram of the polcystic ovary. A large number of small cystic structures are 'crowded' and stand out from the surface of the enlarged ovarian stroma (left). Pulsed wave Doppler analysis of the intraovarian blood flow showed low resistance index (right)

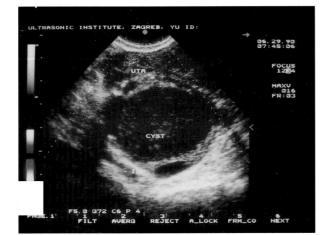

Figure 20.11 Endometriotic cyst in a primary infertility patient: note the regular shape of the cyst and internal echoes

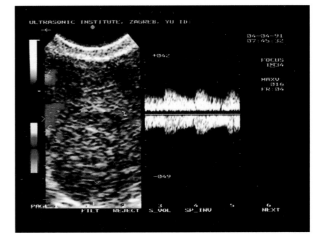

Figure 20.12 Transvaginal scan showing uterine myoma in a patient suffering from secondary infertility. Transvaginal color Doppler detected a good vascular supply to the uterine tumor. The diastolic component of the cardiac cycle was increased

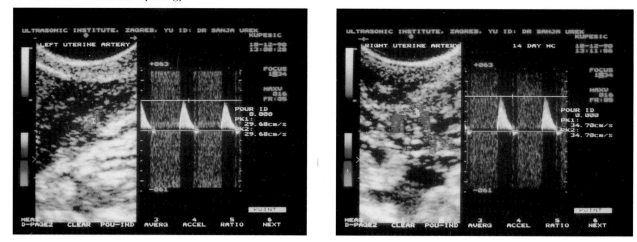

Figures 20.13 and 20.14 Absent diastolic flow was noted in the both uterine arteries during the 14th day of the menstrual cycle

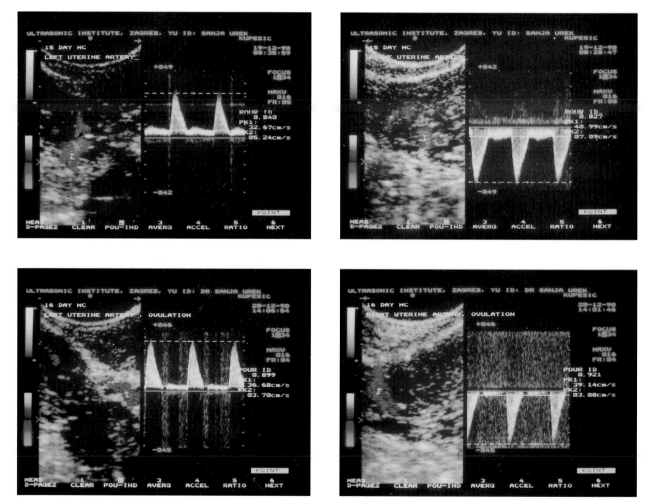

Figures 20.15–20.18 Blood velocity of the uterine arteries tended to increase until the follicle had ruptured. There was no apparent difference in blood velocity between the left and right uterine arteries

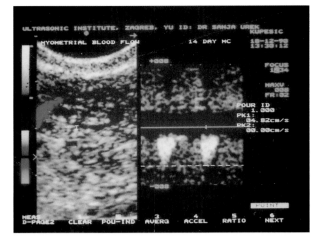

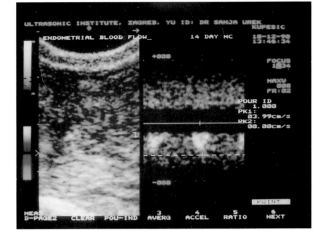

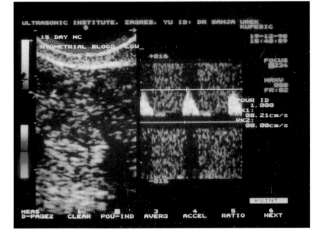

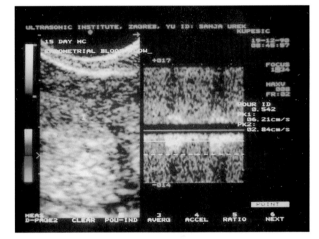

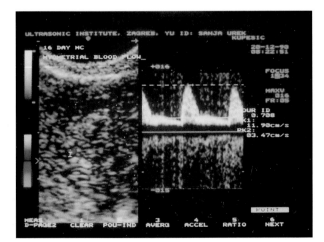

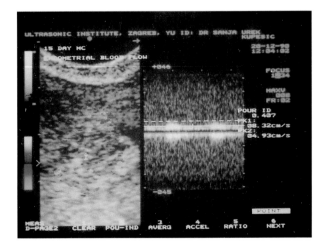

Figures 20.19–20.21 Blood velocity of the myometrial blood flow tended to increase, while the value of resistance index tended to decrease during the day of the follicular rupture

Figures 20.22–20.24 Flow velocity waveforms were obtained from the endometrium during the preovulatory period. Decreased resistance index (increased flow velocity) of the endometrial blood flow occurred during the day of ovulation

21 Ultrasound and Infertility

A. Kurjak and S. Kupešić-Urek

Ultrasound plays an important role in the diagnosis and treatment of infertility. Today ultrasound is widely accepted as a technique in the investigation and detection of pelvic pathologies that may be the causes of infertility. The main advantages of ultrasound include monitoring of the growth and development of Graafian follicles, ovulation detection and demonstration of uterine endometrial changes during the menstrual cycle. It has become the standard modality for monitoring ovulation induction and for follicular puncture in *in vitro* regimens.

In any assessment of the ovarian function the techniques used should be non-invasive, have a high degree of patient acceptability and provide readily accessible information to the clinician. Although radioimmunoassays for steroid hormones are available, their levels reflect the changes within the ovary indirectly, and give no information about the number and nature of the follicles which may be developing.

Using real-time transabdominal sonography one of the requirements for clear visualization of the pelvic anatomy is a full bladder. Because serial ultrasound assessment of follicular growth and maturation is necessary, it is important that each patient establishes her own bladder regimen. Despite a good knowledge of pelvic anatomy, and excellent scanning technique, there are still some occasions when identification of the ovary is not possible. This is particularly likely in obese patients, or in those patients unable to tolerate the degree of bladder filling required for the procedure. The introduction of transvaginal sonography has transformed this situation. Transvaginal sonography provides better resolution because the proximity of the probe to the pelvic structures permits the use of higher ultrasound frequencies. The great practical advantage of vaginal sonography is that it obviates the need for a full bladder.

From the 9th or 10th day, the growing follicle can be easily recognized as a small anechoic cystic structure with well-defined borders, usually measuring 8–10 mm in diameter (Figures 21.1 and 21.2). Depending on the cycle length, serial examinations may start a few days earlier or later (Figures 21.3–21.6). During the next few days the leading follicle undergoes rapid growth, such that by day prior to ovulation it has reached a diameter between 19 and 23 mm. The mean daily growth rate of the follicle is 2–3 mm and represents an indicator of normal follicular development. This constant increase in follicular size parallels the rising estradiol levels that occur in the late follicular phase of the cycle.

In the assessment of follicular maturation, one of the basic parameters used is the diameter of the dominant follicle (Figure 21.7). Follicle measurement should be made in three orthogonal planes. This approach most closely reflects the follicular size, because the follicle is ovoid or elongated in its shape due to the pressure caused by a full bladder. The round shape of the follicle remains unaltered on a transvaginal scan, thus allowing the use of simplified measurement techniques. The measurement is performed by positioning two bright calipers on the inside wall of the follicle. In order to avoid confusion with artifacts only echo-free areas with clear borders and a mean diameter over 8 mm are measured.

There is, as yet, no reliable ultrasonic sign of imminent ovulation, although there are some helpful signs such as a minor change of follicular shape or a crenation pattern within the follicle due to the advanced separation of the granulosa cell layer. Sometimes it is possible to observe a small echoic structure bulging from the inner wall of the dissociated cumulus oophorus in the preovulatory follicle. Visualization of the cumulus oophorus is the most reliable sign of forthcoming ovulation. However, its practical use as a predictor of ovulation is limited by a low visualization rate of 15–20%.

Ovulation and rupture of the preovulatory follicle occur as a result of biochemical changes that are induced by the midcycle luteinizing hormone (LH) surge. After ovulation has occurred, a sudden change in the appearance of the follicle can be observed (Figure 21.8). As early as 1 h after the rupture, the corpus hemorrhagicum may be seen. The early corpus luteum has a varying appearance on the ultrasound image. The most common feature includes complete collapse of the follicle or its modification into an irregular and more solid structure. Sometimes corpus luteum is seen as a small residual thick walled cyst, usually filled with echogenic blood clots. In some cases, the decrease in follicular size is not so obvious and inhomogeneous, intrafollicular echoes which represent a reaccumulation of the fluid and blood within the follicle are present. A careful observation of changes in the amount of fluid in the pouch of Douglas seen by ultrasound may help to confirm a diagnosis of ovulation.

Simultaneous sonographic assessment of follicular growth and uterine endometrial changes provides for a better evaluation of ovarian function than the monitoring of follicular development alone (Figures 21.9–21.14). In the immediate postmenstrual phase the endometrium is seen as a thin, highly echogenic linear echo (Figures 21.9 and 21.10). During the second week of the proliferative phase it becomes thicker, more hypoechoic as compared to the myometrium, and is characterized by a thin, well-defined boundary in the basal layer (Figure 21.11). In the preovulatory phase of the cycle the endometrium is 3.5–7 mm thick as measured by ultrasound. In the preovulatory period the echogenicity of the basal portion of the endometrium increases (Figure 21.12). The central echo is now less pronounced, but still present. This feature of the endometrium has been named the 'ovulation ring' because of its similarity with an early gestational sac (Figure 21.13). It has been suggested that this sign can be used as an additional sign of forthcoming ovulation in spontaneous cycles. During the secretory phase the endometrium becomes homogeneous and hyperechoic as compared to the myometrium (Figure 21.14).

Correlation between endometrial thickness and peripheral estradiol levels has been reported. In the late proliferative phase of the cycle there is a significant increase in endometrial thickness, with a mean daily growth rate of approximately 1 mm/day. Comparative studies have confirmed the crucial role of estradiol in promoting normal development of the endometrium in the proliferative phase. In the luteal phase of the cycle there is no further increase in endometrial thickness. It seems that the increase in the progesterone levels seen in the periovulatory period is a major factor responsible for the marked increase in endometrial echogenicity. A significant rise of progesterone above baseline levels causes glycogen incorporation into glandular elements. Glycogen is a strongly echogenic substance and it contributes to the high echogenicity of the secretory endometrium.

Various cycle abnormalities can be easily diagnosed on the basis of the ultrasound monitoring of follicular growth. Ultrasound remains particularly helpful for making the diagnosis of polycystic ovary syndrome (Figures 21.15–21.18). The criteria to identify polycystic ovaries by ultrasound are the presence of multiple small cystic structures and an increase in the ovarian stroma. The cysts may be distributed predominantly around the periphery or scattered throughout the enlarged stroma. It has been demonstrated that the typical polycystic appearance of ovaries on ultrasound, characterized by bilateral symmetrical ovarian enlargement and microcystic changes in their internal structure, is associated with polycystic ovary syndrome in 75–95% of cases.

A characteristic example of an ultrasonically detectable ovulation disorder is luteinized unruptured follicle syndrome (Figures 21.19 and 21.20). The main characteristics of this disturbance are complete luteinization of the follicle without ovulation and oocyte release. Possible etiological causes of this syndrome are a primary oocyte abnormality, abnormalities in prostaglandin synthesis and low progesterone and midcycle LH levels. The ultrasound diagnosis of luteinized unruptured follicle is based on daily observations of normal follicular development and on normal diameter of the preovulatory follicle. The ovulation does not occur and the follicle remains the same size. Luteinization of the unruptured follicle is seen as a progressive accumulation of the strong echoes located predominantly on its periphery. At the same time the endometrium becomes echogenic and thick, and a small amount of fluid can be detected in the pouch of Douglas. A particularly high incidence of luteinized unruptured follicle has been reported in patients with endometriosis, pelvic adhesions and unexplained infertility.

Other ultrasonically detected abnormalities of the follicular growth include abnormally slow growth rate, rupture of the small follicle and premature atresia of the preovulatory follicle. In the majority of cases with disturbed ovulation elevated progesterone levels and biphasic temperature are present.

Sonography in the induction of ovulation is used for evaluating the patient's response to the therapy, detecting the number of developing follicles, predicting the ovulation, timing the administration of human chorionic gonadotropin and detecting hyperstimulation (Figures 21.21–21.24). It is equally important to repeat the examinations every day starting from day 9 of the cycle. The follicle growth

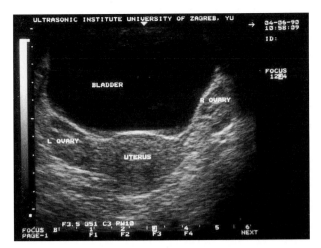

Figure 21.1 Transverse sonogram of the uterus and both ovaries in the postmenstrual phase of the cycle: small cysts affecting ovarian texture homogenicity can always be seen. The dominant follicle cannot be distinguished from the other antral follicles in this phase of the cycle

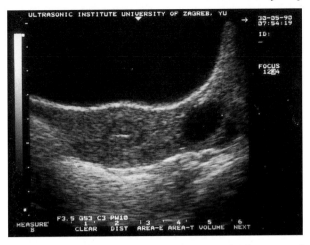

Figure 21.2 Transverse, B-mode, real-time scan showing a normal uterus and left ovary. The left ovary contains a developing follicle that appears as a small and ovoid cystic structure with well-defined walls and clear fluid within

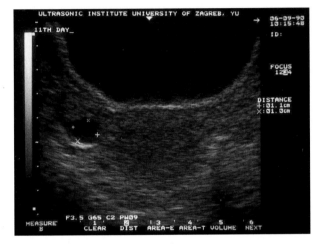

Figure 21.3 Ultrasonic diagnosis of ovulation after serial daily scanning: the dominant follicle is seen here in the right ovary on day 11 of the cycle

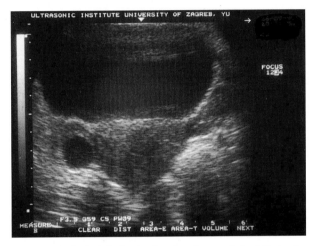

Figure 21.4 On the following day there is an increase in the follicular size

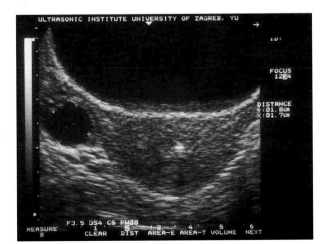

Figure 21.5 On day 13 the mean diameter of the follicle has reached 18 mm

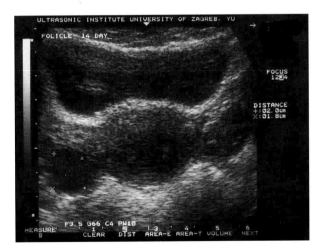

Figure 21.6 Mature preovulatory follicle on the 14th day of the menstrual cycle: the mean diameter of the follicle is 20 mm

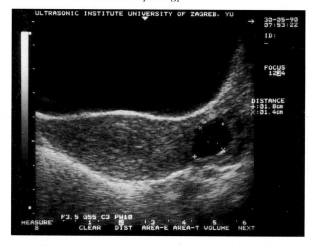

Figure 21.7 An illustration of the ovarian follicle measurement technique. Diameter of the follicle should be measured in three orthogonal planes by placing the calipers on the inner wall of the follicle

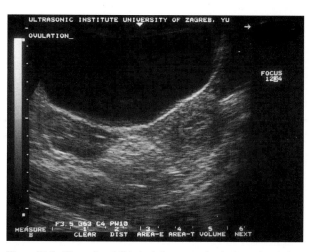

Figure 21.8 The mature follicle had almost completely disappeared when examination was repeated on the following day

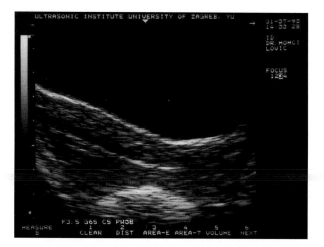

Figure 21.9 Longitudinal sonogram of the uterus in the early proliferative phase of the cycle showing a strong uterine cavity echo. This represents the thin endometrium with attached superficial layers and can be seen regularly in early proliferation

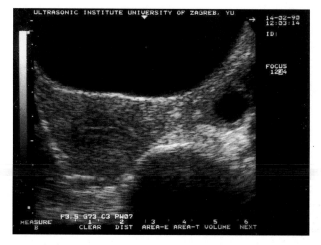

Figure 21.10 Transverse sonogram of the uterus and left ovary showing a developing follicle on the 12th day of the menstrual cycle. The central echo of the attached superficial layers of the endometrium is clearly visible

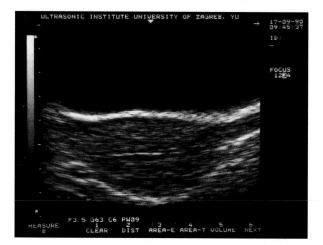

Figure 21.11 Transverse sonogram showing the endometrium in the late proliferative phase. The endometrium is hypoechoic compared to the myometrium and its boundary within the latter is well-defined. The central echo of the attached superficial layers is also clearly visible

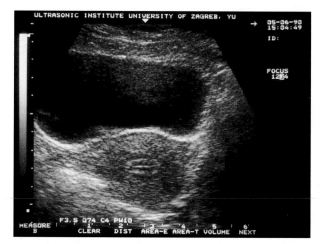

Figure 21.12 Typical appearance of the preovulatory endometrium exhibiting increased basal layer echogenicity

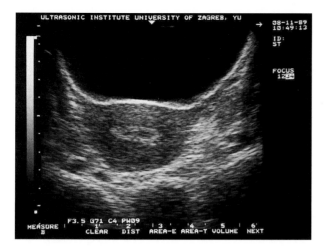

Figure 21.13 Ultrasonographic demonstration of the 'ovulation ring' resembling an early intrauterine pregnancy

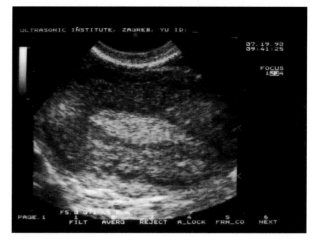

Figure 21.14 Transvaginal scan of the echogenic endometrium in the secretory phase. The endometrium is thick and the central echo is lost

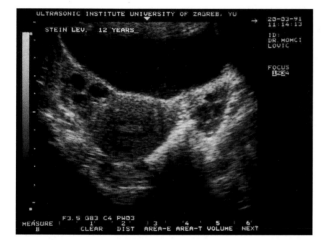

Figure 21.15 Transverse sonogram of a patient with amenorrhea and hirsutism: both ovaries are enlarged and polycystic. The uterus is small and hypoplastic

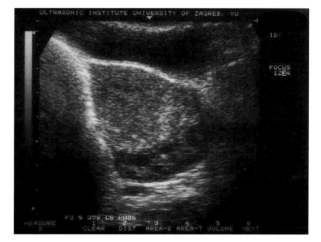

Figure 21.16 Large polycystic ovary in a patient suffering from primary infertility: the ovary is filled with numerous small cysts and increased stroma is also visible

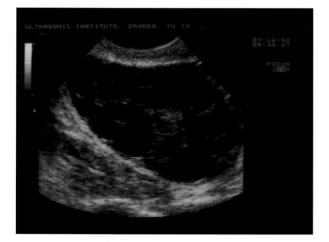

Figure 21.17 Transvaginal sonogram of the polycystic ovary of the same patient

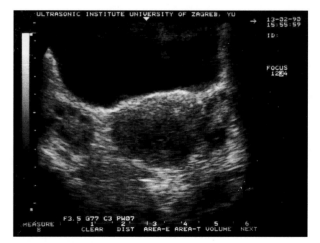

Figure 21.18 A large number of small cystic structures stand out from the surface of enlarged ovarian stroma in a patient suffering from primary infertility

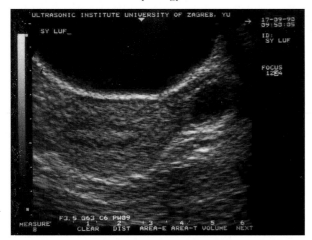

Figure 21.19 Ultrasonic finding in a case of luteinized unruptured follicle syndrome: note the presence of intrafollicular echoes within apparently normal preovulatory follicle and increased endometrium echogenicity

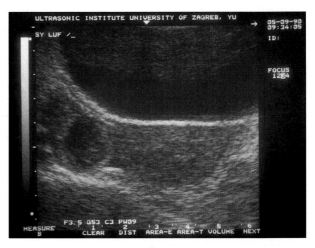

Figure 21.20 Another case of luteinized unruptured follicle syndrome

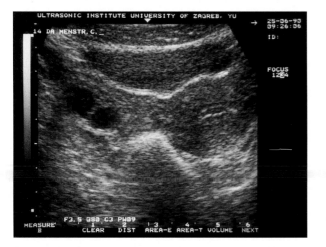

Figure 21.21 Transverse sonogram performed on day 14 of the cycle in a patient receiving clomiphene stimulation: the right ovary contains two follicles

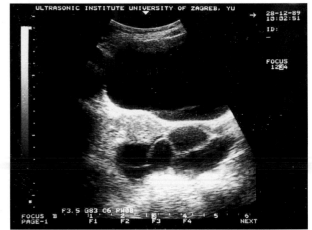

Figure 21.22 A case of severe ovarian hyperstimulation after human maternal and human chorionic gonadotropin ovulation induction: this transverse sonogram shows the left ovary extremely enlarged and filled with cystic structures

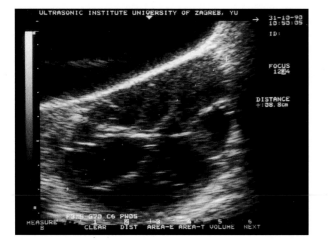

Figure 21.23 Longitudinal scan displaying the left ovary more than 8 cm long (hyperstimulation)

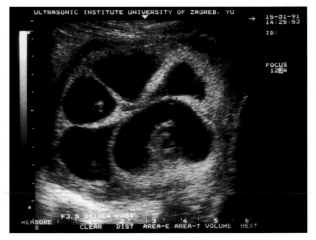

Figure 21.24 Quintuplet pregnancy in an infertile patient after induction of ovulation with human maternal gonadotropin

rate in stimulated cycles is similar to that in spontaneous cycles and the mean diameter of the preovulatory follicle is not significantly larger. However, there is a poor correlation between the peripheral estradiol levels and the diameter of the leading follicle in stimulated cycles. Peripheral estradiol levels may reflect the production of a single large preovulatory follicle or multiple immature follicles. Much better results are obtained when peripheral estradiol levels are correlated with the total follicular volume or with the number of the follicles larger than 10 mm in diameter.

The most important complication of the ovulation induction is hyperstimulation. It is characterized by the development of multiple follicles and luteal cysts after ovulation. While mild or moderate hyperstimulation is an acceptable consequence of ovarian induction, severe hyperstimulation represents a potentially life threatening condition. In severe hyperstimulation significant ovarian enlargement (usually more than 10 cm in diameter), peritoneal and pleural effusions and symptoms of cardiovascular and renal failure are present.

Ultrasound monitoring of the follicle growth in stimulated cycles is necessary in patients undergoing *in vitro* fertilization therapy. Transvaginal ultrasonically guided puncture of the follicles represents the most successful and most convenient way of collecting oocytes for *in vitro* fertilization. There are numerous advantages of the transvaginal route for egg retrieval, among which reduced cost, avoidance of general anesthesia and eliminated laparoscopy are the most important.

READING LIST

1. Kurjak, A. (ed.) (1989). *Ultrasound and Infertility.* (Boca Raton: CRC Press)
2. Haeckeloer, B.J. (1984). The role of ultrasound in female infertility management. *Ultrasound. Med. Biol.,* **10**, 35
3. Funduk-Kurjak, B. and Kurjak, A. (1982). Ultrasonic monitoring and ovulation in normal menstrual cycles and ovulation induction. *Acta Obstet. Gynecol. Scand.,* **61**, 329
4. Fleischer, A.C., Kalemeris, G.C. and Entman, S. (1986). Sonographic depiction of normal and abnormal endometrium with histo-pathologic correlation. *J. Ultrasound Med.,* **5**, 445
5. Katz, E. (1988). The luteinized unruptured follicle and other ovulatory dysfunctions. *Fertil. Steril.,* **50**, 839
6. Rankin, R.N. and Huton, L.C. (1981). Ultrasound in the ovarian hyperstimulation syndrome. *J. Clin. Ultrasound,* **9**, 473
7. Feichtinger, W. and Kemeter, P. (1985). Transvaginal sector scan sonography for needle guided transvaginal follicle aspiration and other applications in gynaecologic routine and research. *Fertil. Steril.,* **45**, 722

22 Magnetic Resonance in Visualization of Fetal Anatomy

Z. Alfirevic and A.S. Garden

INTRODUCTION

There is little doubt that the use of ultrasound has dramatically changed obstetric practice. The ability to examine the fetus *in utero* has enabled the development of prenatal diagnosis and biophysical investigation has had a major impact on clinical practice. The standards set by present ultrasound equipment are high, although there are a few instances in which application of ultrasound is limited by technical factors such as gross obesity or oligohydramnios.

The search for improvements in fetal imaging, however, continues. Imaging techniques used in obstetrics should be safe and non-invasive. At present, the only other imaging technique that can match these criteria is magnetic resonance imaging (MRI).

The independent discovery of the nuclear magnetic resonance phenomenon by two American scientists, Felix Bloch and Edward Purcell, for which they were awarded the 1953 Nobel Prize for Physics, was the basis of the clinical application of MRI. The methods for obtaining images using the magnetic resonance phenomenon are quite complex and beyond the scope of this review. The article of Pykett is recommended for those who wish a comprehensive explanation of the physics[1].

In a clinically orientated review it is sufficient to say that atomic nuclei, which normally act as small bar magnets in the body, will re-emit radio waves when placed within an external magnetic field and resonated choosing appropriate radio wave resonance frequencies (MHz) specific to the nuclei of interest. The most frequently used nuclei are hydrogen (^{1}H) because of their very high MRI sensitivity and abundance in water and fat in the human body. Construction of an image from the magnetic resonance signal is a complex computerized process.

MRI has no known adverse biological effects despite exhaustive *in vivo* and *in vitro* research[2]. However, possible biological effects of static magnetic fields, rapidly changing electromagnetic fields and radio frequency radiation can not be ruled out. At present, the guidelines laid down by the National Radiological Protection Board in Great Britain state that the static magnetic field should not exceed 2.5 T to the whole body or a substantial part of the body, and radio frequency exposure should be such as to avoid a temperature rise of more than 1°C in any part of the body[3]. Imaging in pregnancy is not permitted during the first trimester unless the pregnancy is going to be terminated.

IMAGING OF THE FETUS

The major limitation of MRI, especially in obstetrics, is the lack of real-time images. Conventional spin-echo MRI requires around 15 min to produce a single MR image[4]. Fetal movements with consequent movement of the amniotic fluid result in image distortion. In some instances the image can be so distorted as to resemble an empty uterus with no fetal parts visible. To overcome this problem several researchers have used fetal sedation via the mother or even by injecting vencuronuim or pancuronium directly into fetus. This is obviously not acceptable as routine procedure. This problem may be overcome using high-resolution, rapid-imaging techniques[5,6].

Magnetic resonance imaging is well tolerated by pregnant patients. Claustrophobia is rarely a problem. Easily recognizable fetal features, especially in sagittal planes (Figure 22.1), are much appreciated by expectant mothers[7].

Central nervous system

In our series of 26 fetal MR scans which were performed using a fast-scan imaging technique in the third trimester, fetal brain was visualized in 25 cases. In eight cases intracranial details such as falx cerebri and posterior fossa were recognized (Figures 22.2 and 22.3). We were unable to differentiate gray and white matter probably because most myelination

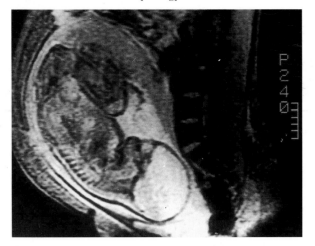

Figure 22.1 Sagittal section image of normal third trimester fetus (35 weeks gestation): fetal profile is easily recognizable

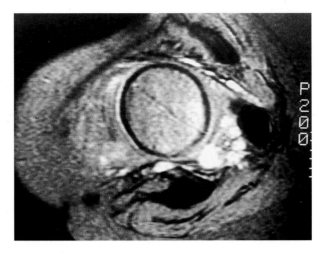

Figure 22.2 Cross-section of fetal head at 39 weeks gestation: falx cerebri is clearly seen. Biparietal diameter and head circumference could be measured

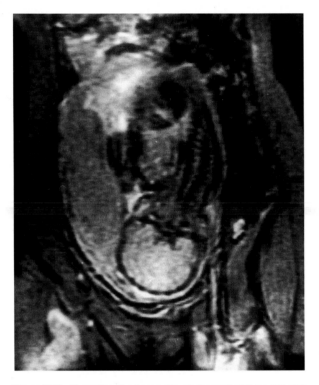

Figure 22.3 Coronal section image of posterior cerebral fossa and neck at 37 weeks gestation

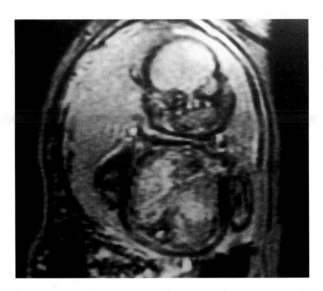

Figure 22.4 Details of fetal face at 37 weeks gestation: eyes, bony part of the nose and tongue are visualized

occurs in the first year of postnatal life. The fetal face including orbits could be easily seen in the third trimester (Figures 22.4 and 22.5). However, the value of MRI in diagnosing facial abnormalities such as cleft palate is difficult to assess because of lack of experience and real-time capabilities.

The vertebrae could be accurately assessed in 50% of cases in the third trimester. The spinal cord was more difficult to assess, although a large portion could be seen on a single sagittal image (Figure 22.6).

Thorax

The fetal heart was easily recognizable in the third trimester, although the anatomical details such as ventricles, septa and major vessels were visible in less than 5% of scans (Figure 22.7). The role of MRI in fetal echocardiography will undoubtedly change with the introduction of real-time MRI with blood flow measurement capabilities.

In contrast, fetal lungs were better seen on MRI than on ultrasound scans. In 15% of our MRI images the fluid-filled fetal lungs were seen with all details enabling accurate antenatal anatomical assessment (Figure 22.8). It has been suggested that intensity characteristics of fetal lungs using conventional imaging could provide information about lung maturity[8]. Further work is needed to confirm this interesting hypothesis. At present, MRI seems to be

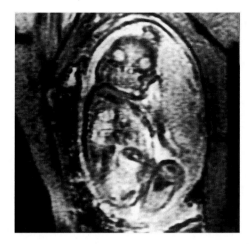

Figure 22.5 Fetal orbits at 37 weeks gestation

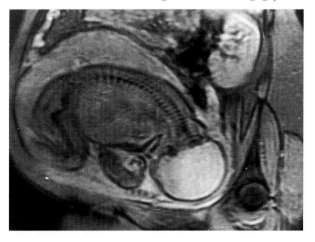

Figure 22.6 Sagittal section of normal fetus at 38 weeks on which thoracolumbal part of fetal spine can be studied

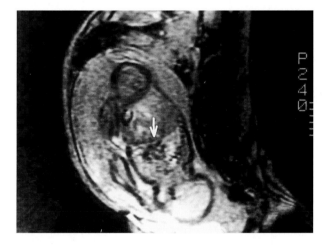

Figure 22.7 Coronal section of fetal thorax: both lungs and heart (arrow) are clearly visualized

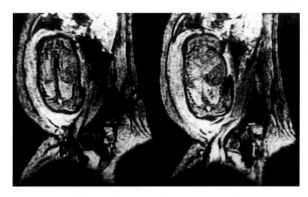

Figure 22.8 Fetal lungs at term

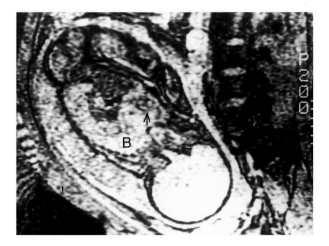

Figure 22.9 Right-sided congenital diaphragmatic hernia with bowel (B) in thoracic cavity: anatomy of thoracic cavity is distorted with heart (arrow) shifted to the left

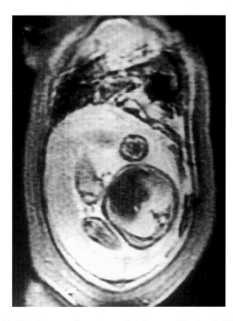

Figure 22.10 Cross-section of normal abdomen at the level of fetal liver (34 weeks gestation): intrahepatic circulation is not visualized and therefore the exact level of the cross-section is difficult to determine

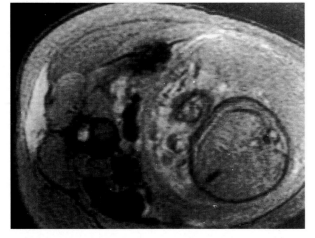

Figure 22.11 Intrahepatic part of umbilical vein within fetal abdomen at 34 weeks gestation: fetal subcutaneous tissue is also clearly visualized

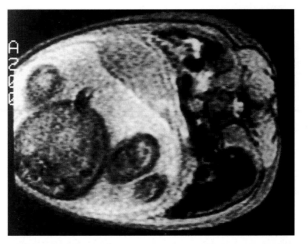

Figure 22.12 Fetal umbilicus with umbilical cord in the normal fetus at 38 weeks gestation: umbilical vein can be seen within cord

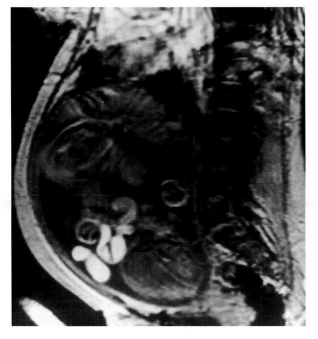

Figure 22.13 Fetus with gastroschisis at 38 weeks gestation: loops of fetal bowel are clearly seen floating free in the amniotic fluid

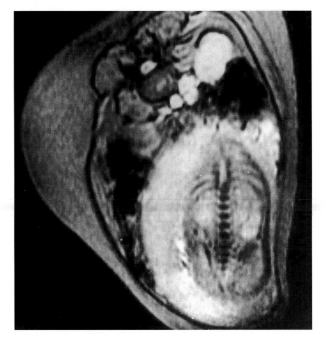

Figure 22.14 Fetal kidneys are usually poorly visualized on MR scans. This is an exceptionally good longitudinal section image of fetal kidneys at 40 weeks

a useful adjunct in ultrasound diagnosis of anomalies that distort lung anatomy such as diaphragmatic hernia (Figure 22.9).

Abdomen

The fetal liver, bowel and subcutaneous tissue are easily recognized on both sagittal and transverse sections of the fetal abdomen (Figures 22.10–22.12). In addition, fetuses with anterior abdominal wall defects can be further investigated to obtain information which is complementary to ultrasound[9] (Figure 22.13). The images obtained also enable accurate measurement of subcutaneous tissue. It has been suggested that thickness of subcutaneous tissue

together with phosphorus-31 spectroscopy of the placenta may provide MRI clues for accurate diagnosis of abnormal fetal growth and identification of jeopardized fetuses[10,11].

In our experience the fetal kidneys, bladder, stomach, spleen and pancreas are poorly visualized with MRI and ultrasound is the technique of choice if their abnormalities are suspected (Figures 22.14–22.16).

Extremities

Fetal extremities are clearly seen on MRI (Figures 22.17 and 22.18). Assessment of both bones and soft tissue is feasible. In our experience the quality of images matches those obtained by ultrasound. After

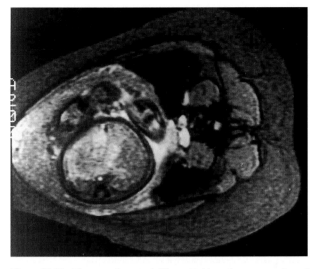

Figure 22.15 The same fetus as in Figure 22.14: on the cross-section of the fetal abdomen the transverse section of both kidneys is clearly visualized

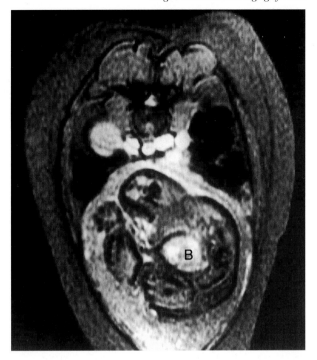

Figure 22.16 Fetal bladder immediately before emptying at term, B = bladder

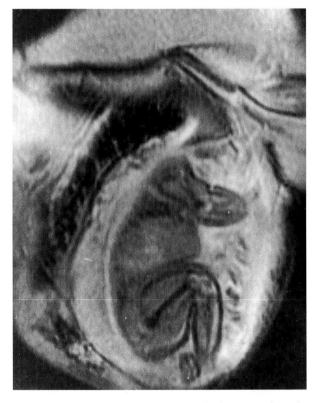

Figure 22.17 Fetal leg at term: femur is clearly seen and can be accurately measured. Note both distal femoral and proximal tibial epiphyses

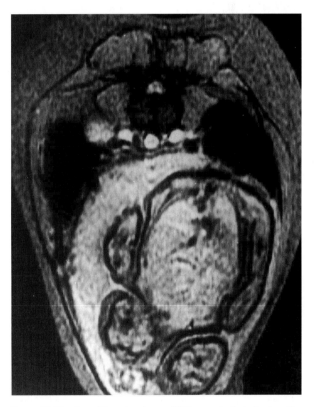

Figure 22.18 One of the advantages of MR scans is that all extremities can be seen on the single image. Orientation is easy, although lack of real-time capabilities is an obvious disadvantage

34 weeks gestation MRI is in fact superior to ultrasound in visualization of fetal limbs. Unfortunately the lack of real-time capabilities of MRI scans presents a significant problem for the assessment of musculoskeletal disorders.

IMAGING OF PLACENTA, AMNIOTIC FLUID AND CORD

The value of MR placental imaging lies in the ability to visualize the whole placenta, uterus and cervix on

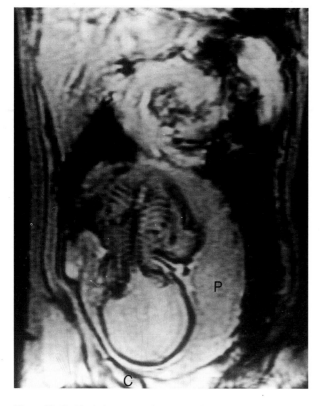

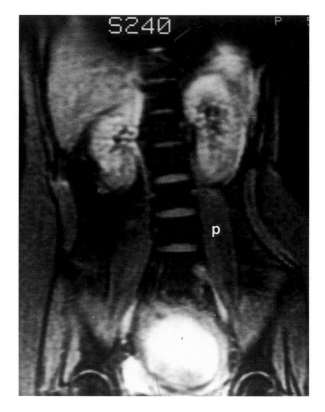

Figure 22.19 Total placenta previa at 38 weeks gestation: the degree of placenta previa was underestimated on ultrasound scans due to a posterior placenta and posteriorly tilted cervix. On MR scans it is possible to visualize internal cervical os, lower pole of placenta and fetal presenting part with great accuracy; P = placenta, C = cervix

Figure 22.20 Assessment of maternal anatomy is a rare indication for imaging in pregnancy. However, visualization of maternal kidneys, lumbosacral spine, muscles and pelvis could be useful in order to exclude organic cause for common low abdominal and back pain in pregnancy. This image shows normal maternal kidneys, normal spine and no pelvic masses; p = psoas muscle

the same sagittal plane. The relation of lower pole of placenta to the cervical internal os is crucial for the diagnosis and grading of placenta previa (Figure 22.19). Therefore it is not surprising that MR scans have proved their superiority to ultrasound, especially when placenta and cervix are both lying posterior[12]. The ability of MR to diagnose placental abruption and/or intrauterine bleeding has not been assessed.

The umbilical cord can be seen in the majority of third trimester MR images, but the resolution is largely insufficient to distinguish fetal vessels and/or cord anomalies.

IMAGING OF MATERNAL ANATOMY

During fetal MR scanning exceptionally clear images of maternal anatomy are obtained (Figure 22.20). Pelvimetry is possible and not infrequently maternal hydronephrosis and pathology of the lumbosacral spine are encountered. MRI also enables precise localization and sizing of uterine fibroids and ovarian masses which can be quite difficult with ultrasound, especially in the second half of pregnancy[13].

REFERENCES

1. Pykett, I.L., (1982). NMR imaging in medicine. *Sci. Am.*, **246**, 54–64

2. Saunders, R.D. and Smith, H. (1984). Safety aspects of NMR clinical imaging. *Br. Med. Bull.*, **40**, 148–54

3. NRPB ad hoc Advisory Group on NMR clinical imaging. (1983). Revised guidelines on acceptable limits of exposure during nuclear magnetic resonance clinical imaging. *Br. J. Radiol.*, **56**, 974–7

4. Powell, M.C., Worthington, B.S., Buckley, J.M. and Symonds, E.M. (1988). Magnetic resonance imaging (MRI) in obstetrics. II. Fetal anatomy. *Br. J. Obstet. Gynaecol.*, **95**, 38–46

5. Garden, A.S., Griffiths, R.D., Weindling, A.M. and Martin, P.A. (1991). Fast scan magnetic resonance imaging in fetal visualization. *Am. J. Obstet. Gynaecol.*, **164**, 1190–6

6. Stehling, M.K., Mansfield, P., Ordidge, R.J., Coxon, R., Chapman, B., Blamire, A., Gibbs, P., Johnson, I.R., Symonds, E.M., Worthington, B.S. and Coupland, R.E. (1989). Echo-planner magnetic resonance imaging in abnormal pregnancies. *Lancet*, **2**, 157

7. Alfirevic, Z., Garden, A.S., Griffiths, R.D., Weindling, A.M. and Martin, P.A. (1991). Comparison between ultrasound (US) and magnetic resonance imaging (MRI) in visualization of fetal

anatomy. *Ultrasound Obstet. Gynecol.*, **1** (Suppl. 1), 51

8. McCarthy, S.M., Filly, R.A., Stark, D.D., Hricak, H., Brant-Zawadzki, M.N., Callen, P.W. and Higgins, C.B. (1985). Obstetrical magnetic resonance imaging: fetal anatomy. *Radiology*, **154**, 427–32

9. Garden, A.S., Weindling, A.M., Griffiths, R.D. and Martin, P.A. (1991). Fast scan magnetic resonance imaging of fetal abnormalities. *Br. J. Obstet. Gynaecol.*, in press

10. Garden, A.S., Weindling, A.M., Griffiths, R.D. and Martin, P.A. (1991). Assessment of fetal growth using fast-scan magnetic resonance imaging. *J. Matern. Fetal Invest.*, **1**, 7–13

11. Weindling, A.M., Griffiths, R.D., Garden, A.S., Martin, P.A. and Edwards R.H.T. (1991). Phosphorous metabolites in the human placenta estimated *in vivo* by magnetic resonance spectroscopy. *Arch. Dis. Child.*, **66**, 780–2

12. Powell, M.C., Buckley, J., Price, H., Worthington, B.S. and Symonds, E.M. (1986). Magnetic resonance imaging in placenta previa. *Am. J. Obstet. Gynecol.*, **154**, 565–9

13. Weinreb, J. (1988). Obstetrics. In Stark, D.D. and Bradley, W.G. (eds.) *Magnetic Resonance Imaging*, pp.1297–1322. (St. Louis: C.V. Mosby Company)

Index